ETHICS AND THE BUSINESS OF BIOSCIENCE

Ethics and the

Business of Bioscience

Margaret L. Eaton

STANFORD BUSINESS BOOKS
An Imprint of Stanford University Press
Stanford, California 2004

Stanford University Press
Stanford, California

Printed in the United States of America
on acid-free, archival-quality paper.

Library of Congress Cataloging-in-Publication Data

Eaton, Margaret L.
    Ethics and the business of bioscience / Margaret L. Eaton.
        p.   cm.
    Includes bibliographical references and index.
    ISBN 0-8047-4249-9 (alk. paper)—
ISBN 0-8047-4250-2 (paper : alk. paper)
        1. Medical ethics.   2. Medicine—Research—Economic aspects.
3. Business ethics.
        [DNLM: 1. Biomedical Research—ethics.   2. Ethics, Business.
3. Commerce—ethics.   4. Equipment and Supplies.   5. Industry—ethics.
6. Research Design.   W 20.5 E14e 2004]   I. Title.
R725.5 .E25   2004
174.2—dc22   2003017561

Original Printing 2004

Last figure below indicates year of this printing:
13   12   11   10   09   08   07   06   05   04

Designed by James P. Brommer
Typeset in 10.5/13.5 Caslon

To Ron, my best friend, who supported me through this work more than I deserve.

Contents

Contents

Contents

Acknowledgments

As with any textbook, this one was completed with the help of many others. Although it would take too much space to name them all and to say how they helped, some deserve individual mention as well as my deepest gratitude.

First, to the people who funded this project. My fellowship, which led to the development of the project, was funded in part by SmithKline Beecham. Thane Kreiner of Affymetrix, Inc., in Santa Clara, California, first understood the importance of the project and gave what I call my "angel funding." Full funding came from the Human Genome Project, specifically the National Human Genome Research Institute's Program on Ethical, Legal, and Social Implications (ELSI). The ELSI Program, funds for which come from the Department of Energy and the National Institutes of Health, exists to identify, analyze, and address the ethical, social, and legal implications of human genetic research prior to the time that scientific information is integrated into health-care practice. This business ethics project is intended to emulate the "heads up" vision of ELSI, and I was funded because the ELSI program managers at the DOE and NIH recognized the need to include industry executives in the wider dialogue about the consequences of new genetic advances.

Second, to the Stanford University principal investigators of this project. Barbara Koenig gave me a fellowship and a home in the Stanford University Center for Biomedical Ethics and provided continual support for this project. David Brady at Stanford's Graduate School of Business is my teacher, challenger, supporter, and friend. He gave more time to this project than anyone else. His help is impossible to repay. I also had a wonderful advisory board of professionals, whose names are listed below. Although they all gave much needed direction and contributed beyond what I expected, I want to especially thank Steve Holtzman, Don Kennedy, and Karen Bernstein for their extra effort and guidance.

Third, to the students who worked on the initial stages of the project with me. Julie Juergens did groundwork with me and helped to set up the experimental workshop course that started the project. This workshop was a case writing class where mixed teams of Stanford University M.B.A. and medical science students were assigned cases and issues, conducted interviews, prepared the first case study drafts, and then presented them in test classes so that the value of the case studies could be assessed. Although the case study material has substantially changed since then, without the work of these students I could not have shaped the case studies into effective educational material. This was a great group of students, and their individual contribution to the project is noted in the first footnote of each case study. The case studies of students Jonathan Dugan, David Socks, Birgit Voigt, Sonja Ho, and Cynthia Leung do not appear in this book because either I could not determine how to teach the material adequately or the company did not grant its permission to publish. Nonetheless, these students' work was excellent, and the enthusiasm of all of the students and their eagerness to learn was one of the best aspects of this work.

Thanks also to all of the industry executives from the companies featured in this book. These individuals, who are also listed in the opening footnote of each case study, participated graciously in interviews and follow-up clarifications, patiently reviewed case study drafts, and provided the insights necessary to gain an understanding of each company and the decision-making processes involved in managing the complicated issues of this industry. At times, people related to the company and the issues also gave us their time and information. I have expressed my gratitude to them all in the case study footnotes, but two stand out for the extra effort given: Wili Gruissem for the Novartis case and Elliott Hillback for the Genzyme case. Also, two remarkable patients, Jim Finn and Steve Schalchlin, participated enthusiastically in the development and teaching of two of the case studies (Genzyme and Merck). These men remind us what this industry endeavor is for.

Others who helped enormously and who gave generously of their time include Margot Sutherland, who is responsible for case study writing at the Stanford Graduate School of Business. Margot was an excellent teacher and gave many helpful comments on each case study. Raina Glazener and Kathi Hanna were a great help with editing. Albert Jonsen, one of the pioneers in the field of biomedical ethics, provided many insights for the general ethics discussion. Finally, two faculty members from the Stanford University School of Law, Professor John Barton and Visiting Professor Rebecca Eisenberg, also provided valuable time and teaching advice for a Celera case study, which unfortunately does not appear in this book.

I am deeply grateful for all of this assistance.

ADVISORY BOARD

Karen Bernstein, Ph.D.
Vice President and Editor-in-Chief, Biocentury Publications, Inc.,
Belmont, California

Brian Cunningham, J.D.
President, Rigel, Inc., Sunnyvale, California

A. Grant Heidrich III
General Partner, The Mayfield Fund, Menlo Park, California

Steven H. Holtzman, B. Phil.
Founder, President, and CEO, Infinity Pharmaceuticals, Inc.,
Cambridge, Massachusetts

Donald Kennedy, Ph.D.
Editor-in-Chief, *Science* Magazine
Bing Professor of Environmental Sciences, Stanford University,
Stanford, California
President Emeritus, Stanford University

Thomas Raffin, M.D.
Professor and Chief, Division of Pulmonary and Critical
Care Medicine
Department of Medicine, Stanford University School of Medicine,
Stanford, California
Co-Director, Stanford University Center for Biomedical Ethics

Mickey C. Smith, Ph.D.
Professor of Management and Marketing, School of Pharmacy,
University of Mississippi, University, Mississippi

Albert I. Wertheimer, Ph.D.
Professor, School of Pharmacy, Department of Pharmacy Practice,
Temple University, Philadelphia, Pennsylvania
Director of the Temple University Center for Pharmaceutical
Health Services Research

MARGARET L. EATON
STANFORD BUSINESS SCHOOL
FEBRUARY 2004

Preface

Questions about the ethical nature of business activity have existed for ages. Perhaps the first business ethics case study question was posed by the Roman orator and statesman Cicero (106–43 BCE). In "A Practical Code of Behavior (On Duties III)," he posed the following case to foster a discussion about the proper course of action when a businessman is confronted with a conflict between doing what is personally advantageous and what is right:

> Suppose that there is a food-shortage and famine at Rhodes, and the price of corn is extremely high. An honest man has brought the Rhodians a large stock of corn from Alexandria. He is aware that a number of other traders are on their way from Alexandria—he has seen their ships making for Rhodes, with substantial cargoes of grain. Ought he to tell the Rhodians this? Or is he to say nothing and sell his stock at the best price he can get? I am assuming he is an enlightened, honest person. I am asking you to consider the deliberations and self-searchings of the sort of man who would not keep the Rhodians in ignorance if he thought this would be dishonest but who is not certain that dishonesty would be involved.
>
> —*From*: "Cicero, Selected Works," translated by Michael Grant, Penguin Books, 1971

ETHICS AND THE BUSINESS OF BIOSCIENCE

PART I   INTRODUCTION

Introduction

In the fall of 2002, over six years after genetically modified (GM) foods and crops had been on the market without showing evidence of toxicity, the government of Zambia had accepted the advice of its science advisors and decided that no GM foods would be distributed in the country because the long-term health effects of GM foods had not been studied to their satisfaction. This decision occurred during a widespread famine and, despite the need for food, led the government to reject thousands of tons of corn donated by the United States because some of it was likely to be genetically modified. According to the United Nations Food and Agricultural Organization, the decision to reject the U.S. corn increased the risk of starvation for about 2.9 million people.[1] What was going on to produce such an anomalous decision?

In her book *Licensed to Kill?* (University of Pittsburgh Press, 1998), former U.S. Nuclear Regulatory Commission senior policy analyst Joan Aron describes why the nuclear power industry is at a standstill. She makes clear that nuclear technology was employed long before consideration was given to the political, ethical, and social implications of its use as a source of energy. According to the author and many others, this lack of attention has been a significant reason for the continuing political and consumer opposition to nuclear power. Critics believe that the public has been less than fully informed about nuclear safety, that nuclear scientists are overconfident and fail to question many aspects of a dangerous technology, and that those who promote the use of nuclear power serve their own and not society's interests. As a result, the technology is feared, the nuclear power industry is mistrusted, and nuclear power plants (the relatively few that still exist) have been built and run in an atmosphere of conflict and resistance. In an attempt to prevent the same type of criticism and fear from undermining the promise of biotechnology, many science policy makers advocate that the overall implications of innovative or "frontier" discoveries be studied concurrently with the development of new technologies. This approach was taken at the beginning of the biotechnology revolution when scientists and policy makers met at the Asilomar Conference Center in 1975 and agreed voluntarily to halt work on recombinant DNA techniques until safety measures and oversight programs were put into place. Similarly motivated, the architects of the Human Genome Project created the ELSI Program in 1990 to anticipate and address the *e*thical, *l*egal, and *s*ocial *i*mplications that arise as the result of human genetic research.[2] ELSI Program topics have included access to genetic information, privacy and fairness in the use and interpretation of genetic information, research ethics, responsible application of the new technologies to prevent misuses and promote the well-being of patients, and public education. By studying such issues in advance, problem areas can be anticipated and solutions developed before the scientific information is integrated into health care practice.

The educational project that led to this textbook was based on the same premise. From the start, ethical and social questions have been raised about biotechnology's impact on people (both sick and healthy), the environment, and society. If anything, commercialization—to produce products such as gene tests, drugs, vaccines, cell therapies, and genetically modified foods—has added to the complexity of these ethical and social issues. As a consequence, business executives in these companies have been and will continue to be compelled to deal with ethical and social issues, something usually considered to be outside of their ken. Yet if bioscience business managers can obtain the skills that allow them to anticipate and address the ethical and social aspects of their work, benefits similar to those anticipated by the ELSI Program can be obtained. These include avoiding the problems such as seen with the nuclear power industry, improving corporate performance, promoting the commercialization of products, and advancing the positive social use of these technologies. This textbook is intended to promote these ends by facilitating instruction in the effective business management of the ethical and social ramifications of commercializing new medical and biotechnology products.

For the purposes of this book, the term *bioscience industry* is used to include bio-agricultural, pharmaceutical, biotechnology, genomics, and medical device companies.[3] The educational material here is a look at this industry from an ethics point of view and is intended for bioscience business managers and future managers (that is, students), whether from science, medical, business, or legal disciplines. Students of this topic using both the background material and case studies of this textbook should gain the following: (1) an understanding of how bioscience corporate activities generate ethical and social issues; (2) familiarity with the basic set of ethical principles that can guide business decisions; and (3) an improved ability to make reasoned and defensible moral choices and thereby an improved managerial competence when dealing with business activities that raise ethical and social issues. This material does not advocate any specific behavior as "ethical" but operates on the belief that an ethical analysis will provide a fuller appreciation of business problems so that creative solutions can be achieved that are more likely to benefit the company, those directly affected by the actions of the company, and society at large.

WHY STUDY BIOSCIENCE BUSINESS ETHICS?

Seminal events in biology and medicine led to the decision that education in business ethics for the bioscience industry would be useful; for example,

- the $3 billion government-sponsored effort to map and sequence the human genome
- the cloning of Dolly the sheep
- the marketing of the first gene tests for breast cancer and Alzheimer's disease
- the marketing of genetically modified foods

These and other medical and biotechnology advances were occurring at such speed that by the early 1990s it was common to hear that a biotechnology revolution was underway. Geneticists were beginning to discover how human genes caused or prevented disease. Embryologists were gaining insight into reproduction at the molecular level and were working on techniques to create and manipulate embryos to produce cloned human tissue. Gene tests were being marketed that, for the first time, could detect risks for future diseases. Research promised to deliver remarkable improvements in medical therapy, including cancer cures, infertility treatments, cloned human tissues and organs, which would overcome the chronic organ shortage and tissue rejection problems, and gene therapies for currently incurable diseases. Biotechnologies were being developed to extend human longevity. In addition, genetic modification of seeds promised to improve the yield and quality of foods, ameliorate environmental hazards from pesticide and herbicide use, and even create plant sources for plastic, thus reducing our dependence on oil.[4] These and other medical and biotechnology discoveries were providing an unprecedented opportunity to improve the human condition. Few doubted that the benefits could be immense and some even went so far as to consider these advances central to the future of humanity.

As these genetic and biotechnology innovations were speeding ahead, however, they were challenging society's readiness to cope with their consequences. Increasingly, research was creating possibilities for application in society before the accompanying ethical, social, and legal uncertainties could be resolved. While scientists were beginning to grapple with these ramifications, they dealt many times with the theoretical. What would happen if a certain technology was used in a certain way? However, when corporations translate these scientific advances into marketed medical products, the ethical and social ramifications become real. Therefore, any consideration of the ethical and social impact of genetic and other biotechnologies needs to include the role played by the bioscience industry. According to Elliott Hillback Jr. of Genzyme Corporation, a biotechnology company based in Cambridge, Massachusetts, "I don't think you can be involved in genetics and not in ethical issues."[5]

Some of the questions resulting from the ethical and social issues that surround the new genetics and biotechnologies include: What are the acceptable limits to corporate patent ownership of human genetic material? How can DNA data banks preserve patient privacy and still obtain maximal benefit from the stored information? Should scientists stop all efforts at human embryo cloning even if it is intended to treat lethal diseases? Is it appropriate to offer abortion to a woman before the full consequences of an *in utero* gene test are known? Should tests for genetic predisposition to a disease be marketed before interventions to prevent or treat the disease are available? Should gene tests be made available before there is legal protection to prevent insurance and employment discrimination? Is it safe to implant modified animal tissue into humans for therapeutic purposes when there is a possibility that the tissue could harbor an undetectable infectious agent? Would it be acceptable to perform the type of gene therapy that eliminates the possibility of a patient's offspring developing an inherited lethal disease? Should gene therapies be used for enhancement purposes or to prolong life? Is it acceptable to exclude from a food label information that the product had been derived from the genetic modification of a plant or animal? Should we create new life forms? Does it matter if advanced medical products are available only in developed countries?

These questions and many more are circulating in scientific, medical, government, and public circles and, sooner or later, must also be addressed by corporate managers in charge of commercializing the products of the biotechnology revolution. In all likelihood, commercializing these new products will further complicate the associated ethical and social dilemmas, given the increasing expectation that businesses should assume responsibility for the larger consequences of their activity beyond just increasing shareholder value. It will take some effort to meet this challenge since there are reasons to believe that businesses are not living up to this expectation.

Public trust in business has been low for decades. Since 1973, when the Gallup organization began polling Americans about their confidence in major institutions, big business has consistently ranked close to if not at the bottom. In each survey, less than one-third of responders claim that they have a high degree of confidence in big business.[6] Furthermore, the public has been wary about biotechnology. Surveys in the late 1990s by several public and private organizations showed that U.S. public opinion increasingly has been resembling that of Europe, where there is significant opposition to biotechnology.[7] According to a telephone survey by the Public Policy Research Institute at Texas A&M University, the percentage of responders who thought that biotechnology would be deleterious in the next twenty years approached the percentage who thought the same about nuclear power, an institution that had lost a significant amount of public trust.

More and more people are beginning to believe that public trust is critical to the future viability of the bioscience industry. Reasons for this include the fact that there are perhaps no products more important to people than medical therapies and devices because of the fundamental role they play in saving lives and maintaining and prolonging health. In addition, people need to believe in the safety and integrity of the food they eat and feed to their children. In an environment of wariness about big business and biotechnology, bioscience corporate missteps can easily generate harmful repercussions, including regulatory restrictions and public backlash sufficient to hinder or halt product marketing and acceptance.[8]

Some of this backlash and public protest has already occurred. For example, there have been widespread public protests against genetically modified foods, including burning crops in the field and vandalizing laboratories. After Dolly the cloned sheep was born there were immediate calls for a ban on all cloning research. More recently, in the late 1990s, polarizing debates followed the news that corporate scientists had used cloning techniques to create an embryo out of human and cow cells and, later, had attempted to produce the first cloned human embryo as the first step to produce transplantable human tissue. Bills have repeatedly been introduced in Congress that would ban human embryonic stem cell research, despite the promise of these cells to solve the most resistant medical problems, such as how to regenerate nerve tissue. Federal funding for such research has been banned for years. For the past decade there has been a persistent public fear that gene tests will be used in a discriminatory fashion to deny people medical insurance or employment. An ongoing debate concerns the use of patents to own and control genetic information. Fears have also been fueled with disclosures of tragic consequences involving human genetic research. The death of a relatively healthy teenager in a gene therapy experiment resulted in the enforced closure of an entire research program at a top-tier medical school, certainly not the first closure of such a program for infractions of research ethics. Corporations were involved in all of these events (all of which are discussed in this book), and corporate executives have become involved in the struggle to address the moral and social implications of this activity and their responsibility for the consequences of the application of biotechnologies.

Not only are bioscience corporations involved in these specific issues, but they also operate in an arena of the larger debate about science's role in society, a debate with two polarized refrains. On the one hand are groups who say that "science cannot and should not be stopped." On the other hand, others argue that science should be allowed to progress only when the risks and other social consequences are understood. Adherents to the idea that science advances best without heavy outside constraints believe that science benefits society by generating knowledge, which is seen as inherently good. They argue that it is society's responsibility to use, misuse, apply, or misapply that knowledge. This view is shared by many in science and in business.[9] One such scientist is Dr. James Watson, who shared a Nobel Prize for the 1953 discovery of the structure of DNA. Watson was also the first director of the Human Genome Project and currently serves as president of Cold Spring Harbor Laboratory. Known for his sharply stated beliefs, he said the following:

> Never postpone experiments that have clearly defined future benefits for fear of dangers that can't be quantified. Though it may sound at first uncaring, we

can react rationally only to real (as opposed to hypothetical) risks. Yet for several years we postponed important experiments on the genetic basis of cancer, for example, because we took much too seriously spurious arguments that the genes at the root of human cancer might themselves be dangerous to work with. Unlike many of my peers, I'm reluctant to accept such reasoning, again using the argument that you should never put off doing something useful for fear of evil that may never arrive. The first germ-line gene manipulations are unlikely to be attempted for frivolous reasons. Nor does the state of today's science provide the knowledge that would be needed to generate "superpersons" whose far-ranging talents would make those who are genetically unmodified feel redundant and unwanted. Such creations will remain denizens of science fiction, not the real world, far into the future. When they are finally attempted, germ-line genetic manipulations will probably be done to change a death sentence into a life verdict—by creating children who are resistant to a deadly virus, for example, much the way we can already protect plants from viruses by inserting antiviral DNA segments into their genomes. If appropriate go-ahead signals come, the first resulting gene-bettered children will in no sense threaten human civilization. They will be seen as special only by those in their immediate circles, and are likely to pass as unnoticed in later life as the now grownup "test-tube baby" Louise Brown does today. If they grow up healthily gene-bettered, more such children will follow, and they and those whose lives are enriched by their existence will rejoice that science has again improved human life. If, however, the added genetic material fails to work, better procedures must be developed before more couples commit their psyches toward such inherently unsettling pathways to producing healthy children. Moving forward will not be for the faint of heart. But if the next century witnesses failure, let it be because our science is not yet up to the job, not because we don't have the courage to make less random the sometimes most unfair courses of human evolution.[10]

This kind of confidence in science is sometimes deplored, leading to calls for restraints or even bans on certain types of biotechnology research. Leon Kass falls in this group. Dr. Kass is a physician and biochemist who has held many medical ethics positions, including currently the chair of President George W. Bush's Council of Bioethics. In his book *Toward a More Natural Science*, Kass commented on the question of whether babies should be created for infertile people by any and all available means (for example, *in vitro* fertilization, cloning, parthenogenesis):

> Drawn by the promise of fame and glory, driven by the hot breath of competitors, men do what can be done. Biomedical scientists are no less human than anyone else. Some of them are unable to resist the lure of immortality

promised, say, to the scientific father of the first test tube baby. Moreover, regardless of their private motives, they are encouraged to pursue the novel because of the widespread and not unjustified belief that their new findings will probably help to alleviate one form or another of human suffering. They are even encouraged by that curious new breed of technotheologians, who after having pronounced God dead, disclosed that God's dying command was that mankind should undertake its limitless no-holds-barred self-modification by all feasible means.[11]

This "green light, caution light, red light" debate about research also applies to the commercialization of products and services developed from genetic and biotechnology research. Carl Feldbaum, the president of the trade group BIO (Biotechnology Industry Organization), acknowledges that ethical and social issues are deeply embedded in the commercial development of new biotechnologies. He told the audience at one of BIO's annual meetings that, because of the connection between biotechnology and ethics, he had been asked questions never before addressed to an industry representative; for example, What is the industry position on the day of development that a human embryo gets a soul? Will gene therapy lead to a brave new world of genetically engineered children who can do advanced calculus by age five and run four-minute miles soon thereafter? Is it morally right to develop animals so we can mine them for replacement body parts? How does biotechnology change our place in the universe—are we usurping God by attempting to improve upon God's creatures? Can we trust any human beings with such power?[12]

Because they increasingly are drawn into the larger debates, bioscience companies and the organizations that represent them have started to consider the strategic need to address the ethical and social implications of what they are doing. Feldbaum even went so far as to state his belief that the greatest threat to emerging biotechnology companies would be from industry mishandling of troubling ethical problems.[13] He told one science reporter that "bioethics has become a major component of what we do at BIO. The watershed event which put biotechnology on the frontlines was the birth of Dolly. Since then, it has become more apparent to those in the industry that if a company handles a controversial issue well, the public will be more likely to accept it, and the company's stock price will reflect that."[14]

Increasingly, the managers of large pharmaceutical companies are expressing the same beliefs. Although still focused primarily on developing traditional chemical-based drugs, these so-called Big Pharma companies are starting to develop new biotechnology products of their own or those acquired from smaller biotechnology companies. Consequently, these managers are also facing the same debates as their counterparts in the smaller biotechnology and genomics companies. This situation is not entirely new to pharmaceutical business managers. Whether they were recognized as such, ethical and social issues have always attended the process of commercializing any medical treatment:

- Will patenting medical discoveries limit access to them?

- How can a company decide when product research data are mature enough to safely proceed with human testing?

- How should companies remunerate physicians who conduct clinical trials on their behalf without creating a conflict of interest or undermining their objectivity?

- How can companies accommodate the rights and interests of people used as human subjects in studies of experimental treatments?

- How can companies ensure that human subjects are fully informed about research risks and give free and voluntary consent?

- When are there sufficient data to assure that a product is safe and effective enough to market to the general public?

- How does a manager weigh and balance current scientific limitations and the unknown risk of products with long-term benefits?

- To what degree should companies take into consideration the potential social harms of the products they develop?

- How should companies disclose research data findings without creating false expectations in sick patients that a cure is imminent?

- What constitutes the appropriate use of medical treatments, and what obligations does industry have to prepare physicians to use new products wisely?

- How should companies responsibly market and advertise medical products to physicians and the lay public?

- How should the industry respond to the increasing demands of patient activist groups who want access to experimental treatments and a voice in how research is performed?

- What constitutes fair pricing of a medical product?

- What role, if any, should companies play in making its products accessible to the poor and uninsured, both in the home country and in developing nations?

Since the lines that demarcate biotechnology, genomics, and pharmaceutical companies have blurred, business managers in all of these companies face these larger questions as well as many that are specific to biotechnology. How well they manage these issues makes a difference in how well medical and biotechnology products are received and, therefore, whether companies marketing these products will succeed. Commenting on this connection, BIO's Feldbaum likes to use the nuclear power industry's failure to heed the public concerns as a cautionary tale for biotechnology. "The result can be seen in the towers of nuclear power plants standing idle that dot the American landscape," Feldbaum said. "They are testimony to the hubris of the scientists who thought that the public was too ignorant to be brought into the discussion about the technology. If the [biotechnology] industry can't learn from a graveyard of nuclear power plants, there's not a lot of hope."[15]

Some corporate chief executive officers (CEOs) have been more aware of these challenges and ready to respond to them than others. On the one hand, Monsanto (as can be seen in the case study in Chapter 3) has been pilloried for its past research and marketing practices, which ignored public fears about its genetically modified foods and crops. On the other hand, Randy Scott, CEO and chairman of Genomic Health, Inc., of Redwood City, California, understands the social and economic complexity created by the continuous announcements of biotechnology advances. According to Dr. Scott, "The future is accelerating toward us at a pace that will shake the very foundations of human thought and understanding. If we had not experienced the change of the past 30 years in the computer industry, the coming force of biological change would not be believable."[16] Scott makes it clear in his writings and public statements that he recognizes that the biotechnology breakthroughs will have significant impact on companies developing them into products and that these companies are obliged to address the ethical and social aspects of the use of those products:

> Although the potential of genomics is vast, so too are the concerns. Genomic technology in the hands of intelligent beings has infinite possibilities—from human cloning to genetic manipulation of the human race. If the future of genomics depends on consumers, then it will be dependent on their education, trust, and support of the consumer as well. Consumers will embrace genomic products only if there is a strong basis of trust and a foundation built on bioethics. Genomics is not like computing; it is personal and emotional. Individual privacy and control over one's own genomic information will be critical to engaging consumers in genomics at any level, whether for research, for medical treatment, or for business.[17]

Public trust and support might be hard to come by given the uncertainty and even fear about what will happen when biomedical technologies enter the hands of corporations. Responding to this problem, Carl Feldbaum said that "we will never overcome all objections [to the commercial development of biotechnologies] and satisfy every concern. Fear of the unknown is powerful and persistent, and so we hear protests over biotech foods long after they are proved safe. We can't simply dismiss people's misgivings: There's something primal in people's relationship with their food, their bodies, and we should be thoughtful in responding to that."[18]

Until recently, however, a thoughtful response to ethical and social ramifications was not a significant part of the bioscience company product development process. This is not to say that executives in these companies ignored the larger consequences of what they did and kept their eye solely on the bottom line. Rather, the approach was more related to following the laws and regulations, attempting to stay out of legal trouble, hiring public relations personnel to manage the public face of the company, and doing what was "right" based on customary corporate practice and perhaps on intuition derived from life experiences and religious teaching. This approach has not been uniformly successful. More often than not, the way that ethical issues arise in companies is after management has faced some negative consequence to a course of action. Because of this, ethical dimensions are often by-products of corporate action, not explicit determinants of business strategy. This situation is lamentable because companies that fail to anticipate ethical issues lose opportunities to prevent problems, both for the company and those who are affected by its actions.

BENEFITS OF ADDRESSING ETHICAL AND SOCIAL ISSUES

As described more fully in Chapter 2, there are many potential benefits to including an ethical and social dimension to business decision making. Sensitivity to the ethical aspects of business problems can help managers avoid mistakes that may otherwise result from a narrow focus on the firm's interests. Businesses that adopt reasonable ethical business practices can forestall burdensome government regulation and oversight and prevent customer or public relations problems that can negatively affect the ability to market new products. Ethical analyses applied to problem solving can also allow managers to understand how others view corporate behavior, to predict public reactions, and to prepare appropriate responses. Finally, ethical analyses can prompt managers to make decisions that serve the long-term interests of society, which can ultimately benefit business.[19]

The best business decisions, like all decisions, come from a careful and comprehensive assessment of all of the implications of alternative courses of action in the attempt to choose an optimal solution. An ethical perspective, therefore, can only add value to the decision-making process. When a manager incorporates an ethical aspect to decision making, a different and complementary set of questions is asked than when dealing with the financial, political, legal, or public relations aspects of the question. When different questions are asked, decision making is approached from a broader perspective. With this perspective, managers can more creatively formulate strategy and accept or reject alternative courses of corporate action with a better understanding of the consequences. An ethics analysis prompts managers to ask, "What is the right thing to do?" which complements the typical business question, "What is the action that will maximize the interests of this company?" Legal assessments force managers to ask how they can avoid litigation or promote legal advantages, and in public relations and investor relations, managers ask how the company reputation can be preserved or enhanced. An ethical approach tends to be more outward looking and considers broader consequences, both to the company and the individuals and entities directly affected by corporate action. When companies ask questions about such things as the consequences of their actions, the rights of others, and the fairness of outcomes, they tend to operate in ways that promote the well-being of more than just shareholders.

Ethical analysis, however, should not be expected to result in clear-cut solutions to business problems. On the contrary, as this book will show, there is seldom a "right" answer to an ethical question. Business managers must therefore become comfortable with ambiguity in order to effectively manage business ethics issues. What an ethical analysis can do is help the business manager achieve insight and implement business decisions with a fuller understanding of the consequences of those decisions.

TOUR OF THE BOOK AND SUGGESTIONS FOR USE OF THE MATERIAL

Background Material

The book begins with background material about business ethics principles that can be used as a guide to resolve ethical and social dilemmas. Provided are a set of analytical principles and a system of application intended to make sense to a business manager who does not have training in philosophy and is not an ethics scholar. As a result, the presentation is not "pure" ethics, if there is such a thing, and there is no attempt to cover all schools of ethical thought. In the next chapter, the suggested approach to business ethics analysis is applied to a short case study (Monsanto's labeling of rbST) as an example of how the analysis can be performed.

Following this chapter is a chapter devoted to human and animal research ethics, a topic that cannot be ignored by any manager of a company that engages in this activity. This chapter serves as a background to all of the case studies dealing with clinical research—Genzyme, Adiana, and VaxGen. Another short chapter is also included on the Food and Drug Administration (FDA) regulation of the bioscience industry. It was important to include this information as background for all the case studies since the FDA regulations often govern and restrain corporate decision making.

Case Studies

The main section of the book contains a series of case studies that can be used in discussions of the management of the ethical and social dilemmas involved in developing and marketing medical and biotechnology products. Business case studies are most useful when they detail events that have actually occurred at corporations using information provided by those directly involved in and affected by the events. This approach was used for the case studies presented here. Except for the OncorMed/Myriad case, executives at each company provided interviews to the authors and otherwise assisted in the preparation of the case studies. Knowledgeable outsiders also provided information about various topics, such as the underlying science, the business environment, and particular situations faced by each company. These case studies are perhaps longer than many in business education since most management problem solving involving ethical and social issues is heavily influenced by the myriad facts and circumstances at play. The intent, as much as possible, therefore, was to present the facts and circumstances as accurately as possible, along with details sufficient to allow for an appreciation of the complexity faced by company managers. To facilitate teaching, each case study is preceded by background material about the general subject matter of the case and followed by discussion questions and suggestions for a general ethics analysis approach.

The case study method was chosen to teach this subject because of the time-tested value of this style of learning. Case study teaching is a form of mediated group discussion using the case study as the focus of the discussion. For many reasons, it is the primary method employed in business education.

Students typically are required to place themselves in the shoes of the company manager and asked to resolve the conflict or otherwise address the issues involved. In so doing, students must make decisions, create alternative strategies, and defend the reasoning behind a chosen course of action. As a result, case study methodology requires active participation by the student, encourages independent thinking, forces participants to analyze the various aspects of the problem, encourages the harmonizing of conflicts, and fosters the development of judgment. The case study technique has advantages over other teaching methods such as textbook reading about ethical theories or lectures. Because they are required to perform an independent analysis of the issues and develop alternative strategies, the participants are actively engaged in real corporate problem solving and are therefore better able to remember and apply these techniques later. Also, because case analysis is done in a group setting, this method encourages a constructive exchange of ideas and promotes peer cooperation.[20]

Another reason that case studies are valuable is that they allow students and managers to learn from the experience of others. To enhance this kind of learning, the background material in this book is dotted heavily with small descriptions of how various companies became involved in particular events such as patent litigation, research conflicts, regulatory enforcement actions, and resolution of manufacturing problems. Some of these stories have become industry lore invoked so as to warn others not to repeat past mistakes. Other stories are used to explain how various conflicts have played out, often with unexpected results. An additional reason to use these small histories was to make the reading less dry and to provide details that are difficult to supply in straight text. Real life examples are therefore included as a feature of this book to provide a greater perspective on the industry, its history, and the complex situations that can occur.

The selection of case studies included in this book was based on several criteria. To maximize an understanding of each sector of the industry, the case studies include a mix of company type—pharmaceutical, biotechnology, bioagricultural, genomics, vaccine, and medical device. The companies are also of various sizes since company size can determine the nature of ethical and social questions that arise, what resources are available, and what constrains management. The types of executive officers also vary, which is intended to illustrate the different management approaches taken by those with science versus business backgrounds. Each case study also focuses on one aspect of company endeavor that spans the product development continuum, including research discovery collaborations with academia, human research, regulatory strategy, marketing, postmarketing, and advertising. The case studies feature important products with large or potentially large markets, making what happens to these products vital to patients and to the company. The selected case studies also involve enduring issues common to many types of companies so that, as much as possible, the lessons learned can apply broadly across the industry. Finally, case studies feature ethical or social questions for which there were no obvious right or wrong answers. Ethical issues involve true dilemmas and often place managers in situations where it is difficult to make choices between competing claims. Each case can lead to reasonable differences of opinion about the appropriate course of action, and there is no intent to suggest that one option is preferable to another. Consequently, these case studies are presented in a neutral manner with no personal judgments made about corporate conduct.

Teaching Suggestions

Unless the teacher of this material has provided students with ethics instruction, the chapter on ethics (Chapter 2) should be read prior to any case study discussion. The cases are meant to be studied in the order presented since many concepts are introduced sequentially. Basic information about certain subjects (for example, research and development [R&D] processes, regulations, human subjects protections) is contained in the earlier cases because this information is useful in considering the later case questions. For example, information about human research processes is introduced in the Adiana case and is important to all four of the subsequent cases, which add material specific to the company circumstances. To avoid a rigid requirement to use all of the case studies, however, the cases were also written to be sufficiently useful as "stand alones." Each case study should be comprehensive enough to allow for an adequate understanding of the general business issues, the underlying science, the regulatory aspects of the product, and the ethical and social dilemmas involved. Depending on who is teaching the material and who the students are, other background chapters can be used or omitted. For instance, if the students are unfamiliar with the industry, the chapters on research ethics (Chapter 4) and industry regulation (Chapter 5) are important to an understanding of the environment in which these companies operate. If the teacher has a preferred method of ethics analysis, the chapter that applies an analysis method to the Monsanto case (Chapter 3) can be skipped. Hopefully, the way that the material has been divided makes this text flexible enough for all interested audiences.

CONCLUSION

Given the power of new biotechnology and medical discoveries and the degree to which these discoveries have become a matter of public discourse, bioscience company managers are beginning to appreciate the need to consider the larger consequences of their work. The public is struggling to accommodate itself to the rapid technological changes in biology and medicine. Polarized opinions are frequently published about the impact these new discoveries will have on the human condition. Conflicts exist between those who yearn for the benefits that bioscience can provide and those who fear the consequences of unfettered scientific and corporate license. In such an atmosphere, bioscience companies can be harmed by the perception that they are focusing on economic advantages and ignoring the ethical and social consequences of their work. The most satisfactory way to deal with the conflicts that exist is to anticipate them and decide in advance how they should be managed. In this way, it is more likely that business decisions will benefit the company and those impacted by corporate action. Enlightened business management also makes it more likely that the products of bioscience will maximally benefit the public. This book is an attempt to provide students and business executives with educational material that will help them achieve these goals.

Notes

1. Bohannon J. Zambia rejects GM corn on scientist's advice. *Science* 2002; 298: 1153–54.

2. Information about the National Human Genome Research Institute's ELSI Program is available from www.nhgri.nih.gov/ELSI/aboutels.html#Issues.

3. The term *bioscience industry* was chosen for lack of a better one in the changing nomenclature of this industry sector. Other terms used for the same grouping of companies include *life sciences* and *bio-pharmaceutical*.

4. Carey J. The biotech century. *Business Week* 1997 Mar 10; 78.

5. Day K. Genetics research begets questions; Biotechnology industry seeks ethics advice to deal with complex issues. *Washington Post* 1996 May 8; Sect. A:1.

6. Newport F. Military retains top position in American's confidence ratings. Gallup Organization. 2001 June 25. Available at www.gallup.com/poll/releases/pr010625.asp.

7. Priest SH. U.S. public opinion divided over biotechnology? *Nature Biotechnology* 2000; 18:939–42.

8. Young JH. *The medical messiahs*. Princeton, NJ: Princeton University Press; 1967; Morrison SW, Giovannetti GT. *The twelfth biotechnology industry annual report, new directions 98*. Palo Alto, CA: Ernst & Young LLP; 1998.

9. Don't be afraid of genetic research [editorial]. *Business Week* 1997 Mar 10; 126.

10. Watson JD. All for the good; why genetic engineering must soldier on. *Time Magazine* (The future of medicine) 1999; 153:91. Used with permission.

11. Kass LR. Making babies. In *Toward a more natural science*. New York: The Free Press; 1985. p. 47.

12. Feldbaum CB. *Keeping the faith*. Proceedings, Biotechnology Industry Organization Annual Meeting. San Diego, CA; 2001 Jun 25.

13. Hoyle R. Arrogance on human cloning may pose a threat to biotechnology. *Nature Biotechnology* 1998; 16:6.

14. Brower V. Biotech embraces bioethics; but are they being exemplary or expedient? BioSpace.com 1999. Accessed 2000 Nov 11. Available at www.biospace.com/b2/Articles/061499_bioethics.cfm.

15. Ibid.

16. Ernst & Young LLP. Focus on *fundamentals: The biotechnology report*. Washington, DC; 2001. p. 87. Available at www.ey.com/global/vault.nsf/US/Focus_exec_summary/$file/FocusExecSum.pdf.

17. Scott R. Genomics: The forces of acceleration are upon us. In *Focus on fundamentals: The biotechnology report*. Washington, DC: Ernst & Young LLP; 2001. p. 26.

18. See Note 12.

19. Baron DP. *Business and its environment*. 2nd ed. Upper Saddle River, NJ: Prentice-Hall; 1996.

20. Stiles P, Jameson A, Lord A. Teaching business ethics: An open learning approach. *Management Education and Development* 1993; 24:256–61; Barnes LB, Christensen CR, Hansen AJ. *Teaching and the case method*. 3rd ed. Boston: Harvard University Business School Press; 1994; Pemberton JM. Bringing ethics to life: case study method and ARMA International's code of professional responsibility. Records *Management Quarterly* 1995; 29:56–62; Donaldson T, Gini A. The case method. In *Case studies in business ethics*. Upper Saddle River, NJ: Prentice-Hall; 1996. pp. 11–20.

PART 2   ETHICS AND INDUSTRY OVERVIEW

2

Ethics and Business Activity[1]

The purpose of this chapter is to explain the discipline of business ethics in such a way as to serve the needs of business managers whose positions demand that they make practical decisions when confronted with ethical conflicts. To achieve this purpose, various ethical principles will be discussed followed by a suggested method of applying the principles so as to arrive at responsible business decisions. The next chapter provides an example of how this method can be applied to a business dilemma that faced Monsanto when marketing a genetically engineered product. Certain trade-offs are necessary in an attempt to apply ethics to business decision making, and these trade-offs will be apparent to those who devote their careers to philosophy and ethics and who might deplore in this presentation the lack of abstraction, depth, or disciplinary precision required in their field. However, since it is not common for business managers to have systematic training in philosophy or ethics, this discussion of business ethics is intended to pare down concepts to make them straightforwardly applicable to real business situations. As much as possible, references are supplied for those who seek more in-depth understanding of this topic.

When beginning any discussion of "business ethics," it is important to understand that the term is used here as a shorthand expression for the use of ethical principles to guide an analysis of business activity and not because there is something different about ethical theory in a business context. Ethics is generally considered to involve analysis and reasoning based on moral principles and standards. Ethical reasoning attempts to determine whether the results of a decision are morally right or wrong.[2] Moral principles are no different whether they are applied to a physician treating a patient, a teacher grading a paper, a business manager developing a marketing plan, or any other human endeavor. Differences of opinion do arise, however, in deciding which moral principles should govern a given situation. In that regard, this book deals with the predominant moral principles and ethical standards that are used by ordinary persons as well as philosophers and which, over time, have proved most useful in business circumstances. These moral systems include utilitarianism, rights and duties, and various formulations of justice, all of which are commonly applied in our society and are considered fundamental to our collective morality.[3] Each of these systems has its strengths and weaknesses; none alone is broad or flexible enough to cover most situations, but together they can generally provide a comprehensive approach to moral reasoning that can guide the business manager.

Business managers in the bioscience industry also need to appreciate that companies often interact with two other fields that have developed their own set of ethics codes and that apply ethical principles in ways unique to their endeavor. The first field is academia, where many companies seek faculty with expertise to advise on R&D and to conduct research on products. Universities operate under deeply entrenched canons of academic freedom and duty and have developed codes of conduct that companies need to understand to avoid conflictual relationships and prevent the erosion of the academic purpose.[4] This topic is discussed in Chapter 6. The second field of corporate interaction is medicine or, more specifically, medical research. Because most bioscience industry products are studied in animals and humans prior to marketing, business managers also need to be familiar with the codes of ethics and ethical thinking that have been adopted for and applied to these kinds of research. An entire chapter (Chapter 4) has been devoted to the ethical issues in animal and human research since this activity is central to the success of most bioscience companies and because the field of ethics for human research especially has become highly evolved. The evolution has resulted in the selection of a set of ethical principles that apply to human research and in the development of many ethics codes and guidelines that specify appropriate conduct. Understanding research ethics also aids in the understanding of the law since many of the ethical principles and codes have been incorporated into the statutes and regulations that govern this activity. Further, the primary principles of ethics that have been employed in human research have also been applied to the practice of medicine.[5] Thus, bioscience business managers who become knowledgeable about human research ethics will not only be better able to navigate through this ethically difficult terrain but also have a useful understanding of the ethics involved in the practice of the physicians who are their customers. Again, it is not that there are fundamental differences between business, academic, and medical ethics, but over time these three fields have developed distinct ways of applying ethical principles to guide their various activities. Any business manager interacting with the other two fields should understand these differences.

Another aspect of any business ethics discussion is the consideration of what ethics is not. For example, ethics is not a question about resisting temptation. Ignoring a burdensome regulation because it is not enforced and therefore poses no threat of punishment is not an ethical dilemma; it is simply wrong. Although lack of enforcement invites disdain for the law, these and other questions of legal propriety should be handled by corporate lawyers skilled in resolving such conflicts. In addition, the study of business ethics is not value imposition or a search for consensus on personal values, because different people have different values, and majority rule is not advocated as a method of ethical problem solving. Also, resolving ethical problems should not be a reverse engineering process; that is, one should not determine a desired outcome and then search for an ethical principle that comes closest to justifying that choice. Finally, ethical reasoning is not simply the search for direct mutual advantage. While it is valuable if all parties to a transaction benefit, this exercise does involve ethical analysis.[6]

Another preliminary question that is commonly asked is why adhering to the laws and regulations does not alone meet a company's obligation to act ethically. That the two are often equated is fostered by the fact that many business ethics codes of conduct and business ethics audits involve primarily legal compliance. So as not to unduly burden the introduction to this chapter, the appendix (Appendix 2.1) contains a fairly detailed description between legal and ethical systems and explains why business managers need to adhere to both.

The remainder of this chapter will discuss the importance of business ethics and the various ethical principles typically used in a business context. Next, a system for business ethics analysis is presented, which, in the following chapter, is then applied to a bioscience case study as an example of how managers can analyze business problems that have ethical and social implications.

BENEFITS OF INCORPORATING ETHICS
INTO BUSINESS DECISION MAKING

Isn't business ethics an oxymoron? This common reaction is sometimes borne of mistrust of big business and a belief that, for instance, businesses tell the truth only when or only because it is financially rewarding to do so. A more moderate view is that business does not concern itself with ethics, since to do so would require that company managers (at least sometimes) act against corporate financial self-interest and thus undermine their overriding fiduciary responsibility to make profits for shareholders. When the financial incentive is restrained, the argument continues, investors and business managers lose motivation to start and run companies, overall productivity suffers, and society is denied beneficial products and services. Under this reasoning, business and ethics are often incompatible. The view that companies benefit society when they maintain a self-interested focus on profits is most often attributed to the philosopher and economist Adam Smith (1723–90) and was further legitimated by the 1976 Nobel Prize-winning economist Milton Friedman (b. 1912). Their views are still prevalent today.

Other points of view, however, encourage managers to make decisions that take into account the ethical and social implications of business action. To begin with, Adam Smith qualified his endorsement of unrestrained self-interested business activity by noting in his treatise "The Wealth of Nations" that "every man, *as long as he does not violate the laws of justice*, is left perfectly free to purse his own interest his own way, and to bring both his industry and capital into competition with those of any other man, or order of men" [emphasis added]. If Adam Smith believed that justice has a role in business, this suggests that he was concerned about how business activity affected others. That notions of justice should temper business action is a minor and little-appreciated aspect of Adam Smith's business philosophy.[7] Still, it is important given the strength with which he argued for the free pursuit of business profits.

There are other views about the role of business in society that contrast with the traditional views of Smith and Friedman. One has become known as the stakeholder theory, which is advocated by those who believe that corporations are obliged to behave in a socially responsible manner toward those who have an interest, or a "stake," in their relationship with the business. Corporate stakeholders are those affected by the decisions of businesses and can include shareholders, employees, customers, suppliers, lenders, the local community, and society. In the case of bioscience companies, stakeholders could also include farmers, physicians and other health care providers, human subjects, patients, and medical payors.[8] For those who adhere to notions of corporate social responsibility, business managers have an obligation to treat corporate stakeholders fairly and to avoid harming them. Further, corporate self-interest should be restrained when it operates at the expense of others and would lead to an injustice. Justifications for a philosophy of corporate social responsibility come from the view that because businesses have become powerful social institutions, they need to maintain a positive role in society. If businesses abuse their power or fail to meet changing social expectations, they will lose their legitimacy. Included in these expectations are that the products of businesses and business action will benefit and not harm society and that business will otherwise adhere to ethical standards prevalent in society. Issues included on the corporate social responsibility agenda include fair wages, adequate benefits, high-quality products and services, consumer safety, responsible dealings with vendors, avoiding environmental harm, contributing to the local community, and fair marketing practices. Even further out on the liberal spectrum are those who believe that corporations should be agents of social improvement and that a business best serves its shareholders by being responsible to society.[9]

Milton Friedman entered the debate about corporate social responsibility when he published an article in 1970 and stated that "there is one and only one social responsibility of business—to use its resources and engage in activities designed to increase its profits so long as it stays within the rules of the game, which is to say, engages in open and free competition without deception or fraud."[10] Friedman deplores expansive notions of corporate social responsibility and believes that if a manager uses company resources for the benefit of society, especially without also contributing to the economic performance of the company, then that manger fails to adhere to fiduciary obligations by improperly taxing shareholders and misusing their resources. Public institutions or individuals can work for the betterment of society, but Friedman believes that this is not a proper direct focus for business.

However, even Friedman believes that there are circumstances when it is not only acceptable but required for company managers to become socially involved and act according to ethical precepts. These are situations where behaving in an ethically and socially responsible manner benefits shareholders by avoiding corporate harm or by promoting profits. Unethical corporate behavior can result in legal or regulatory sanctions or in retaliation from business partners. Also, negative reactions can come from any number of external entities, including employees, public institutions, foreign governments, trade groups, the media, professional organizations, activist groups, and other members of the public. These reactions can harm companies financially. Customers can also retaliate against a company for perceived unethical conduct by refusing to buy product or by boycotting the company. Issues that have generated such negative reactions include environmental protection, health and safety, advertising, product pricing, international trade policy, globalization, legislative politics, labor practices, and unjust treatment of other stakeholders. Managers have come to appreciate that failing to address the ethical and social aspects of these and other corporate issues can have important bottom-line consequences. In such cases, managers are compelled to adopt strategies to address ethically sensitive subjects.

Ethical behavior can also be justified because it is good for business. In some cases, a company attuned to social issues can position itself strategically to generate better investor, consumer, and media reactions. Companies that are routinely ethical gain a reputation that can improve organizational effectiveness. Employees prefer to work for companies with ethical standards and will work harder and better when they believe they serve a good company. Companies also usually prefer to do business with other companies they can trust. Looking out for customer interests creates long-term relationships by promoting customer satisfaction. This leads to increased sales. Consumers also like buying products from reputable companies, and chambers of commerce welcome such companies into their communities. Therefore, ethical and socially responsible behavior promotes mutually beneficial business exchanges and relationships. Like the avoidance-of-harm reasoning above, this view of the value of business ethics is a utilitarian justification in that it is a strategic approach that seeks to improve bottom-line results.[11]

There are times, however, when adhering to an ethical practice will not produce win/win scenarios as described above. There are circumstances where the moral choice will be difficult, expensive, or will harm the company somehow. In such cases, why take the ethical road? How a business manager handles such situations is an age-old question that can sometimes be answered solely by appealing to the view that there is intrinsic value in ethical behavior.

In Cicero's grain merchant hypothetical presented in this book's preface, he uses the case to discuss the following questions:

Is a thing morally right or wrong?

Is it advantageous or disadvantageous?

If apparent right and apparent advantage clash, what is to be the basis for our choice between them?

Cicero responded to the last question by claiming that it is incorrect to contrast morality and advantage. What is perceived as advantageous is, on reflection, usually illusory since nothing unethical is ever advantageous. In Cicero's view, "you can never gain advantage from an improper gain, regardless of whether it was detected or not."[12] Loss of integrity, honor, and good repute and (secondarily) the advantages that go with them are the result of unethical behavior. Under this view, managers are obliged to question whether the morally suspect act is advantageous and to strive to obtain a result that is both ethical and beneficial for the company.

More modern versions of the appeal to the intrinsic value of ethics takes into account common human experience, an appeal to rationality, and the psychic benefits that can come from doing the fair or right thing. Aspects of ethical behavior pervade the life experience of most people. It is common for people to want to be treated fairly and to protest when someone does them wrong. Consequently, we have long been socialized to treat others in ways that are considered fair or right, ways in which we want to be treated. We are also prone to use our ability to reason to come to conclusions about what constitutes right behavior. We reason, analyze, and judge other people's actions and motivations based on our concepts of right and wrong and thus develop moral expectations for ourselves and others. For instance, it is common to believe that circumstances can alter decisions about what is right action or that between two choices that can both cause harm, it is better to select the action that produces the lesser harm. It is also rational to think that people who are alike in all relevant ways should be treated alike. While there might be arguments about what counts as "relevant," no one disagrees with the concept that "like should be treated in like fashion."

It is also natural and rational to generalize from personal experience to consider some things right or wrong in any context, including an institutional one. Despite a modern tendency to disparage their motivations, business managers are no exception. Although we come to understand that circumstances can change what is considered right or wrong conduct, many people do not want to live a life where what is right is determined by their contingent desires and the contingencies of their situations. Hence, the notion that people's personal moral views should change when they leave home and go to work does not make sense without substantial justification. It has also been argued that it is psychically detrimental for people to feel compelled to check their moral beliefs at the door of the workplace. Most people do not want to do this, and they suffer if they are made to. Although promoting people's psychic well-being may be considered a consequentialist appeal to ethics, it also indicates that there is something fundamental about people's need to live a moral life, no matter what the context. Adhering to this notion, James A. Autry, former CEO of Meredith Corporation, wrote that

> I take seriously the role of business and its impact on society. I shudder when I hear some businessperson say, "It's just business," because that usually means something is being done in the name of business that would not be done if that person were doing it in the name of himself or herself. Always remember this: If we can commit an injustice in the name of business, we can commit an injustice in the name of anything.[13]

It is interesting that Milton Friedman also shares this view and has said, "If I'm employed in a business that I think is unethical, I have a clear choice. I can get out of that business and find something else to do. It doesn't seem to me it's ethical for me to do unethical things because the business can let me do it."[14]

As further evidence that ethical behavior has intrinsic value for people, there are even studies that suggest that people will act in an ethical manner even when it is against their self-interest. Employee studies have shown, for instance, that when workers think they are paid more than others for the same amount of work, some will attempt to negate the injustice by working harder. Employees who believe they are unfairly paid also tend to react negatively by working less, complaining, sabotaging the work effort, or quitting.[15] Two other studies routinely taught in business schools also show that justice tends be ingrained in the way people behave. In the first study, one person was given a set amount of money to divide with another person who could either choose to accept the portion offered or negate the transaction such that neither person got any money. Because neither subject had done anything to earn this money, the study was intended to assess the extent to which the distribution of money is affected by people's intrinsic sense of fairness. The study data showed that most of the time the first subjects would split the money more or less equally rather than take substantially more for themselves. When the first subject did give substantially less, the second subject would most often forgo the money that was offered and negate the transaction. In both cases, the subjects tended to act against their self-interest for the sake of fairness.[16] In the second study, subjects were given money and told that they could distribute as much of it as they wished to another and that their decision could not be influenced in any way by the second person. In other words, the second subject could not negate the transaction. In only 36 percent of the cases did the subjects keep all of the money for themselves.[17] The study is cited as an even stronger indication that many people will relinquish personal gains for the sake of justice.

Manuel Velasquez, professor of business ethics at Santa Clara University, cites several other workplace and psychological studies that show that, for instance, justice promotes harmony and order among members of a group; procedurally just institutions are accorded more respect and are valued above those using unfair processes; and the decisions reached using fair procedures are also more likely to be accepted by affected parties.[18] These findings support the view that people value the integrity that comes from ethical behavior and that there is something essential about the desire to be treated ethically and to reciprocate in kind. Preserving this sense of integrity can have powerful influences making it more than worthwhile for managers to seek business decisions that are both beneficial and right.[19]

MORAL SYSTEMS

As with any business endeavor, strategizing about ethics requires principles for reasoning about issues and methods for applying the principles to arrive at alternatives for action that are ethically acceptable. This book relies on the primary moral systems that have become widely adopted in business ethics education. These systems are classified as *teleological* or *deontological*, terms that were devised by the British philosopher Charlie Dunbar Broad (1887–1971) to describe ways to reason about moral questions.[20] The teleological (also called *consequentialist*) approach proposes that right action can be judged in terms of the overall consequences of actions.[21] An action is right if it produces a good result for as many as possible. *Utilitarianism* is the principal teleological ethical system, and modern concepts of this principle hold that duty in any given situation is to perform the action that will result in the greatest overall balance of benefit over harm compared with alternative actions.[22] A utilitarian analysis therefore closely resembles a business risk-benefit analysis. Teleological ethical systems are useful to apply in business and most other situations in which determining whether an action would produce benefit or inflict harm is generally a relevant consideration. For instance, giving the press an interview about company events could lead people to invest in the company, conduct business deals, or buy its products. If the press interview contains true statements, people are more apt to make informed decisions and beneficial choices about their dealings with the company. In contrast, untruths could mislead people, cause them to make harmful choices, and ultimately lead to a loss of trust in the company. Under this scenario, teleological reasoning explains why truth telling (which produces an overall benefit) is the right action and lying (which ultimately produces more harm than good to all involved) is generally wrong.

In contrast, deontological systems stress one's duties or obligations to act in a morally acceptable manner.[23] Actions are justified by their conformance to moral or right rules (Kant called them maxims); if the rules are followed, the result of the action is considered right. Deontological systems therefore seek to develop universal rules and principles (such as the Golden Rule) that guide actions without considerations of the consequences of actions. For example, an unregulated dietary supplement is widely believed by the public to prevent cancer. It is entirely safe and quite inexpensive, but despite people's perception, there is no definitive medical proof of any anticancer effects. How does a company decide to market such a product? A consequentialist might argue that the product should be marketed with no statement about efficacy since selling the product to as many people as possible would benefit many (for example, the company, its shareholders and employees, consumers experiencing peace of mind) while causing only minimal economic harm to consumers. Disclosing that the product might not prevent cancer would stifle sales and detract from the benefit side of the equation. In contrast, a deontological rule might be "do not deceive." Reasoning from this rule, a company might conclude that simply marketing the product would mislead some consumers to believe that the product prevented cancer. To avoid this misapprehension, the company would disclose that the supplement lacks medical proof of efficacy. If this disclosure would so seriously undermine the market for the product, the company may decide not to market it.

One of the primary difficulties encountered in the ethical analysis of business problems is in deciding whether to use a teleological or deontological approach. The two systems can often lead to opposite conclusions about right behavior, such as when considering the rightness of truth telling and lying. An unconditional adherence to the requirement to tell the truth can, on certain occasions, result in harmful consequences, as can be seen with both of the above examples. When incompatibilities like this occur, how does one choose between them? Adhere to one and reject the other depending on the circumstances? Consider both and attempt to determine if there are modifications (for example, become a "modified deontologist" and develop rules open to exception—"always tell the truth unless ... ") that can lessen the harm of truth telling? Modern philosophers who have considered this problem of incompatibility have tended to blur the distinction between teleology and deontology to make ethics analysis more flexible. The approach suggested here is to consider both types of reasoning and then attempt to harmonize conflicting conclusions to arrive at optimal solutions. This process will leave the business manager with an appreciation for the harm that can result from different courses of action and, when one course of action is selected, better able to understand the consequences of the action selected and to address critics.

Justice is a third moral system applied in business contexts. Justice can be retributive (punishment for wrongdoings), compensatory (righting past wrongs), or distributive (ensuring a fair distribution of the benefits and burdens of society). Some theories of justice combine elements of teleological and deontological systems.

UTILITARIANISM

The most prominent teleological or consequentialist system of ethical reasoning used in a business setting is utilitarianism. In a utilitarian approach, an action is ethical if it is likely to produce better consequences overall for human well-being (that is, maximizes aggregate social utility). Utilitarian reasoning is like a risk-benefit calculus (maximize the good and minimize the harm), but what makes it moral is the fact that it seeks to achieve an ethical endpoint. In other words, the social utility sought is some particular human good.[24]

To engage in a utilitarian analysis, facts must be gathered to determine who might benefit from or be harmed by contemplated actions. As described in the example above, telling the truth to a reporter can be justified as meeting utilitarian requirements. However, utilitarian analysis can also justify lying to a reporter if one were to conclude that the harm of truth telling would outweigh the good, for example, because it would needlessly damage the reputation of a valued scientist. Thus, utilitarian reasoning can recommend an action (here, deception) in a particular circumstance that some would think unethical. For this reason, two forms of utilitarian theory have developed, called *act* and *rule* utilitarianism. Act utilitarianism focuses on increasing aggregate social utility for that particular situation and accepts that facts can change the conclusions for other similar situations. Rule utilitarianism focuses on a general rule of behavior intended to be applied by all individuals in similar situations. In rule utilitarianism, a rule of behavior is chosen, which, if followed by everyone, maximizes aggregate social utility across the majority of situations over time. Hence, a rule utilitarian might conclude that deceiving a reporter would not be acceptable because in most situations it causes more harm than good. The rule utilitarian accepts that application of the rule will result in a less than optimal utilitarian result in some few circumstances. There are other philosophers who take a middle ground and hold that rules can be justified in most circumstances but that in particular cases when their application would produce overall harm, they should be ignored so long as doing so does not undermine general conformity to moral rules.

The persuasiveness of utilitarianism comes from the fact that it is self-evident to most people that actions that maximize good outcomes for all affected persons necessarily benefit society. One of the reasons that utilitarianism can be so readily applied is that most people in everyday life engage in utilitarian deliberations to make optimal choices for themselves and those close to them. In a business situation, utilitarian reasoning feels comfortable because it is similar to the risk-benefit decision-making practices used by most managers. Because this type of analysis is applicable to most business situations, utilitarian analysis is relevant to most of the case studies in this book.

Although utilitarian analyses are usually easily applied in the business setting, several aspects of utilitarianism can make this exercise difficult. These include deciding what facts are relevant, defining the benefits, selecting measurements to determine benefits, and setting the scope of the analysis, that is, how wide the net should be cast in assessing potential risks and benefits.

Gathering and Assessing Relevant Information

Utilitarian analysis requires that the decision maker diligently search for all facts relevant to the particular circumstance. Otherwise, incomplete information can lead to faulty reasoning and an inability to accurately predict the consequences of a decision. Making accurate predictions can also be hampered if managers are not able to obtain all of the needed facts. For example, regulatory managers at a cash-constrained start-up company launching a first product are always under the gun to obtain Food and Drug Administration (FDA) approvals as fast as possible. In such circumstances, these managers could persuade themselves that a negative manufacturing test finding was so insignificant or idiosyncratic that they could decide not to include it in a filing intended to obtain FDA approval for full-scale manufacturing. Leaving aside the question of whether such reasoning is improper "strategic innocence," managers need to strenuously and objectively assess all facts relevant to the consequences of such a decision and not allow the need to arrive at any particular outcome drive these determinations.[25] Otherwise, excluding problematic information can result in a failure to arrive at the optimal utilitarian out-come, that is, failure to take into account all of the pertinent benefits and harms for each possible action. In the example cited, ignoring the test data might lead to more harm than good—the company could lose the opportunity to improve manufacturing, the FDA might force the company later to recall a faulty product, or patients could be injured. A decision to include the data in the report could lead company managers to develop creative options to address the manufacturing problem and to take other actions that result in maximiz-ing benefit for all concerned. In any case, all relevant facts need to be consid-ered so that managers can accurately predict the consequences that flow from various possible courses of action.

Defining Benefits

A second difficulty in utilitarian analyses is deciding what is beneficial and what is harmful in any given situation. A corollary consideration is whether the benefit in question is considered a human good. In utilitarian theory, it is difficult many times to define utility clearly and to achieve consensus on that definition. Differences of opinion can easily exist, for example, on whether so-ciety is better off having seeds that are genetically modified to resist pesti-cides. Proponents see the benefits of reducing agricultural chemical use and increasing crop yield. Both can be considered ethical endpoints since they im-prove the human condition by reducing toxic chemical exposure and con-tributing to food supplies. But detractors can argue that these benefits are not real or are exaggerated. They can also believe that the seed use is harmful. What if the seeds pollute the natural environment with mutant plants? Since the health and environmental risks for such a result are largely unknown, this prospect is frightening to some people. Thus, seed companies can view the products as beneficial while "Green" activists view them as harmful. Neither camp can agree with the other's point of view. The analytical process of utili-tarianism considers these differences of opinion in choosing the action that would tend to produce aggregate utility, even if the company does not agree with the opinions of its detractors. A utilitarian approach would prompt a company that contemplates the development of such a product to gather in-formation about the perceived or potential harms and take actions that pre-serve the benefits for companies, farmers, and consumers and minimize as much as possible the perceived or potential harms of the genetically modified seeds. To achieve the most utilitarian outcome in such a situation, a company could decide, for instance, to develop only the most useful seeds, extend safety testing and monitoring, or provide additional information to concerned consumer groups.

Measuring Risks and Benefits

Modern applications of utilitarian ethics have tended to adopt an economic approach to measuring benefits and comparing them to harms. Monetary numbers can produce easily comparable alternatives, but many consequences of business action cannot be measured precisely, nor are they valued equally among people. Drug companies may be able to predict such things as the amount of money it costs to develop a drug and the amount of profit to be gained once the product is sold; the economic impact of the product on medical treatment; or the subsequent costs of product liability claims. However, not all consequences of the drug development process lend themselves to economic or precise measurements. How do you measure, for instance, the suffering of a research subject who becomes sterile as a result of receiving an experimental drug? Or the impact on a child whose mental processes are dampened with drug treatment for hyperactivity? The answer is that there is no way to place a monetary value on such life events that will indicate their true worth in society. However, despite the difficulty, the monetary value of non-economic events is routinely assessed by economists so that governments and businesses can make plans and predictions. Moreover, courts and insurance experts are accustomed to assigning monetary values to such things as personal injuries, taking into account the economic impact of an injury (for example, cost of medical care and provision of services the injured person can no longer perform, lost earnings potential of a spouse, costs of raising a disabled child) and non-economic losses (for example, emotional distress, or the loss of "love, comfort, and society" provided by a spouse). Pharmacoeconomists routinely assess the financial and nonfinancial impacts of the use of drugs (for example, adverse drug reactions). There are, therefore, sources of guidance to measure non-economic benefits and harms. For those events that have undergone no such measurement, reasonable application of a utilitarian analysis requires only that educated approximations be made relying on common experience.[26]

Care also must be taken to recognize that these assignments of value be as objective as possible and not driven by personal views. Moreover, majority rule should not govern here; that is, small or moderate benefit to many does not necessarily outweigh great harm to a few. For example, a company should ask if it is ethical to market a hair growth drug for bald men that has a small potential for lethal side effects.

Scope of Analysis

A third difficulty with utilitarianism is called the scope or boundary issue. How broadly should the net be cast to include those affected by a business decision in order to determine if an action can produce maximal aggregate benefit over harm? Obviously, a company must consider the impact of its actions on its shareholders, customers, managers, and other employees. In the biomedical industry, affected individuals also include physicians who use and prescribe medical products and patients treated with these products. Beyond these obvious groups, who else, if anyone, should be included? Companies, for example, could consider the concerns of patient or environmental activists, but these groups are usually small or less organized compared with other groups, and it is not always easy to determine the extent to which they represent a broader constituency. Examples of other questions that can raise a boundary issue include:

- Should the company consider the impact on the overall cost of health care when it introduces an expensive new product?

- Should the company consider the social impact of a product? Judging by the enormous number of newspaper articles written about Viagra®, the introduction of this drug appeared to have had a huge impact on American society, ranging from saved to ruined marital relationships, new opportunities for sexual abuse, widespread discussions of male sexuality, and new questions about the meaning of sex in old age. But how much of this impact is the concern of the drug's manufacturer?

- Should a drug company that engages in direct-to-consumer prescription drug advertising factor in the effect of these ads on the demands on physician time by patients asking about drugs they have seen advertised?

- To what extent should a bio-agriculture seed company consider the possibility that use of its product might put farmers at risk of field destruction by environmental activists?

- To what extent should a pharmaceutical company consider the public health impact of its product? Antiretroviral drugs that could reduce HIV levels to nondetectable levels were linked to an erosion of safe-sex practices in the gay community. Selling antibiotics as a poultry feed supplement was feared to cause a rise in life-threatening antibiotic-resistant infections in people who ate antibiotic-contaminated meat. Are these legitimate concerns for pharmaceutical companies?[27]

Time is another dimension of the scope issue, and managers need to ask whether only short-term or long-term consequences should be considered in a utilitarian analysis. To respond to uncertainties about who to include in the aggregate of those affected by corporate activity, prudence suggests that, when in doubt, companies lean toward setting larger boundaries and relax the utilitarian standard so as to make utilitarian-tending choices.

Rights and Justice in the Utilitarian Framework

Perhaps the most serious weakness of the application of utilitarianism is that, because it focuses on overall consequences, there is a tendency to ignore the rights of individuals or considerations of justice by allowing the interests of the majority to override those of the minority. For example, using humans to learn about the effects of experimental drugs can usually be justified from a utilitarian perspective. If the drug is more effective than harmful, large numbers of sick people (including the human subjects) will benefit, and if the drug is more harmful than beneficial, the injuries incurred by the research subjects will prevent the drug from being marketed, thereby sparing many sick people in the general population from suffering the adverse reaction. Either way, medical science is advanced and companies are either in a better position to make a profit or are spared the costs of marketing an ineffective or harmful drug. In the worst case, a few are harmed to serve the interests of many, which is an acceptable utilitarian outcome. In another example, for companies considering whether to use American or third world country patients to test a new drug, the utilitarian argument can even go so far as to attempt to justify the third world research by concluding that subjecting wealthier sick Americans to research risk produces more overall harm than using patients in the indigent society because the latter contribute less to society. Such reasoning ignores the rights of individual research subjects, tends to allow them to be used solely as a means to an end, and places the burdens of society on the minority. The immorality of using people solely as a means to a research end was affirmed long before the atrocities of medical experimentation that occurred during Germany's Third Reich. But how to achieve the utilitarian goal of human research while fully respecting and protecting the rights of subjects continues to be not only a relevant question but also an unsettled matter.

To some extent, utilitarianism can address these questions and, if long-term consequences are taken into account, might produce the conclusion that if the rights of research subjects are routinely abused, eventually no one will agree to become a research subject. Such a result will bring this useful activity to a halt.

For this reason, rule utilitarians would adopt rules that certain research rights must be respected at all times. Viewed in this light, such rights are deemed "instrumental" and justified under consequentialist systems because, in more cases than not, respecting these rights results in benefits that exceed their associated costs. But most human subjects' rights, such as the right of the subject to consent before being experimented upon, are considered "intrinsic" in that they are to be respected because they have moral standing independent of the consequences. Utilitarianism cannot account for these rights, and it would be inappropriate to ignore the added dimensions that a rights and a justice analysis can bring to business activities such as human research.

KANTIAN ETHICS, RIGHTS, AND DUTIES

Concepts of rights and duties exist in the deontological realm of ethics. Broadly defined, a right is an entitlement to act in a certain way and, implicitly, to have others act in a particular way toward you. Rights have corresponding duties. For instance, a right to privacy of medical information collected in medical research requires that companies have a duty to refrain from disclosing medical information. What makes a right moral is not that it is granted by law (for example, some laws, such as forced sterilization, existed in the United States in the early 1900s, but were immoral), nor by widespread consensus (until recently, it was common practice that researchers did not disclose whether they had a significant financial interest in the company whose product they were researching). What makes a right moral is its consistency with principles, the most authoritative of which were developed by the philosopher Immanuel Kant.

Kant believed that morality should be derived from a recognition that we share a common human condition, that what makes us valuable as humans is our ability to reason, and that moral rules grounded on reason should govern human behavior. According to Kant, this view was preferable to rules grounded in tradition, intuition, desire, conscience, emotion, or sympathy. Kant believed that free will comes from our ability to reason and prompts people to develop rules for moral behavior that are universally applicable regardless of any utilitarian consequences. These moral rules should recognize that all people have a certain human dignity and deserve respect as autonomous beings.

From his beliefs, Kant formulated an overarching canon for the acceptability of all moral rules that he called the "categorical imperative." The validity of moral rules is determined by testing them against two related formulations of the categorical imperative.

(1) An act is ethical if it can be applied
universally to all and is reversible.

This first formulation of Kant's categorical imperative is similar to the Golden Rule and, in its modern version, can be stated as follows: an action is morally right for a person in a certain situation if, and only if, the person's reason for carrying out the action is one that he or she would be willing to have every person act on, in any similar situation.[28] This formulation is universal since it requires every similarly situated person to do the same thing for the same reason. The formulation is also reversible since it requires a willingness to have others treat you for the same reasons that you treat them. Kant intended that an action be considered morally worthy only if performed by someone motivated by a morally valid reason, that is, that it was the right way for all people to behave. Conversely, moral worth would not be attached to an action motivated solely to advance personal interests or for pleasure and that, if an act is wrong for other people, it is wrong for any one person unless there is some compelling difference that justifies making an exception.

As an example of how Kant's formulation can be applied, consider the following question. In order to avoid refusals and to obtain as much data as efficiently as possible, should Dr. Golda be able to use hospital patients in an experiment without their knowledge? To answer the question according to Kant, Dr. Golda needs to ask what it would be like if all researchers were similarly motivated and behaved in this way and whether she would want to be used in this way if she were hospitalized. If Dr. Golda is not willing to have all researchers behave this way, even toward her, then the act is morally wrong.

(2) Persons should be considered as ends
and not only as means to an end.

According to Kant, all people have equal dignity and treating people as ends requires that each person's freedom or autonomy be respected and that people will be treated only as they freely consent to be treated.[29] Respecting this formulation of the categorical imperative means that, for instance, it would be wrong to obtain the consent of a patient to participate in human experimentation without telling the patient beforehand of the risks and other consequences of participation. Without this information, patients cannot choose freely whether or not to participate, and without the ability to exercise free choice, patients are allowed to be used merely as a source of research data. Furthermore, research physicians should be motivated to obtain fully informed consent out of respect for the freedom of the individual patient and not because of the good or bad consequences of providing the information. The fact that disclosing a particularly frightening risk, for instance, would likely dissuade many patients from agreeing to the research should not be a factor in deciding whether to make the disclosure.

From Kant's categorical imperative, it is easy to see how the concepts of moral rights and duties developed. If everyone is to be treated as a free person equal to everyone else, then it follows that people have a right to such treatment and that others have a corresponding duty to operate in such a way as to respect, protect, and refrain from violating those rights. Rights developed from this position, such as the right to free speech or to be free from deception, arise from agreement about essential human interests.

Frequently, there are several different competing rights and duties involved in managing a business situation. Rights can be specific to certain individuals (such as rights granted by contract), general (rights belonging to all persons), negative (creates an obligation for others to refrain from acting in ways that interfere with the freedom of action of others), or positive (obliges others to provide whatever is necessary to implement the right). When more than one right is involved, which has priority over others is usually determined by whether the right has been legally granted or claimed. Legally granted rights are considered mandatory, and claimed rights need to be justified before they create a corresponding duty to uphold the right. While it may seem that a legally granted right might be easily identified compared to one that is claimed, the distinctions present some complications for those who attempt to sort out any conflicts in the priority of rights at stake.

Legal Rights

Many rights are legally granted, many laws having been enacted after instances of abuse. For example, legal protections were enacted to stop using prisoners as subjects of unduly risky research and to stop coercive inducements to participate.[30] Legal rights are protected entitlements that legally require others not to infringe on the right. Yet although legal rights are obligatory, they are not easily or uniformly applicable for several reasons. Legal rights are specific to a particular jurisdiction or country and are not shared by all people, so that prisoners will not have the same legal protection everywhere. Another difficulty with legal rights is that, even when regulations specify what constitutes prisoner protection, there can be continuing debates about what conduct falls within the ambit of the law. For instance, prison research review boards are required to ensure that "any possible advantages accruing to the prisoner through his or her participation in the research, when compared to the general living conditions, medical care, quality of food, amenities and opportunity for earnings in the prison, are not of such a magnitude that his or her ability to weigh the risks of the research against the value of such advantages in the limited choice environment of the prison is impaired."[31] It is easy to see how there can be disagreements about what aspects of a research protocol will impermissibly impair a prisoner's ability to weigh the risks and benefits of research. Sometimes the courts have settled such disputes after lawsuits are brought. Often however, there is no court opinion that is "on point" with the practice in question.

At times, some rights, while not legally granted, have been informally promulgated in codes of ethics and can be authoritative in guiding conduct or future legislation. Like legally granted rights, many ethics codes and guidelines were developed in response to abuses, such as when the Nuremberg Code and the Declaration of Helsinki (described further in Chapter 4) were developed to prevent abusive medical experiments like those that had occurred under the Third Reich in Germany. Similarly, in the United States, human subject protection laws were passed after disclosure of several instances of research abuse. For example, the 1963 Jewish Chronic Disease case in Brooklyn, New York, involved researchers injecting live cancer cells into patients without their knowledge. The Tuskegee syphilis study, halted in 1973, involved physicians observing the natural course of syphilis in four hundred African American men for decades after it was known that penicillin cured the disease. These and other mistreatments led to the first U.S. research protection law, the 1974 National Research Act. This act created the National Commission for the Protection of Human Subjects of Biomedical and Behavioral Research, which published its recommendations in what is known as the *Belmont Report*.[32] Shortly thereafter, the President's Commission for the Study of Ethical Problems in Medicine and Biomedical and Behavioral Research also made recommendations on how the rights of research subjects were to be protected.[33] These documents have had a substantial impact on American human research practice and policies, and many of the concepts, especially those from the national commission, were subsequently incorporated into U.S. federal and state laws and regulations.[34] However, the research protection laws did not adopt all aspects of the recommendations in these documents, and there are also differences between the American laws and research commission reports and those from various other countries. Debates continue to exist, therefore, about whether recommended research rights qualify for protection. Nonetheless, rights enumerated in ethics codes or by government commission, while they may not have been accorded legal status, deserve considerable respect so long as they were promulgated by an objective, authoritative, and deliberative entity.

Claimed Rights

Given the ambiguities and lack of uniformity of laws, many rights in a business situation will be claimed and not granted. Claimed rights are moral entitlements whose legitimacy stems from general agreement that the right exists to promote a fundamental human interest. Unlike legal rights, under a Kantian view, all people should have the same moral rights. However, there are disagreements about whether claimed rights are Kantian and valid. Debates have existed for years in the United States about whether there is a right to a minimum level of health care and whether laws should be passed to protect such a right. Engaging in a Kantian analysis and applying the categorical imperative requirements does not automatically result in a definitive answer to this debate.

Other Difficulties and Limitations in a Rights Analysis

There can be other problems in applying a Kantian rights analysis to decide what is moral conduct. For instance, Kant's theory lacks specificity so that defining a right can be difficult. If a patient claims a right to privacy of his medical information, this cannot be considered an absolute right if no one could fulfill a duty to provide absolute privacy. There are many legitimate ways that medical information privacy could be lost, such as when laws require that physicians report the names of patients with specific infectious diseases to the health department. Therefore, the right to medical privacy needs to be redefined to include exceptions created by law. In addition, hospitals allow researchers to have access to medical record information and human biological materials stored in pathology laboratories so long as they do not label the data with any identifying information about the patient. However, so that researchers can subsequently determine the medical relevance of the data (for example, whether patients with a specific gene defect subsequently suffer a given disease), many researchers assign an identification code to the data that is linked indirectly to the patient's identity. Whether this is an impermissible invasion of a patient's right to medical privacy has been hotly debated.[35] A similar problem exists with a right to be free of research harm. It is impossible to ensure complete freedom from harm for a research subject, since research can never be a risk-free endeavor. So the right may be better stated as a right to be reasonably free from harm. The definition of "reasonably" makes this right amorphous and open to interpretation.

Even if there is general agreement on what interests have the status of moral rights, it can be difficult to determine the limits of the right and what action is required to uphold it. For example, in some sense, human subjects are always used as a means to an end, but it is not always clear what it takes to ensure that they are not used *solely* to derive research data. Ideally, all human subjects should be treated as we would wish to be treated in similar circumstances. But business managers can find it difficult to assess how a company's research recruitment strategies affect potential human subjects. Opinions have differed, for instance, on what constitutes undue coercion that can hamper free choice of a potential human subject—payments? free medical care? access to potentially life-saving experimental treatment? The answers would probably differ depending on the group recruited, their age, their economic status, and the extent and severity of their illness. Inducements can influence the behavior of physicians as well, for example, in the incentives offered to physicians by pharmaceutical companies to prescribe a drug. Questionable incentives in the past have included such things as free medical equipment, invitations to meetings in upscale resorts, and frequent-flier miles based on the number of prescriptions written.[36] Distinctions between effective sales effort and unfair pressure are not always clear, and today pharmaceutical companies are frequently asking themselves about the proper limits of sales inducement offers. Under a rights analysis, this question translates to asking what offers would violate a physician's right to be treated as a rational being entitled to make free, informed prescribing choices and not to be treated as a means to a sales end.

Another difficulty is that rights can conflict, and it can be difficult to determine which rights should be limited in favor of others. An intractable conflict that raises this issue is the abortion debate, which has been characterized as conflict between the right to life of a fetus versus the right of the pregnant woman to choose whether or not to bear a child. Or, some AIDS activists have claimed a right to access certain anti-HIV-drug pricing information that a company considers to be a highly sensitive trade secret. Finding alternatives that can satisfy both parties to such conflicts takes especially creative thought. Oftentimes, there will be no fully adequate solution, but choices can be made that respect in part the rights of each party.

Finally, agreements about what rights exist can evolve and change over time. Product advertising was once (and still is in some instances) conducted under the precept of *caveat emptor* (let the buyer beware). Advertising abuses led to truth in advertising laws, passed in recognition of the fact that consumers have a right to be free from fraud and deception. Also, there is a new right of access to investigational drugs being claimed by sick patients who demand enrollment in clinical trials. Researchers are currently trying to reconcile this claimed right with the notion that much research is nontherapeutic and risky and that research takes place primarily to benefit researchers and medical progress, not to provide individual benefit to human subjects.

All of these difficulties can come into play when attempting to analyze whether contemplated business action impacts the rights of others and whether the company has any duties with respect to these rights.

Rights Analysis Method

In order to fulfill a business responsibility to respect the rights of those affected by business decisions, managers must be able to identify and sufficiently define rights, prioritize them, and decide how they influence corporate choices, all the while dealing with the ambiguities and difficulties discussed above. To conduct a rights analysis and to counter some of the problems of engaging in a rights analysis, especially where rights conflict, the following process is suggested:

- Identify the rights at stake: do they have moral standing (that is, are they universal and reversible according to the Kantian framework)? If an interest seems to deserve protection but cannot be considered an "absolute" right, reframe the definition of the interest so that it is possible to respect and protect it as a right. Thus, instead of a right to privacy, say that there is a right to a reasonable degree of privacy, and then define the limits of what is considered reasonable.

- Determine whether the rights at stake are claimed or are granted in law or contract and give priority to granted rights and second priority to those rights enumerated in established codes of ethics before addressing any claimed rights.

- Determine what the moral or legal basis is for the right, acknowledging that a legal basis does not necessarily confer moral status but does require higher priority.

- Determine what interests the rights protect (for example, liberty, opportunity, autonomy).

- Determine what actions are consistent with the identified rights.
- Assign priority to the rights in question. Delete rights that are not universal and reversible, respect granted rights, give priority to claimed rights based on the importance of the interests served, and also give priority to limited (versus broad) claimed rights.[37]
- When rights conflict and call for different outcomes, act consistently with the highest of rights.

Becoming facile with a rights analysis is important for managers in bioscience companies that engage in or sponsor human subject research. The Genzyme, Adiana, and VaxGen case studies in this text all involve aspects of human subject rights.

JUSTICE AND FAIRNESS

Justice is a concept that is widely applied in social, legal, political, and economic practices and institutions. Notions of justice, which are essentially comparable to those of fairness, come into play when dealing with questions of who gets what in society and for what reasons. Justice therefore deals with three main concepts: the fair distribution of the benefits and burdens in society (distributive justice); compensation for harms committed (compensatory justice); and punishment for wrongdoing (retributive justice). The concepts of justice relevant to business ethics primarily involve those dealing with distribution and compensation.[38]

Justice Versus Utilitarianism Versus Rights

Concepts of justice are often considered to be more important than utilitarian outcomes. Therefore, for example, many in the international human rights community believe that the coerced abortion and contraception/sterilization laws in the People's Republic of China are unjust even if forced limitations on the number of children lessen poverty and overcrowding and improve the public health in that country.[39] Under justice and rights principles, achieving greater benefits for a group is not a valid reason to treat some members unfairly, to force them to make sacrifices, or infringe on personal liberties. There are conditions, however, such as with infectious disease epidemics, where the potential gains are sufficiently large or important that a certain level of injustice or rights infringement can be tolerated. Compared to utilitarianism, justice and rights are closer relatives. Because justice principles have been derived in part on respect for the rights of people to be treated freely and equally, justice considerations do not usually override the moral rights of individuals. Only to correct extreme injustice can the rights of certain individuals be restricted.

FORMAL AND MATERIAL PRINCIPLES OF JUSTICE

Common to all theories of justice is a minimal requirement traditionally attributed to Aristotle that equals are to be treated equally, and unequals can be treated unequally so long as the differences between them are relevant to the circumstances under consideration. This requirement is called the formal principle of equality, and it does not identify what groups are equal or what is a relevant difference that can justify unequal treatment. Material principles of justice, however, specify the circumstances that are relevant to justify unequal treatment (for example, merit, effort, need, and so on) and prescribe who is entitled to equal or unequal treatment. As will be seen in the discussions below on distributive and compensatory justice, the formal principle of equality is the same for each category of justice and the material principles provide specifics on how justice can be achieved.

DISTRIBUTIVE JUSTICE

Distributive justice is concerned with the fair allocation of the benefits and burdens in society. Issues concerning distributive justice exist when the demand for beneficial goods and services outstrips supply. The formal principle of distributive justice requires that there be consistency in the way we distribute benefits and allocate burdens to similarly situated people. There are numerous material principles used to determine how we might legitimately treat groups inconsistently, for example, based on equality, merit, need, or contribution. For instance, when human organs are scarce, as they generally are, principles of distributive justice can guide determinations of which patients should have priority to receive an organ. The formal principle of equality requires that similarly situated patients should have equal access. The material principles are used to develop the criteria that are relevant to determine who gets first priority in organ allocation and specify the factors that are relevant to the circumstances. For liver failure patients, for instance, medical need is an obvious criterion as is the patient's ability to make good use of the organ. Therefore, patients with more severe organ failure and whose health is otherwise good will have priority over patients whose liver disease is milder or who cannot refrain from excessive liver-destroying alcohol consumption or who cannot comply with the rigorous post-transplant medical regimen. Other factors, such as the sex or wealth of the patient are agreed to be irrelevant to the decision of where the patient is placed on the transplant waiting list. Other factors have been debated regarding their relevancy to allocation policies; for example, where the patient lives (the organ donation system is regional and some regions have a greater supply of organs), the "worthiness" of the patient (many find it difficult to put a patient on the priority list who is imprisoned for a heinous crime; there were also questions about why Mickey Mantle received an organ when the probability of his post-transplant survival was so limited), or age (younger patients will use this scarce resource longer, and the older the patient is, the more likely the organ will be seen as wasted for the relatively shorter life span it provides). It has taken years and large numbers of people to arrive at the current organ distribution system. Debates about fairness of access continue, however, and the material principles of organ distribution are continually being reassessed.[40] The Merck case study in Chapter 11 involves questions about the fair distribution of a limited supply of life-saving drugs.

Another goal of distributive justice is to fairly allocate the burdens of society, and this can also lead to disagreements, such as when people debate how taxes should be assessed. Another example is the controversy about whether foreign patients should be used as research subjects in preference to U.S. patients. The formal principle of justice requires that we first ask whether the two groups are equal. If they are (for example, same health characteristics), preferring foreign over U.S. patients would unjustly expose the foreigners to the burdens of the research risks. If the two groups are unequal in relevant ways (the foreign group has a much higher incidence of the disease the drug is intended to treat), then there is a justifiable reason to place that population at risk. The Monsanto case study included in the next chapter highlights the various considerations that can come into play when attempting to ensure that everyone bears a fair share of burdens.

The continuing debates surrounding allocation of scarce organs and distribution of tax burdens and benefits illustrate how difficult it can be to agree on what constitutes fair distribution and equitable trade-offs. One of the reasons for the difficulty is that there are several commonly used material principles of distributive justice that are relevant to decision making. The conclusions drawn from their application tend to be inconsistent. Under many of these material distribution rules, allocating benefits to some can create burdens for others. For instance, diseased patients are spared from drug toxicities when research with human subjects demonstrates that a drug is too toxic to market. Also, what is considered just under one rule can be unjust under another. So, while each of the material principles can be useful in resolving distributive justice questions, each also has its drawbacks, and specific circumstances can often determine what rule is appropriate. The following list of common distribution rules allows for an examination of the characteristics that may be relevant when determining what benefits and burdens people should receive.

First Come, First Served

One simple principle that people often use to decide who should receive goods or services in short supply is the principle of first come, first served. This principle operates when waiting in line to receive a limited number of concert tickets or when businesses use seniority systems for managerial advancement. This principle assumes that being first is relevant to determining who should be served first when not all can be served at once or at all. In some cases, this might be justified because the first person should be rewarded when his or her ability, ingenuity, industriousness, or sacrifice contributed to earning this spot. However, first come, first served ignores many factors that might be more relevant, such as need.

Egalitarianism

Egalitarians believe that all humans are fundamentally equal and are entitled to share equally in society's goods and services and should also equally share in the burdens.[41] Many political systems are founded on principles of equality, which require that all people, regardless of their differences, be accorded the same political rights, be treated equally before the law, and have equal duties to refrain from interfering in the rights of others. When it comes to economic systems, an egalitarian distribution of goods and services is easy to administer and tends to cause solidarity, harmony, and cooperation within a group by eliminating the need to compete and by indicating that all people are valued equally. Egalitarianism also eliminates discrimination since all groups are treated the same regardless of racial, religious, sexual, or other traits. However, many find it too difficult to adhere to a system of economic egalitarianism because they cannot ignore the fact that most humans differ in such fundamental characteristics as mental and physical ability, contribution, effort, or need, and these factors can be relevant to deciding what people deserve. Because of these differences, equal distribution of benefits, such as salaries, can result in unfairness. Furthermore, those who are more productive but who get no more than those who contribute minimally are apt to lose motivation, which leads to inefficiency and loss of productivity. To correct for these problems, some egalitarians limit the requirement for equality to a certain level, after which goods and services can be distributed based on need, merit, or other factors. Proponents of such a view might argue that all people are equally entitled to a certain minimum level of health care and that more advanced health care can be obtained by those who have medical insurance or who can otherwise afford it.

To Each According to His or Her Contribution

When goods and services are distributed based on the value of what people contribute, the more people contribute, the more they get, and vice versa. Often compared with capitalism, under this system of distribution, people who pay more, get more. Basing salaries and work promotions on contribution tends to promote business competition and productivity. This proportionality also extends to distributions of burdens. The more that someone contributes to a problem, for instance, the more he or she should shoulder the burden of correcting it. Like other distribution systems, this one ignores need. Also, those who are unable to contribute (because of a disability or illness, for instance) are left out. Paying more to get more can lead to unfairness, such as with campaign contributions or health services, in which those who cannot afford to pay lack access to power and valuable services. It can also be difficult to objectively value various types of contribution. Because of a lack of innate ability, one person may need to work very hard to produce less than a gifted colleague who extends little effort. Some have advocated that market forces determine the value of people's contribution, but market forces do not always seem to correlate with intrinsic value; for example, the low salaries of school teachers as compared to those of professional athletes.

From Each According to His or Her Abilities, to Each According to His or Her Needs

Need-based distribution systems are little used in business but are commonly found in medicine and the health care system. Under the most common formulation of such a distribution system, likened to the socialist teachings of Karl Marx, people should contribute according to their abilities, and these contributions are distributed according to need. If everyone contributes according to their full abilities, groups benefit from the maximal productivity of their members. When need is the only relevant factor in distributing goods and services, the well-being of the group as a whole is served. These notions are difficult to apply in business since the needs of a company are often in conflict with the needs of those related to the company—employees, contractors, business partners, customers—all of whom might assert their needs for the company to pay more money, lower prices, or provide more benefits. Difficulties in applying a need-based distribution system to business also include the fact that such a system dampens the incentive to work harder, to compete, and to produce more, because what one gets is not related to the amount of effort expended. By their nature, businesses are competitive and seek to advance their own interests, and if need is a factor, it comes into play as a recognition of a business opportunity to fill a marketplace need. Businesses could not exist if they priced products based on need. In medicine, however, need is often a primary factor in deciding who receives benefits and who has to wait. Sicker patients get seen first in the emergency room, older patients get first access to the influenza vaccine, poorer patients get government health care support. When bioscience businesses interact with the health care system, these different approaches can lead to conflict, such as when third world countries cannot afford to buy drugs from first world companies and demand price breaks.

Procedures Determine Just Distribution

It is always appropriate to consider procedures when formulating a distribution system, and fair procedures are so important to some that they are the sole determinant of just outcomes. Adherents to this view tend to be libertarian in nature and believe in social and economic liberty. A libertarian approach to distribution values the free and unregulated operation of fair procedures over any result such as equality or utility. Under this view, people should be free to choose what they contribute and free to obtain rewards based on effort. This freedom to act should be preserved even if it eventually results in inequalities in the distribution of benefits and burdens in society. So long as the procedures by which benefits and burdens were allocated were fair and voluntary, any nonvoluntary readjustment in position is considered to infringe on basic liberty. The only circumstance under which interference is tolerated in this system is when government or some other entity seeks to correct or redress an unfair distribution process.

The most widely quoted adherent of a libertarian view of justice is Robert Nozick, who developed what has been called an "entitlement theory of justice."[42] Nozick's theory holds that that there are three principles that ensure just distributions. First, the principle of "justice in acquisition" states that there must be fairness in the way things came to be originally acquired. The principle of "justice in transfer" states that there must be fairness in the way things are subsequently acquired from the original holder or divested to others. The principle of "rectification of justice" states that any unfairness in the process of acquisition and transfer can be rectified. So long as fair procedures were followed, people are entitled to keep what they end up with without outside interference or re-allocation. Nozick asserts that adherence to this theory favors initiative and protects private property, rights, free choice, and legal exchange.

Several problems with a libertarian view of distribution have been identified. It can be difficult to determine what are fair procedures. Also, preserving the individual liberty of one person can often impinge on the liberty of others. In addition, placing such emphasis on being free of involuntary re-allocation of benefits and burdens ignores other freedoms that are important to people. Disadvantaged people also suffer in a libertarian distribution system. People who cannot afford to pay or who cannot work or produce through no fault of their own or lack of effort do not participate in the acquisition and distribution of goods and services and must depend on the voluntary help of others. There will always be differences in economic ability and in opportunities to be productive that create groups of needy people and that prompt governments to re-allocate wealth to assist those in need.

Justice as Fairness: Rawls

Depending on the circumstance, any of the above principles of justice can be applicable and valid. Conflicts among them, however, can create serious priority-setting problems, and sole reliance on any one often leads to unjust results. To compensate for these difficulties, people have naturally tended to use either different theories in different situations or to blend features of two or more principles to arrive at what they consider to be a just result. The most influential, comprehensive, and structured attempt of this nature came from Harvard professor John Rawls.[43] To arrive at just solutions when conflicts develop between people pursuing their self-interests, Rawls places primary importance on basic human civil and political rights and on people's ability to freely choose their own ends. Rawls believes that these rights and freedoms should never be violated to produce greater good for others. To further these rights and freedoms, his theory of justice relies heavily on Kantian concepts of equality. Rawls also attempts to ameliorate the unfairness of applications of libertarian and utilitarian theories. With these beliefs as a foundation, Rawls set about to develop both a method by which people can arrive at a fair distribution of society's benefits and burdens and a set of principles that can be applied using that method.

Rawls's method involves a hypothetical construct in which people are all rational and self-serving and they make distribution decisions not knowing who they are in society. Rawls calls the situation of such an imaginary group of persons the "original position," and he calls their ignorance about who they are the "veil of ignorance." As an example, in deciding whether priority for access to pharmaceuticals should be given to those who can pay, Rawls's group of self-interested, rational people in the original position would not know if they were rich or poor, sick or well, physicians or lay people. Being ignorant of their place in society, it is unlikely that people would agree that ability to pay would be a fair way to get first access to important drugs. If they ended up in society being poor or sick, people would want those factors to be taken into consideration over ability to pay to get access to treatment. Because they are unable to predict who they are, people will be unable to safeguard their own special interests and will be forced to choose principles of access that are fair to all. Rawls argues that using the construct of the original position and making distributive justice decisions behind the "veil of ignorance" is morally justified because the original position incorporates the Kantian moral ideas of reversibility (the parties choose principles that will apply to themselves), of universalizability (the principles must apply equally to everyone), and of treating people as ends (each party has an equal say in the choice of principles).

The principles that Rawls developed to resolve situations of social conflict are as follows:

1. Each person has an equal right to the most extensive basic liberties compatible with similar liberties for all, and
2. Social and economic inequalities are arranged so that they are both
   a. to the greatest benefit of the least advantaged persons and
   b. attached to offices and positions open to all under conditions of fair equality of opportunity.

According to Rawls, if there is a conflict, principle 1 takes priority over principle 2, and within principle 2, part *b* takes priority over part *a*.

Principle 1 is called the principle of equal liberty. Essentially it says that everyone's liberties are equal and all share the duties to protect liberties from infringement. Among the important basic liberties, Rawls included the right to vote, freedom of speech and conscience, and the other civil liberties, freedom to hold property, and freedom from arbitrary arrest. Under the principle of equal liberty, people (and businesses) would refrain from invading privacy, using force, using undue influence or bribery to get their way, committing fraud, breaking contractual promises, or otherwise violating the equal liberties of others or giving them reason to fear they will not be treated equally and fairly. From a distribution standpoint, principle 1 stands for the proposition that if it is possible to share equally, no one should be forced to accept less than an equal share. The only time the principle of equal liberty would be rejected is when everyone is better off with the inequality. In other words, the bar is raised for everyone only under situations of inequality.

Principle 2 is a recognition that equality cannot always be achieved and provides rules for how inequalities can be fairly distributed. The goal of principle 2 is to have everyone benefit from social and economic inequalities. Part *a* of principle 2, called the "difference principle," was founded on the belief that many advantages were not earned but were obtained through the "luck of the draw" (for example, birth, historical circumstances, or natural endowments) and that it is only fair to correct these undeserved advantages by improving the situation of naturally disadvantaged people. Rawls also believed that people in the original position would choose to abide by the difference principle since they would want to protect themselves if they ended up in the worst-off position. Again, the only exception to the difference principle would occur if, in improving the worst-off position, everyone, including the neediest, would be worse off than before.

Part *b* of principle 2 is the principle of "fair equality of opportunity." It says that everyone should be given an equal opportunity to qualify for society's positions, goods, and services. Once given equal access to things like training, education, or information, people can advance themselves through the use of their abilities, efforts, and contributions.

According to Rawls, society should design its institutions based on what choices people will make from the original position and how they will behave once the veil of ignorance is lifted and people begin to pursue their own interests. Similarly, businesses can make policies on matters of moral concerns by applying Rawls's principles and then take actions consistent with the policies developed.

As with other theories of distributive justice, the value of various aspects of Rawls's theory has been debated. Some object that there is insufficient explanation as to how the set-up of the original position and the veil of ignorance would necessarily result in choosing moral principles. It is also not clear that these people would choose the two principles that Rawls did. Many people would prefer to take more risks to get bigger rewards and would eliminate the leveling protection of the difference principle. Others who favor utilitarianism do not believe Rawls provides sufficiently for the greater good. Libertarians think that Rawls's framework is unjust to those who should receive more benefits because they are more capable or hardworking. Finally, others have questioned the priority that Rawls placed on the various principles, such as valuing freedom over need.

Despite the criticisms, Rawls's approach to justice has been widely accepted as a useful business ethics tool since it fits in with our basic economic institutions, accepting the market system in principle 1 and providing adjustments in principle 2 for the unfairness that can result from the unfettered operation of free markets. At the same time, Rawls's theory tends to preserve generally agreed upon basic values of freedom, equality of opportunity, and a concern for the disadvantaged. Third, the theory allows for the expression of both the communitarian and the individualistic tendencies of Western people. The communitarian tendency is furthered in the difference principle, in which those who are better off assist the needy. The principle of equal liberty encourages the free pursuit of individual special interests. Fourth, the difference principle accounts for need and, with the application of the equality of opportunity, would allow for qualities such as ability, effort, and contribution to determine distribution of benefits and burdens. Last, the original position embodies fairness since it forces people to choose impartial principles that take into account the equal interests of everyone.

Despite their differences and the problems that come from their application, each of the theories of justice has its own appeal, and managers are encouraged to find ways to take the best from each theory to find just solutions to moral business problems. The Merck case in Chapter 11 was written for this purpose.

COMPENSATORY JUSTICE

Compensatory justice deals with the ways that people are compensated when they are harmed by others, with justice served if the compensation is adequate and fair. Another aspect of a compensatory justice system is that, if designed properly, it tends to provide incentives to prevent injuries and reduce social costs, such as when child-proof caps were placed on medication bottles to prevent accidental poisonings in children. Outside of contractual arrangements, this issue comes into play in the bioscience industry most often when products harm patients or when human subjects are injured while participating in research. The laws that grew out of product liability and personal injury have drawn heavily on concepts of compensatory justice and are useful in determining when compensatory justice is required and how much is owed. Chapter 8 deals with these issues.

The following set of rules can be applied to decide whether there is a moral obligation to compensate a patient or subject injured by a medical product:

- The company's action was the direct cause for the injury or
- The physician or researcher was the direct cause and the company's action indirectly contributed to the injury and
- The company action that inflicted the injury was wrong or negligent.[44]

For product-related injuries, this last rule has been challenged. For instance, some have argued that, as under product liability law, the fault of the company should not determine whether compensation is required for product-related injuries. Rather, compensation for injury should be paid regardless of whether there was any corporate wrongdoing. Such a "strict liability" system, it is argued, gives incentives to the company to take special care in the design, testing, manufacturing, and marketing (including instructions and warnings) of products so as to ensure as much as possible the safety of those using the product. Assuming that these incentives are effective, societies may want to place the entire burden of product safety on the company that produced and marketed the product. Therefore, a single alternative rule for compensating the injured victim can simply be that the company's product caused injury to the patient.

The goal of compensatory justice is to restore the victim to his or her original position as much as possible. Determining how much compensation is required to meet this goal can also be determined by a set of rules, some of which may conflict with each other.

- The compensation should return what was lost
- The compensation should restore the victim to his or her original position
- The amount of compensation should be reduced proportionate to the degree to which the victim or others contributed to the injury

Problems in applying these rules for medical product injury include the fact that some losses are impossible to measure or to restore, such as loss of sight or life. In such cases, money is used as a substitute and given to the injured patient or family. Placing a monetary value on these events is often a process of negotiation guided by what juries or insurance companies have paid in the past under like circumstances. Another problem, however, is that the amount of compensation demanded or required in some cases can be so high that the company cannot afford it. This has happened often in the pharmaceutical and medical product industry, where mass tort litigation, such as for the drug Bendectin and the Dalkon Shield intrauterine device, has resulted in damage awards so high that companies declare bankruptcy or pull the product from the market. Finally, deciding how much other parties have contributed to a specific injury and involving them in compensation can be difficult.

METHOD FOR ETHICS ANALYSIS AND DECISION MAKING

Each of the moral systems described above has been touted as being sufficiently comprehensive to apply to the full range of ethics problems. However, too often a single system fails to address all factors that should be considered when making business choices. Consequently, it is more common to see a more pluralistic business ethics analysis approach—either to determine that a particular situation dictates which moral system applies or to integrate all relevant moral systems in each case. This book relies on the latter approach. The situational approach seems to invite a selection of the moral principles that most conforms with the desired outcome. Thus, the choice of principle determines the answer to the problem, and the essence of moral reasoning becomes an exercise for justifying why Kantian or utilitarian principles, for instance, should apply to the question at hand. This is a difficult exercise because there are relatively few rules or generally acceptable guidelines for making this choice. In contrast, the integrative approach suggested here attempts to obtain insights from all relevant points of ethical views, including maximizing the beneficial consequences of action, honoring the legal and moral rights of those affected by a decision, fulfilling duties based on those rights, and fairly distributing benefits and burdens resulting from the business decision. These key elements can be used to create a process for a business ethics analysis that requires the business manager to do the following:

• Review the relevant facts thoroughly

• Generate alternatives and identify obvious moral concerns

- Analyze alternatives (as discussed above)
  - Examine the type and degree of the benefits and risks under a utilitarian analysis and decide which action maximizes aggregate benefit
  - Consider questions about potential rights of those affected by corporate action and decide what duties the company has to honor those rights
  - Consider the degree to which justice requires that the company, rather than other parties, should accept the burden of intervention
- Make and implement decisions
- Attempt to reconcile conflicting conclusions
  - Identify the optimal solution
  - Attempt to rectify and/or address the concerns of those who will have objections to the corporate decision

An example of how such an analysis might be applied follows the case study in the next chapter.

CONCLUSION

Reasoning from the three moral systems of utilitarianism, rights, and justice allows for a structured approach to guide business action, especially when conflicting claims and needs are involved that are not completely resolved legally. The preceding discussion shows that ethical analysis can be complicated and can result in conflicting conclusions. Ethically justified conclusions can also conflict with the law or can recommend action that is economically inefficient. As for many other business endeavors, managers must expect that disagreement about decisions and actions is a common feature of ethical reasoning. However, when managers develop analytical competence in applying ethical principles to specific situations and account for the conflicts and inconsistencies, ethical analysis can broaden the scope of inquiry and allow for the development of more creative and responsible solutions to business problems. Arriving at an ethically justifiable position will also allow managers to anticipate the actions of others whose motivations stem from moral concern. The company can then better understand and anticipate how others will respond to business decisions. For managers in an industry deeply involved in modern ethical and social issues, the inclusion of this type of ethical reasoning in decision making can become a valuable managerial skill.

Appendix 2.1

The Limits of Law as an Ethical Guide

One question that comes up frequently in discussions of business ethics is why adhering to laws and regulations does not sufficiently satisfy a company's obligation to act responsibly and ethically. After all, laws are based on commonly shared notions of what constitutes acceptable human and corporate conduct and these notions are usually derived from moral principles. The two systems, however, are different in nature and do not cover the same ground. Laws are derived in political systems, are enforced, have predetermined punishments for action that deviates from what is prescribed, and use judges and a judicial system to interpret and say what the law is. Laws can also violate moral principles. Voting laws that exclude groups of citizens are an example. Ethics, on the other hand, operates in a broader sphere and is self-determined, voluntary, unenforced, and unenforceable. Aside from being different in nature, the law does not adequately address ethical questions for the additional reasons listed below.[45]

MANY LAWS EXHORT BUT DO NOT DEFINE ETHICAL BEHAVIOR

Laws often employ ethical concepts that are imprecisely defined, such as "good faith," "due diligence," "due process," "adequate consideration," and "reasonable," making it difficult in some situations to decide what is legal without also considering what is ethical. The definitional imprecision forces business managers to operate in an arena of legal uncertainty because it is often unwise to wait until legal certainty exists. When certainty does develop, moral considerations and an assessment of "good" or "bad" business conduct have often shaped the development of laws. Thus, training in ethics can give a business manager a better perspective on what legislators and judges might consider legal conduct.

THE LAW IS NOT COMPREHENSIVE

The law does not and cannot deal with all conduct, but much conduct has an ethical dimension that should be considered. Companies often are financially rewarded for bold and aggressive maneuvering and it is not uncommon to hear that a company succeeded because it "pushed the envelope" of what was considered legal conduct. According to many business analysts, direct-to-consumer prescription drug advertising was typical of this aggressiveness. As an example, the ethical conduct of one company was publicly called into question when it used a pharmacy and a third-party mail house to send promotional material to patients taking its drug or its competitor's product. This program was not illegal but did raise questions about whether the company was improperly invading the privacy of patients' prescription records.[46] Similar censure was directed to another company that failed to consider the patient privacy issues when it legally negotiated with three teaching hospitals to obtain samples of left-over patient tissues to create a tissue bank business.[47] These examples highlight the fact that although the conduct in question is legal it still deserves consideration of whether it is ethical.

LAWS ARE SLOW TO EVOLVE

The law often plays catch-up with technology, especially when regulating new and challenging medical and biotechnology issues, such as embryonic stem cell derivation, human cloning, assisted reproductive technologies, xenotransplantation, or the production of human-animal chimeras. In these realms, judges, lawmakers, and regulators generally operate in a reactive rather than a proactive mode. In addition, the different branches of government can often play "hot potato" with some of these issues. For instance, in the Massachusetts Supreme Judicial Court case involving the question of whether children born of a dead man's sperm can be his legal heirs and receive Social Security survivor benefits, the judge who authored the opinion deplored the fact that too many new reproductive technology cases were coming to the courts without statutory guidance.[48] Rather than forcing people to sue and go to court, legal questions about medical technology and their associated ethical and social issues are more appropriately addressed, said the judge, in the comprehensive and deliberative legislative process. In essence, the court was asking the state legislature to "get on with it." Many times, the legislative response to such an exhortation is that comprehensive statutes cannot be written for such contentious and idiosyncratic matters. Most lawmakers have no medical or scientific training and therefore can be reluctant to wade into these complicated waters, preferring to gauge public opinion before taking a position or proposing new laws. When these issues become politically divisive, legislators often hesitate to sponsor new laws that will alienate at least some of their constituencies. Current congressional and state legislative wrangling over genetic testing, human cloning, and embryonic stem cell research are all examples of the legislative uncertainty caused by the shifting political climate that surrounds these new technologies.

Companies that have already developed business plans based on these technologies are therefore caught in a bind. There are no statutes or regulations to guide them. Neither can courts act rapidly enough to give companies timely legal guidance. Courts need a "case or controversy" before they can adjudicate a matter, therefore judges must wait until a lawsuit is brought. Contentious court cases can take years before the highest level court sets legal precedent. And when it is set, court-made legal precedent is limited to the facts of that particular case and is therefore often too limited to be broadly useful. Most companies intending to develop products based on new technologies cannot afford to wait for settled legal opinion to guide their activities. Ethical reasoning in management can serve to guide responsible behavior in the absence of legal authority.

THE LAW IS NOT UNIFORM

Laws governing research and business practices are not uniform across all jurisdictions. For instance, human research laws differ from state to state and country to country. There have been instances where companies were accused of engaging in "forum shopping" to conduct research in a country with the fewest legal restrictions. Such a practice can invite questions of why a company feels it is ethical to conduct research in one country that would be considered illegal and/or unethical somewhere else. Using an ethics approach to resolve such legal conflicts and inconsistencies can help managers decide on the responsible course of action. Chapter 9 deals with this issue.

LAWS AND REGULATIONS CHANGE

Laws can lose their legitimacy over time and legislative bodies and courts have been known to alter what was once considered legally settled. The need for legal change is often apparent long before new laws can be enacted. For example, long before there were any regulations requiring gender balanced medical research, numerous medical articles had been published about the negative consequences to women's health of failing to include them in clinical research.[49] In another example, the courts were being asked to change the law and make pharmaceutical companies responsible for failing to warn patients about drug safety hazards. It took more than ten years before the first court ruled that companies have this legal obligation under some circumstances.[50]

NEW LAWS ARE OFTEN WRITTEN TO STOP UNETHICAL CONDUCT OR TO PROMOTE ETHICAL CONDUCT

Because laws and regulations are frequently enacted to curb what is considered unethical or irresponsible conduct (e.g., research abuses, inadequate safety disclosures, overly aggressive marketing practices), an exclusive reliance on what is currently legal invites new legislation and litigation to control questionable conduct. For instance, there are no legal restrictions on the amount of money an American pharmaceutical company can charge for a new medical product. However, what has been viewed as overly aggressive and unfair pricing has fueled legislative efforts to impose drug price controls, as had been done in Europe.[51]

On the other hand, laws and regulations are sometimes designed to impose the good conduct of one company, industry, or profession on others. This occurred in the 1970s when a group of scientists convened at the Asilomar Conference Center in Pacific Grove, California, and called for an international moratorium on recombinant DNA research until scientists developed responsible research standards to ensure that the technology could be safely handled. Many of these scientists were convinced that the new technology was safe and were eager to continue their research work but were willing voluntarily to accept research restrictions in response to public safety concerns that were likely to result in government regulation. The Asilomar guidelines were adopted by the National Institutes of Health (NIH), which instituted the Recombinant DNA Advisory Committee (RAC) to enforce them.[52]

PPL Therapeutics also decided to self-regulate when it made the expensive decision to exceed the purification safety standards that the FDA's Center for Biologics was considering imposing on transgenic a_1-antitrypsin, the company's first human protein derived from transgenic animals. Even though there was no known risk of transmitting animal infections to humans from this product, the extra safety precautions were considered socially responsible, given the public fear of animal infections that resulted from the tragedy of the Mad Cow Disease outbreak in Britain.[53] Companies that want to avoid legal sanction and regulatory interferences or see their conduct widely adopted can benefit from a decision-making process that includes ethical considerations.

LAWS ARE NOT ALWAYS ENFORCED

The FDA suffers mightily from criticism that it is understaffed to enforce all of the food and drug laws and regulations. Even if the Agency was fully staffed, it is unlikely that it would be able to detect all illegal conduct in the industries under its jurisdiction. Consequently, illegal conduct can take place without sanction.

THE LAW DOES NOT ALWAYS CLARIFY
THE BOUNDARIES OF RESPONSIBILITY

How should industry operate as a socially responsible entity in a health care system that does not directly link companies to the patients who are ultimately benefited or harmed by industry products? The roles of the FDA and industry are to ensure that products are properly tested, manufactured, labeled with appropriate use instructions and warnings, and marketed in a responsible manner. Physicians, who are the company customers, are professionally and legally accountable for the proper use of the product. The FDA does not regulate the practice of medicine nor can medical product companies dictate to physicians how their approved products are to be used. Also, so long as medical product companies properly design, test, manufacture, and label their products, they have been insulated from liability to patients injured by those products. But are the legal and professional responsibilities of the FDA and medicine sufficient to relieve companies from a duty to take actions beyond what is legally required?

The so-called "learned intermediary" doctrine is the legal provision that allows a company to fulfill its duty to warn of medical product risks by supplying doctors and pharmacists with the FDA-approved product use and risk information. Once fully informed, a physician can decide how best to use or prescribe a product and what product information to pass on to the patient. Despite this legal protection, questions have been raised about the ethical obligation of companies to patients if the companies know, for instance, that physicians improperly prescribe their products. Industry, FDA, and physicians each have a role in the medical product approval and prescribing process, but there are sometimes differences of opinion about where the responsibilities of one entity ends and the other begins. Some companies prefer to rely on the judgment and integrity of FDA and physicians to fulfill their roles in the system. Other companies have assumed broader responsibilities to patients, especially if it is clear that either FDA or physicians have not or cannot adequately protect the patient from product harm and the company is in a position to do so.

This issue came up with Genentech's recombinant human growth hormone (rhGH), approved and labeled for use in children with a rare form of dwarfism caused by lack of natural growth hormone. So few children (an estimated 12,000 to 15,000 nationwide) had this condition that early questions were raised about how Genentech could ever recoup the considerable expenditure it made to bring this product to market.[54] After the product was launched, physicians began prescribing rhGH to make short healthy children grow taller, to improve athletic performance in adults, to treat obesity, and for other so-called "off label" uses, the markets for which were all much larger than the approved use to treat pediatric dwarfism. Little was known about the efficacy or safety of the product for these other uses and concerns existed about the potential for harm from this off label use of the product. FDA regulations required that Genentech market its product only for the approved use, meaning that it could not provide information about the safe use of rhGH for any "off label" use. Nonetheless, commentators asked whether Genentech or any company should financially benefit or be able to hide behind the legal protection of the "learned intermediary" doctrine by taking no action to control potentially harmful physician prescribing.[55]

Similar questions were raised when it was discovered in 2000 that OxyContin®, a sustained-release narcotic painkiller, was being widely abused in certain areas of the country by addicts who would crush and then inhale the tablets to achieve an opium-like high. In some small towns in eastern United States, OxyContin abuse was rampant and incidents of drug overdose and death were climbing. The market for the product was large to begin with but was enhanced by excessive and illegal prescribing or illegal diversion to street sellers and addicts. Like Genentech, OxyContin's manufacturer, Purdue Pharma, was faced with some difficult decisions about the extent to which it should continue its sales and marketing campaigns, and whether it should attempt to control and monitor physician prescribing, and prevent illegal sales and use.[56] And also like Genentech, Purdue Pharma had to adhere to regulatory restrictions for drug marketing and needed to decide whether and to what extent it had any obligations to patients who needed the drug while considering others who could be harmed by its unauthorized use.

Medical device manufacturers also face a similar question when developing devices that require new skills in physician users. No laws exist to guide corporate behavior in this area, leaving managers with many questions to address. To what extent is the company responsible for ensuring that physicians are skilled in the use of the new device? Should companies rely on physician judgment about their skills? Should the company refuse to sell its product to physicians unless they pass a skills test? Should the company monitor actual use in patients before allowing unlimited purchases? Ultimately, it is the patients who will be harmed if a physician, eager to expand his or her practice, makes an error in judgment about his or her ability to use a new drug or device.

For any of these situations, eschewing ethics and relying on a legal approach to problem solving can get a company into trouble and harm patients. Adherence to the law is required but does not set the limits of responsible business conduct. Ethics can serve this purpose. Decisions about which action is right can be guided with an analysis of the consequences of corporate action, the interests of those affected by what companies do, and whether companies have acted in a fair manner to all those involved.

Notes

1. This chapter is a modified and truncated summary of the material presented in the business ethics section of the preterm course taught to incoming M.B.A. students at the Stanford University Graduate School of Business taught by Professor David Brady. The principle textbook for this course is Stanford University professor David Baron's *Business and Its Environment*, 2nd Edition, Prentice-Hall, 1996. Secondary textbooks relied on for this chapter are (1) Beauchamp TL. *Philosophical ethics: An introduction to moral philosophy*. 2nd ed. New York: McGraw-Hill; 1991; (2) Beauchamp TL, Bowie NE. *Ethical theory and business*. 4th ed. Upper Saddle River, NJ: Prentice-Hall; 1993; (3) Peery NS. *Business, government, and society: Managing competitiveness, ethics, and social issues*. Englewood Cliffs, NJ: Prentice-Hall; 1995; (4) Velasquez, MG. *Business ethics: Concepts and cases*. 4th ed. Upper Saddle River, NJ: Prentice-Hall; 1998; and (5) Rachels, J. *The elements of moral philosophy*. 3rd ed. New York: McGraw-Hill; 1999. Dr. Albert R. Jonsen, professor emeritus of ethics in medicine, School of Medicine, University of Washington, contributed significantly to the ethics discussion in this chapter. The contributions of Drs. Brady and Jonsen are greatly appreciated.

2. It is common for the terms *moral* and *ethical* to be used interchangeably as is done frequently in this book; however, moral philosophy and ethics scholars point out that that they are different. According to many, moral philosophy seeks to discover axioms or self-evident principles and from them deduce moral principles and standards. For instance, a self-evident principle could be "human well-being is good" and from that comes the moral principle that aggregate well-being should be maximized. Ethics is concerned with the study of moral principles and analyzing and reasoning from them to develop rules of behavior or right actions. Reasoning from the principle that aggregate well-being should be maximized, for instance, would lead to a conclusion that an action is right if it will result in the greatest overall balance of benefit over harm compared with alternative actions. An example of such reasoning is when a research manager concludes that using human subjects to obtain efficacy and safety data on an experimental drug is ethical. The activity maximizes aggregate well-being since the data help the company derive income from marketing a drug useful to physicians, who can better treat thousands of sick people. In general, such benefits outweigh the harm suffered by the relatively few human subjects who experience adverse effects from the experimental drug.

3. Other moral and ethical principles and approaches, most of which were developed more recently because of dissatisfaction with the traditional ethical theories, will not be included here. These other theories include *virtue ethics* (which focuses on the

virtuous character of the actor), *communitarianism* (which focuses on community interests), *feminist ethics* (which concerns itself with the differences that men and women use to approach moral issues, men being more focused on rights and justice and women being more focused on relationships and caring); the *ethics of care* (which focuses on the moral responsibilities we have to those with whom we have valuable and close relationships, especially if that relationship involves a dependency); and, except for Nozick's theories of justice, *libertarianism* (in which freedom from the coercion of others is valued above all other rights and values). Neither will contemporary notions of casuistry be applied to resolving ethical problems in business since this approach provides answers based on cumulative experience with moral authority based on precedent, which in business is not considered a reliable way to determine how companies should handle modern emerging ethical issues.

4. For a discussion of academic freedom and duty, see Kennedy D. *Academic freedom*. Cambridge, MA: Harvard University Press; 1997.

5. In situations based on relationships between health-care professionals and patients or research subjects, four principles are usually invoked to guide ethical reflection. These principles are: respect for patient autonomy (the obligation to respect the decision-making capacities of autonomous persons), beneficence (doing the good that can be done), nonmaleficence (avoiding causing harm), and justice (obligations of fairness in the distribution of benefits and risks). For a primary text on the subject, see Beauchamp TL, Childress JF. *Principles of biomedical ethics*. 4th ed. New York: Oxford University Press; 1994. The subject of research ethics is further discussed in Chapter 4.

6. Baron DP. Ethical systems and management. In *Business and its environment*. Upper Saddle River, NJ: Prentice-Hall; 1996. pp. 543–69.

7. Duska R. Business ethics: Oxymoron or good business? *Business Ethics Quarterly* 2000; 10:111–29.

8. The more stakeholders there are, the more companies can have problems prioritizing their interests and adjudicating between them. In addition, stakeholders are not always easy to identify.

9. Freeman RE, Reed DL. Stockholders and stakeholders: A new perspective on corporate governance. *California Management Review* 1983; 25:88–106; Phillips, RA. Stakeholder theory and a principle of fairness. *Business Ethics Quarterly* 1997; 7:51–66.

10. Friedman M. The social responsibility of business is to increase its profits. *New York Times Magazine* 1970 Sept 13; 32–3, 122–26.

11. Velasquez M. Why ethics matters: A defense of ethics in business organizations. *Business Ethics Quarterly* 1996; 6:201–22; Does it pay to be ethical? *Business Ethics* 1997 Mar/Apr:14–17; see also Note 7.

12. On duties *III*. In *Cicero, selected works*. New York: Penguin Books; 1971. pp. 157–209.

13. Autry JA. Life and work: a manager's search for meaning. New York: Avon Books; 1994.

14. Friedman M. A question of ethics. *Stanford Business* 2000; 69. Available at www.gsb.stanford.edu/community/bmag/sbsm0011/feature_ethics2.html.

15. See Note 11.

16. Guth W, Schmittberger R, Schwarze B. An experimental analysis of ultimatum bargaining. *Journal of Economic Behavior in Organizations* 1982; 3:367–88.

17. Ochs J, Roth AE. An experimental study of sequential bargaining. *American Economic Review* 1989; 79:335–84.

18. See Note 11.

19. Messick DM. Why ethics is not the only thing that matters. *Business Ethics Quarterly* 1996; 6:222–26; see also Note 7.

20. Beauchamp TL. *Philosophical ethics: An introduction to moral philosophy*. 2nd ed. New York: McGraw-Hill; 1991; see also Note 6.

21. The word *teleological* is derived from the Greek word *telos*, which refers to an end or a result.

22. Utilitarianism concepts were developed most prominently by philosophers Jeremy Bentham (1748–1832) and John Stuart Mill (1806–73).

23. The word *deontological* is derived from the Greek word *deon*, which refers to duty or obligation. The most prominent proponent of a deontological ethical system was Immanual Kant (1724–1804) and his approach to ethics is sometimes called Kantian.

24. Both Bentham and Mill conceived utility or the human good to be achieved in terms of personal happiness since this was something universally desired. Later, philosophers (called pluralistic utilitarians) who were dissatisfied with a hedonistic approach of defining all right actions as those that maximized personal happiness, broadened the definition of right actions to include those that maximized other things that had intrinsic worth and were desirable, such as friendship, knowledge, or health. Still later, because of disagreements about the superiority of one good over another, concepts of preference utilitarianism developed, in which what was valued was what individuals preferred. Debates exist about which notion of utilitarianism is preferable, and this book does not attempt to resolve these debates but to point out the differences, since questions about how to define what is "good" may come up in discussion.

25. *Strategic innocence* is a term that has been applied, for instance, to the tobacco companies that went to great lengths to avoid "learning" about the cancerous and addictive properties of cigarettes.

26. Boatright JR. Utilitarianism. In *Ethics and the conduct of business*. Upper Saddle River, NJ: Prentice-Hall; 1993. pp. 29–49; Bovbjerg RR, Sloan FA, Blumstein JF. Public policy: Valuing life and limb in tort: Scheduling "pain and suffering." *Northwestern University Law Review* 1989; 83:908–76; Bootman JL, Townsend RJ, McGhan WF, editors. *Principles of pharmacoeconomics*. 2nd ed. Cincinnati, OH: Harvey Whitney Books; 1996.

27. Goode E. With fears fading, more gays spurn old preventive message. *New York Times* 2001 Aug 19; Sect. 1:1; Center for Veterinary Medicine. *CVM responds to citizen petition on antibiotics in animal feeds*. Rockville, MD: Food and Drug Administration; 2001. Available at www.fda.gov/cvm/index/updates/antipeup.htm.

28. Commonly stated, the Golden Rule is "Do unto others as you would have them do unto you."

29. Some philosophers prefer to make the autonomy principle a separate formulation of the categorical imperative.

30. 45 *Code of Federal Regulations* 46.301, et seq.

31. 45 *Code of Federal Regulations* 46.305(2).

32. National Commission for the Protection of Human Subjects of Biomedical and Behavioral Research. *The Belmont report: Ethical principles and guidelines for the protection of human subjects of research.* Washington, DC: Department of Health, Education and Welfare; 1979. Report #GPO 887–809.

33. President's Commission for the Study of Ethical Problems in Medicine and Biomedical and Behavioral Research. Washington, DC: U.S. Government Printing Office; 1983.

34. See generally, 45 *Code of Federal Regulations* 46.

35. Ashburn TT, Wilson SK, Eisenstein BI. Human tissue research in the genomic era of medicine: balancing individual and societal interests. *Archives of Internal Medicine* 2000; 160:3377–84.

36. Scott J. Drug sales practices; is medicine infected by marketing? *Los Angeles Times* 1989 Jun 13; Sect. 1:1.

37. Admittedly, this step might prompt some to engage in consequentialism and invites some value judgment over which there can be disagreement.

38. This section will focus on these two concepts of justice and will not include a discussion of retributive justice, which deals with imposing punishments for wrongdoings and ensuring that punishments are not too lenient nor too severe for the wrong committed. Notions of retributive justice usually have legal implications; for example, when fines are assessed or when punitive damages are awarded by a court or jury against a company for wrongdoing.

39. Reichman JM, Brezis M, Steinberg A. China's eugenics law on maternal and infant health care. *Annals of Internal Medicine* 1996; 125:425–26.

40. United Network for Organ Sharing. OPTN/UNOS board recommends major changes in liver allocation system. Press release. Washington, DC: 2000 Nov 16. Available at www.unos.org/frame_Default.asp?Category=archive.

41. Some ethicists prefer to see the principle of equality as the sole formal principle of justice and thus not treat egalitarianism as if it were a material principle.

42. Robert Nozick's principle treatise is *Anarchy, State, and Utopia*, published in 1974.

43. Rawls's theories were published in his book *A Theory of Justice* in 1971.

44. Negligence here is the same as the legal formulation in that it means that the actor knew or should have known that his or her action would result in injury to the victim.

45. Boatright JR. Ethics in the world of business. In *Ethics and the conduct of business.* Upper Saddle River, NJ: Prentice-Hall; 2000. pp. 16–18.

46. O'Harrow R. Plan's access to pharmacy data raises privacy issue. *Washington Post* 1998 Sept 27; Sect. A:1.

47. Reeves H. The way we live now: 10-22-00: Salient facts, the way of some flesh. *New York Times Magazine* 2000 Oct 22; 40.

48. Woodward v. Commissioner of Social Security, 435 Mass. 536, 557 (2002 Jan 2).

49. The primary reason for excluding women from research was to prevent the possibility of a fetus being exposed to the potential toxicities of investigational drugs. As a consequence, however, insufficient data were available regarding women's responses to many commonly prescribed drugs.

50. Perez v. Wyeth Laboratories, Inc. 734 A.2d 1245, 161 N.J. 1 (August 9, 1999).

51. Griffin MT. AIDS drugs and the pharmaceutical industry: A need for reform. American Journal of Law and Medicine 1991; 17:363–410.

52. Teitelman R. Miracles and money: The evolution of a new industry. In Ono RD, editor, *The business of biotechnology.* Stoneham, MA: Butterworth-Heinemann; 1991. pp. 1–22.

53. Personal communication with Paul Rohricht, PPL Therapeutics, June 18, 1999.

54. Kolata G. Selling growth hormone for children: The legal and ethical questions. *New York Times* 1994 Aug 15; Sect. A:2.

55. Ibid.

56. Rosenberg D. How one town got hooked. *Newsweek* 2001 Apr 9; 48–51; Tough P. The alchemy of OxyContin. *New York Times Magazine* 2001 Jul 29. Available at www.nytimes.com/2001/07/29/magazine/29OXYCONTIN.html.

3

Ethics Analysis Applied to Monsanto and the Labeling of rbST

The following case study and suggested analysis are presenteIGFd as an example of how the analytical process described in the preceding chapter can work.

CASE STUDY: MONSANTO AND THE LABELING OF RBST[1]

In 1999, Monsanto, a company with 131,400 employees worldwide, total sales of $8.6 billion, and a $1 billion-a-year R&D budget, was fighting to create a market for a growth hormone that stimulated milk production in cows. This product, Posilac® (recombinant bovine somatotropin, or rbST, and sometimes rBGH for recombinant bovine growth hormone) had been launched five years earlier. Monsanto was a large life sciences company, which meant at the time that it had business interests in the agricultural, health, and nutrition sectors and had been incorporating genetic technologies into its R&D work in each of these areas to generate new products. To achieve this goal, Monsanto was licensing biotechnologies and buying or merging with seed, plant breeding, genomics, and other biotechnology companies. Posilac was one of Monsanto's and the industry's first genetically engineered products used in food production. Its development corresponded with the launch of the biotechnology industry.

In 1983, Genentech, which had applied its recombinant DNA methods[2] to produce rbST, sold to Monsanto the rights to commercialize the product. Monsanto spent ten years and at least $300 million (and some speculated that R&D costs were as high as $1 billion) studying the efficacy and safety of Posilac for use in boosting milk production in cows. These studies indicated that dairy cows injected with rbST produced up to 20 percent more milk. Posilac was expected to allow farmers to produce more milk or to maintain current milk production levels with fewer cows, thus lowering the cost of milk production and increasing profits. Since the food industry typically operated on very slim profit margins, any production savings were a welcome boon. Wall Street analysts speculated that the product would yield annual sales of $500 million to $1 billion for Monsanto. In 1985, the Food and Drug Administration (FDA) ruled that milk and meat from rbST-injected cows were safe for humans, but more data on the health effects on cows were needed before the product could be approved for marketing. In subsequent FDA-approved animal health studies, farmers using rbST were allowed to sell milk and meat from treated cows to the public. This milk and meat was not labeled to indicate the source from which it was derived.[3]

In 1990, after amassing data from about 120 studies, two physicians from Washington University's Medical School in St. Louis, Missouri, and Cornell University in Ithaca, New York—both of whom had conducted research for Monsanto—published an authoritative article in the *Journal of the American Medical Association* that concluded that the use of rbST in cows posed no threat to human safety.[4] At the same time, FDA published its review of the collected rbST data in the journal *Science*[5] and came to the same conclusion. The National Institutes of Health (NIH) also had conducted a thorough review of the available scientific data on the safety of milk and meat from rbST-treated cows for human consumption and its effect on animal health. In the unanimous judgment of an NIH expert panel, the composition and nutritional value of milk from rbST-treated cows was essentially the same as milk from untreated cows. In addition, as currently used in the United States, meat and milk from rbST-treated cows were as safe as those from untreated cows. The NIH also concluded that rbST administration did not appear to appreciably affect the general health of dairy cows, but the evidence did not permit a conclusion regarding its effect on the incidence of udder infections, known as mastitis, or long-term effects. The panel identified several other areas of research that would be useful in providing information on the long-term use of rbST.[6] However, according to the NIH report, decisions about rbST marketing approval should not be delayed until these studies were completed.[7]

By the end of 1990, the chemical and pharmaceutical companies American

Cyanamid, Upjohn, and Eli Lilly & Co. were competing with Monsanto to obtain FDA approval to market rbST. Monsanto got there first.[8] In November 1993, Monsanto submitted to FDA its extensive animal and human efficacy and safety studies and requested approval to market an injectable version of the product, which they named Posilac. By this time, in addition to the NIH endorsement, the product was endorsed by the American Medical Association and the American Dietetic Association and cleared by the U.S. Department of Agriculture. Monsanto looked forward to FDA approval and a profitable return on its investment. The subsequent course of government product approval and customer and public acceptance, however, was difficult and fraught with controversy.[9]

At the time that the FDA was considering final Posilac approval, many critics of the product were voicing several concerns. The first had to do with human safety. Most of the protests concerned fears that the increased amount of growth hormone (slightly above what is normally found) present in the milk of treated cows could produce harmful human health effects, particularly abnormal growth patterns and high blood pressure in children, and that Monsanto had produced insufficient data to show that milk from rbST-treated cows was safe either in adults or children, especially with long-term use. Groups concerned about the safety of new biotechnology products invoked what was known as the "precautionary principle," which in essence stands for the notion that, in the face of scientific uncertainty about cause and effect, actions taken to protect human health take precedence. A corollary to the principle is that a biotech company sponsor has the burden of proof for showing that its product is safe. These groups invoked the precautionary principle to claim that Monsanto needed to do more to satisfy human safety concerns. Other fears stemmed from studies that showed that rbST-treated cows had a higher incidence of mastitis, which meant that more pus, bacteria, and antibiotics would also be present in the milk of treated cows.[10] Animal welfare groups feared that rbST would induce stress in treated animals, not only from the infections but also from excess lactation, and these groups lobbied for more studies to determine if animal suffering was caused by Posilac use. They argued that there were no offsetting needs, such as a milk shortage, to justify any adverse impact on the animals. A third concern involved the fear that the product could hasten the demise of smaller dairy farms (already suffering from farm subsidy cuts and low market prices) that could not afford to purchase Posilac. These farmers were now at further risk of being shut out of the market by their richer, more efficient corporate farming competitors, who could now produce even more milk per cow. Finally, others feared the economic consequences of Posilac; that an over-production of milk, especially when there was no shortage to begin with, would depress prices and hurt the milk markets.

The critics included consumer, animal welfare, and environmental activists, farming groups, and even legislators in dairy states. Senator Russell D. Feingold, a Democrat from Wisconsin, which had a $10 billion dairy industry, was an early and vocal opponent of the hormone. Feingold, joined by several interest groups, took their combined concerns to government agencies and Congress, protesting Posilac's approval.[11] In March 1993, an investigation by the Government Accounting Office, the watchdog arm of Congress, led to a recommendation to Department of Health and Human Services (DHHS) Secretary Donna Shalala[12] that rbST should not be approved until there was further study on the hazards of any increase in antibiotics in the milk from rbST-treated cows.[13] Just as FDA was in the final stages of Posilac approval, Congress imposed a ninety-day marketing ban on the product in order to further study the complaints.

One of the most difficult problems associated with Posilac was its labeling.[14] When Monsanto submitted its Posilac marketing approval application to FDA, it requested no special labeling for the product; in other words, Monsanto intended that there be no label on milk or meat products to indicate that they came from rbST-treated cows. Monsanto and other dairy industry executives argued to FDA that somatotropins were natural hormones, that milk from rbST-treated cows was no different from traditional milk, that any extra rbST in the milk or meat was negligible and would be destroyed in the stomach, and that studies had shown no human safety risks. Labels, therefore, were not warranted. Furthermore, labeling would be difficult to accomplish and very expensive since milk collection occurred by pooling milk from many sources and there was no infrastructure to segregate milk from rbST-treated cows. Furthermore, labeling would likely detract from milk product sales for no justifiable scientific reason. Consumer and other groups, however, were unconvinced by these assurances and argued that, even if the product was eventually found to be safe, consumers had a right to know what they were eating and to choose nonbiotechnology products. They lobbied for labels that identified milk products that came from rbST-treated cows. FDA suggested that dairy producers who chose not to use rbST be able to label their products as "rbST free." Monsanto objected to such labeling since it would give the impression that the milk products from rbST-treated cows were less safe than milk from untreated cows.

In 1992, FDA had established a policy that its approval of foods developed through biotechnology would be subject to the same regulatory requirements used to ensure the safety of all foods in the marketplace. This meant that products would be judged on their individual safety, allergenicity, and toxicity rather than on the methods or techniques used to produce them. No special labeling would be required for biotechnology foods unless they significantly differed from their conventional counterparts. If the two kinds of food differed, any special labeling should address the difference, not the fact that the food had been derived using biotechnology. Therefore, in considering Monsanto's Posilac application, FDA focused on the characteristics of the milk from treated cows. In 1993, an FDA advisory committee made a final finding that there were adequate safeguards in the milk production process to prevent high levels of antibiotics from entering the milk supply and, with this last barrier down, Posilac was approved for marketing on November 5, 1993.

Monsanto agreed to conduct a postapproval monitoring program in selected herds to check for any unusual increase in animal infections, antibiotic treatment, and the incidence of milk discarded because of high antibiotic residues. Milk and milk products from rbST-treated cows would not be labeled as such, but FDA did work out a compromise with the dairy industry and Monsanto about allowing voluntary labeling of rbST-free dairy products. As a result, FDA interim guidelines issued in February 1994 recommended that any such voluntary labels be "truthful and not misleading" and suggested that labels include language to the effect that milk from rbST-treated cows was no different from, or not inferior to, milk from untreated cows. Also, those making rbST-free claims had to keep detailed records and certify that milk from rbST-treated cows was segregated from other milk.[15] With the labeling issue resolved and following the lifting of the ninety-day moratorium imposed by Congress, Posilac first went on sale on February 4, 1994.

The marketing of Posilac spurred lawsuits, petitions to have Posilac withdrawn, and further protests and calls for product boycotts. In one of the first lawsuits, DHHS and FDA were sued in federal district court in Madison, Wisconsin, by consumer activists who charged that FDA had improperly failed to consider the human health risks of Posilac or to require labeling. Monsanto joined the suit in support of the government and the suit was eventually won by the government.[16] Science and lay activist groups—such as the Union of Concerned Scientists, Consumers Union, which published the influential *Consumer's Reports*, and the Pure Food Campaign (the organization run by biotechnology opponent Jeremy Rifkin)—protested that the scientific data available on rbST were new and short term, and were not sufficient to satisfy fears about safety, especially long-term safety. These groups petitioned FDA to have the hormone withdrawn. Several large dairy cooperatives, milk food producers, and chain retail grocers (including Land-O-Lakes and Marigold Foods and grocery chains Kroger, 7-Eleven, and Pathmark), worried about consumer concerns, announced that they would sell only rbST-free milk products. Groups of chefs motivated by the Pure Food Campaign also refused rbST dairy products, and the Los Angeles County Board of Education refused to purchase rbST dairy products for any of the schools in its jurisdiction. The Humane Farming Association produced ads that mimicked the popular "Got Milk?" campaign that pictured a person humorously stranded with lots of chocolate cake but no milk to wash it down with. Playing on the slogan, the protest ads featured a glass of milk with the caption "Got Hormones?" and these ads were placed in magazines, newspapers, and on billboards. Polls showed that some farmers were not ready to accept the product either. In one 1995 University of Wisconsin poll, about 90 percent of Wisconsin's twenty-eight thousand dairy farmers reported that they were either unlikely to use rbST or were certain they would not use it in the future.[17]

The press actively followed this story. In an article published in the *New York Times*, the dairy manager of a large Madison, Wisconsin, supermarket said of rbST approval, "It's caused a commotion. People don't want the hormone, and they want to know if they're getting it in their food. We're getting 25 calls a day, 6 or 10 letters a day, and if you stand down by the dairy cases, people come up all the time and ask you about it."[18] One *Washington Post* reporter asked in her prolabeling rbST story, "What person in their right mind would choose to ingest a bioengineered hormone—whose long-term effects have not been studied—so cows can produce more milk that we don't need?" and went on to express concern for the cows by saying, "Any nursing mother knows about a certain physiological overload of hunger, fatigue and engorgement with natural lactation. And then to have your chemistry skewed to produce about 20 percent more? No wonder [rBGH-injected] cows suffer from what is called a 'prolonged negative energy balance,' resulting in weight loss, among other things."[19]

As before marketing, labeling remained an important issue of concern. Several states, including Wisconsin, Minnesota, and Maine, passed voluntary laws allowing dairy producers to label their products as containing no milk from cows injected with rbST. Minnesota's law did not require the added FDA guideline clarification, and only some of the dairy producers in the various states used the FDA clarification. One cheese producer in Wisconsin told a reporter that his sales had increased at least 20 percent since he had started using his red "producer certified rB.G.H. free" state-approved labeling. He also stated that he thought Monsanto was "afraid that if labeling becomes widespread, it will kill the hormone, which it would."[20] Monsanto felt that the rbST-free labels amounted to unfair competition because they falsely implied that rbST-free milk was more wholesome. To protect its interests, Monsanto hired two Washington law firms to monitor rbST advertising and labeling that the company believed violated the FDA guidelines or marketing laws. Violators were sent letters warning them that Monsanto considered their labels to be "false and misleading," and in early 1994 Monsanto also sued two milk processors in Iowa and Texas for using such labels. In response, the insurer of one of these defendants vowed to fight the suit, stating, "The main issue, and perhaps the only significant issue, is the right of a food seller to inform the consumer what may or may not be in the food product."[21]

Vermont, home to many small farmers and consumer activists, went further and enacted a law requiring a label on milk products made from rbST-treated cows. Vermont was promptly sued by several national food associations that claimed that mandatory labeling was unconstitutional and violated FDA regulations. Vermont won the suit in the lower court, but the decision was later reversed by a 2–1 decision in the Court of Appeals, and Vermont was forced to rescind its mandatory labeling law in favor of a law allowing the voluntary labeling of rbST-free milk products.[22] Ben & Jerry's Homemade Inc. of Vermont, Stonyfield Farm of New Hampshire, and Organic Valley Farms of Wisconsin ran afoul of these various labeling laws when they included the voluntary label on their products shipped to Illinois, a state that made voluntary labeling illegal. When Illinois prevented the companies from selling their products, Ben & Jerry's sued in federal court claiming that its commercial free speech rights were infringed by the Illinois law and that consumers had a right to know what was in their dairy food. The parties settled in 1997. The dairy producers were still not allowed to label their products rbST-free, but they could use labels stating, "We oppose recombinant Bovine Growth Hormone. The family farmers who supply our milk and cream pledge not to treat their cows with rBGH. The FDA has said no significant difference has been shown and no test can now distinguish between milk from rBGH-treated and untreated cows."[23]

The situation in Europe was worse. In 1990, a moratorium on rbST was imposed in Europe to allow for further study of the human and animal safety issues. Each time the matter came up for reconsideration, the European Union decided that it was not satisfied with the safety data and decided to continue the ban. After one of these votes, David Byrne, the European Union's commissioner of health and consumer protection, stated that the European Union was simply giving health a higher priority over lower-cost milk production.[24]

By 1997, some polls were showing that a majority of U.S. consumers, like their European counterparts, were concerned about the safety of biotechnology foods and wanted genetically modified foods labeled.[25] The International Food Information Council (IFIC), which conducted studies on behalf of the food industry, was taking other polls that showed that 20 percent of consumers did not support the FDA position that food produced though biotechnology should be specially labeled only when biotechnology's use changed the safety or nutritional characteristics of the food compared with traditional foods.[26] However, when the question was worded somewhat differently, 40 percent of respondents replied that they agreed with critics of the FDA policy and that food produced through biotechnology should be labeled even if it has the same safety and nutritional content as nonbiotechnologically produced foods. The number of labeling proponents increased in surveys when, instead of the word "biotechnology," the phrase "genetically modified" was used.

By 1998, Monsanto was directly addressing its critics in various press releases and position papers posted on its Web site. In these documents, Monsanto emphasized that its rbST premarketing studies had not shown any evidence of adverse effects in humans who consumed milk products from rbST-treated cows. In an April 1998 issue paper posted on its Web site entitled "Biotechnology and Consumer Issues: Where We Stand," Monsanto stated that "biotech plants and foods are safe for humans, farm animals and the environment. Monsanto does not believe there is a scientific basis to require labeling of food products simply because they are produced through modern biotechnology. We acknowledge, however, the desire for labeling by European consumers and we will of course be responsive to European regulatory authorities should they require such labeling." Addressing the animal welfare groups, Monsanto posted its belief that Posilac was safe for use in cows but that cows could suffer if farmers did not use Posilac correctly or were not properly caring for their animals. Posilac-treated cows needed to be adequately fed to keep up with the increased metabolic demand from the hormone, and to insure that they ate enough, cows also needed to be healthy and kept comfortable. Monsanto also emphasized that sanitary conditions needed to be maintained to prevent mastitis. The company made considerable efforts to train farmers on the proper use of the drug and on the care of the cows that received it. These efforts included offers of $150 vouchers for consultations with veterinarians.[27]

Monsanto also sponsored (and its Web site linked to) the Life Sciences Knowledge Center, an on-line forum for commentary on, among other things, genetically modified crops and foods. Some of these commentaries focused on the attacks against biotech foods and presented emphatic opinions about Monsanto's detractors. One such article decried the "pestiferous ignorance" of the environmental activists who had been allowed to dominate "the inevitable and necessary public discourse" about biotechnology and foods.[28] This article went on to defend the science behind these products and their safety and pointed out that the detractors were accepting only the science that supported their views and were therefore misleading the public about the value and the safety of these products. To what extent Monsanto agreed with this view is not known. However, Monsanto's beliefs in the worthiness and safety of Posilac led it to focus its efforts on winning further regulatory approvals, preventing regulatory reversals, countering harmful labeling initiatives, and growing its market.

The press continued to follow the rbST controversy. One reason to keep on the biotechnology food story was that public interest in food safety had been increasing over the years. According to conclusions drawn by a Harvard School of Public Health and IFIC Advisory Group,

> 25 yrs ago, chances were slim that a food and health-related study in a scientific journal would make the evening news or greet readers in their morning newspapers. Now, hardly a week goes by when a breaking dietary study doesn't make headlines. There are a number of reasons why. Public interest in nutrition and food safety has increased dramatically. And food stories—because they are inherently so personal—make for compelling news. Just as important, scientists have much to gain from increased visibility. And the same holds true for the journals that first publish the studies or other communicators who have an interest in advancing public understanding of the issues.[29]

Another reason for continuing press interest was the seeming increase in the genetically modified food controversy and the attacks on Monsanto's marketing practices. Despite supportive press releases from Monsanto and IFIC, the press was emphasizing the objectors' points of view.[30] Monsanto did not fare well in these reports and sometimes, selectively quoted or not, contributed to the company's negative reputation. In October 1998, the *New York Times Magazine* published a widely read article called "Playing God in the Garden" about the fears surrounding the growing use of genetically modified crops and food. In this article Monsanto's director of corporate communications was quoted as saying that "Monsanto should not have to vouchsafe the safety of biotech food. Our interest is in selling as much of it as possible. Assuring its safety is the F.D.A.'s job."[31] On December 15, 1998, matters became worse for Posilac when *ABC World News Tonight* aired an rbST story introduced with the tag line "Milk Causes Cancer." This segment dealt with a study by Dr. Sam Epstein, a professor of environmental health at the University of Illinois, who had been researching rbST for several years. Epstein found that milk from rbST-treated cows contained up to six times as much of a growth hormone called IGF-1 or insulin-like growth factor 1.[32] Epstein claimed that these higher concentrations of IGF-1 could stimulate a growth factor for human breast cancer and other cancer cells. These findings led the scientist to call on the dairy industry to stop using Posilac or any other rbST.[33] Both Monsanto and FDA acknowledged that IGF-1 levels were increased in milk from rbST-treated cows but not outside the normal range and that any increase was therefore biologically insignificant.[34] However, this story obviously harmed Monsanto's marketing efforts and gave more ammunition to Monsanto's detractors.

In 1999, Health Canada (the Canadian equivalent of the U.S. FDA) completed more than nine years of review of rbST, including the opinions of two independent advisory panels and many prominent animal health authorities. Their experts had concluded that rbST appeared so far to be safe in humans but that further study was needed. For instance, a ninety-day study of laboratory rats had showed possible invasion of the growth hormone into the prostate, which again would raise cancer concerns. They also urged further study to learn whether rbST was degraded by digestion and whether allergic reactions were possible. There were stronger concerns about animal safety based on a Canadian Veterinary Medical Association report that concluded that cows given rbST suffered weakness and increased mastitis, infertility, and lameness. Largely based on animal health concerns, Posilac approval was denied. Monsanto countered that the animal problems did not occur when rbST was used correctly, and it appealed the decision.[35]

Citing the Health Canada report, a consortium of consumer groups filed a legal petition with FDA to rescind its approval for Posilac.[36] The same Health Canada decision caused two Vermont advocacy groups, the Vermont Public Interest Research Group and Rural Vermont, to send a report to Vermont's two U.S. senators expressing concerns about the safety of rbST, questioning

FDA's review of the product, and requesting that the product be withdrawn from the market. The two senators wrote to DHHS Secretary Donna Shalala, who then required FDA to undertake another full review of all scientific data related to rbST. In March 1999, the European Commission Directorate General XXIV issued the "Report on Public Health Aspects of the Use of Bovine Somatotropin," which stated that the marketing ban on rbST would remain in place until additional exposure data were obtained and an *in vivo* quantitative dose-effect relationship for IGF-1 was established. The following month, FDA's data review was completed, and Shalala reiterated the FDA position that products from cows treated with rbST were safe to consume and that rbST would remain on the market. Undeterred by this conclusion, lawmakers submitted bills that would require manufacturers to label all foods containing genetically modified organisms. These different government positions about the safety of rbST and other genetically modified foods contributed to increased strain in trade relations between the United States and Europe over bioengineered foods and crops.[37] Also, the FDA decision prompted more editorials decrying the "no label" position. One *Washington Post* editorial stated:

> Essentially the regulators are telling us that, as far as science can tell, it's all in the head of the consumer. Therefore, why burden manufacturers with a labeling requirement that can discourage sales? The policy reflects deep respect for science, and it calms the fears of the biotechnology industry, which acknowledges generous government support for research—with generous campaign contributions to both political parties. Nonetheless, the no-labeling policy misuses the authority of science in trampling over the right to know what you're eating. For religious reasons, many Jews and Muslims refuse to eat pork. To guide them in their preference, packaged products indicate the presence of pork, though there is no scientific evidence that it is unwholesome. Package labels also assist vegetarians, as well as persons who are sensitive to particular foods, or who think they are. Scientists are probably right when they insist there's nothing to worry about in genetically modified foods. But in this matter, as well as others, the people have a right to be informed and to arrive at the wrong conclusion. Science can serve as a guide, but it shouldn't perform as a bully.[38]

Several months later, Monsanto was one of thirty-eight signers of an industry letter that reiterated their views on mandatory versus voluntary food labeling but took a more moderate tone. This November 12, 1999, "Open Letter to President Clinton on Science-Based Labeling of Foods," written by the industry group Agri-food Community, stated:

The FDA has vested its considerable credibility with consumers in the veracity of product labels in representing the safety and nutritional value of foods. If the FDA were to change its policy and require special labeling for biotech foods, such labeling could have the effect of misleading consumers into believing that biotech foods are either "different" from conventional foods or present a risk or a potential risk—even though the FDA has determined that the biotech food is safe. Such special labeling of biotech foods could lead to the very kind of consumer confusion that labels are designed to prevent. . . . The FDA's existing policy also allows voluntary label statements that are truthful and not misleading, providing a comprehensive framework for consumer protection as well as choice. In light of that policy, manufacturers are permitted to voluntarily label foods produced *without* the use of modern biotechnology to enable consumers who want this information to make individual choices. We support that right because we believe that consumers who seek specialty foods or foods produced without the use of modern biotechnology should always have a market to serve them.

During all of these legal, regulatory, and public policy negotiations and con-troversies, Monsanto maintained its focus and its considerable skills on the marketing and selling of Posilac directly to veterinarians and dairy farmers. Many industry analysts were interested in Monsanto's progress because, as one put it, "the consensus is that if a deep-pocketed giant like Monsanto cannot make a go of it, Wall Street will shy away from investments in food-industry biotechnology for years to come."[39] Monsanto put together what was consid-ered for the agriculture industry to be an unusually innovative and wide-ranging marketing effort to launch Posilac to over one hundred thousand commercial dairy farmers. In addition to the usual marketing practices and a reliance on a highly trained sales force, the company attempted to ensure that all farmers were well educated on the proper use of Posilac and animal management by providing how-to videotapes and educational seminars. Monsanto even went so far as to provide $150 vouchers toward a consultation with a veterinarian for those farmers who encountered difficulties with product use. Monsanto also re-lied on farmers to convince their neighbors to use Posilac, and farmers were paid $100 for each customer they referred to Monsanto.

While the company has provided few details about Posilac sales or profits, the data it has released have lead analysts to conclude that the early sales were only a fraction of what Monsanto had projected and that the product was still losing money for Monsanto three and four years after it was first introduced in the United States.[40] Some analysts wondered whether Monsanto would ever recoup its huge product development costs. Ultimately, in February 2000,

Monsanto issued a report about its U.S. rbST market experience.[41] Although this report lacked financial sales figures, the company did say that total U.S. and international sales of Posilac from 1996 to 1999 increased annually by 45 percent, 30 percent, 25 percent, and nearly 20 percent respectively.[42] The report also stated that of the nearly nine million dairy cows in the United States, approximately one-third were in herds supplemented with Posilac and that about thirteen thousand dairy producers were currently using the product. Monsanto also reported data showing that the size of herds supplemented with Posilac closely resembled the distribution of herd size in the United States, underscoring the fact that both large and small dairy farmers were using the product. The average dairy operator using Posilac was supplementing more than 50 percent of the herd at any one time and experiencing productivity increases of 5 to 15 pounds of milk per day per cow. By 1999, the company had delivered a total of more than 150 million doses of Posilac, making it the largest-selling dairy animal health product in the United States. Monsanto also reported that FDA had repeatedly confirmed to the company that no unusual or unexpected concerns about cow or human safety had been raised since the introduction of Posilac five years earlier.

Monsanto maintained its optimism that Posilac would eventually be approved in Canada and the European Union, once regulators became convinced, as Monsanto expected they would, of the safety and efficacy of the product. In addition, it made sense for Monsanto to continue its work to deter labeling because farm policy studies were showing that consumer awareness and marketplace pressures were muted in areas where there were no rbST-free and other biotechnology food labels and, conversely, that both consumer awareness and marketplace pressures remained high in areas where there were such labels.[43]

CONCLUSION

As Monsanto continued to grow the Posilac market, commentary about its marketing practices continued apace. The company, many scientists, and industry and technology analysts were convinced that fears about biotechnology products were speculative in nature, much of it having no scientific basis but seemingly founded more on a notion that humans had exceeded what was safe to change in nature. Biotechnology advocates were concerned that allowing irrational fears to deter food technology progress was harmful to the industry and to all of those who benefited from the innovations produced by science and industry. Those benefits included the ability to make farming more sustainable, to feed more people in the world, and to improve health and nutrition. The development of Posilac was just in a continuum of long-standing efforts to improve milk production, which with improved animal nutrition, better medical care, and a trend toward increased milking had nearly tripled annual output per cow from 5,300 pounds in 1950 to 15,500 in 1993.[44] The fact that improvements were now coming from biotechnology should not, in and of itself, be cause for alarm. As Monsanto stated in a December 1999 press release in response to a legal attack, "We believe in biotechnology—its opportunity and its promise. We've invested in it because it is a sound technology of clear and demonstrated value that offers extraordinary benefits to groups throughout society. We remain committed to bringing those benefits forward."

Still, some believed that Monsanto's actions had increased public uneasiness about biotechnology products and corporate behavior. Many people were not predisposed to believe in the efficacy and safety of biotechnology to solve the world's food or medical problems and tended to fear the unintended consequences, many of which might show up years after product introduction. As the Harvard geneticist Richard Lewontin told one reporter, "You can always intervene and change something in [the ecosystem], but there's no way of knowing what all the downstream effects will be or how it might affect the environment. We have such a miserably poor understanding of how the organism develops from its DNA that I would be surprised if we don't get one rude shock after another."[45]

One of the "rude shocks" that Dr. Lewontin was referring to was the 1999 report of a Cornell University laboratory study that found an increase in the death rate of Monarch butterfly larvae when they fed on milkweed dusted with pollen from genetically engineered corn as compared with normal corn pollen.[46] Although the finding later turned out to be a laboratory anomaly, there were immediate attempts by groups such as the Union of Concerned Scientists to halt U.S. testing and regulatory approvals of all genetically engineered crops. The approval of one version of this genetically modified corn was suspended in the European Union, and other versions, including Monsanto's, were placed under regulatory re-review. The Monarch butterfly news was startling for another reason having to do with the realization that the widespread use of biotechnology-derived foods and crops had "snuck up" on the U.S. public. Until the Monarch butterfly story, most of the public was ignorant of the fact that the bioengineered corn in question had been introduced three years earlier and now accounted for more than one-quarter of the nation's corn crop. The stories also informed the public of how many other foods, such as soybeans (commonly found in food oils, salad dressings, margarines, chips, snacks, and many other processed foods), potatoes, and milk, had been bioengineered. Consumer research on the labeling of genetically engineered food conducted by the FDA's Center for Food Safety and Applied Nutrition revealed that consumers wanted mandatory labels, not so much because of safety concerns about genetically modified foods but because they felt "outrage" that such a change in the food supply could happen without them knowing about it.[47]

The fact that Americans were largely ignorant of how much of the nation's crops and foods were produced from biotechnologies increased fears about the "full speed ahead" application of biotechnology and fueled calls for labeling. These concerns combined with a growing distrust of multinational agricultural corporations that were viewed as having developed too much control over the world's food supply and its government regulators. Commenting on the different opinions about rbST among Monsanto, other food producers, farmers, regulators, governments, and the public, Frederick H. Buttel, professor of rural sociology at the University of Wisconsin, said, "This has been a textbook case of how people's views of technology shaped their predictions. People read into it their hopes and fears for a new generation of genetically engineered products."[48] In such an environment, industry analysts and biotechnology commentators questioned whether Monsanto's rbST marketing and labeling approach was good for Monsanto, good for biotechnology, and good for the public.

ANALYSIS OF CASE STUDY

Monsanto has satisfied itself that there are no current scientific, regulatory, or market reasons to label dairy foods derived from Posilac-treated cows. The question here, however, is whether Monsanto has an ethical responsibility to support labeling of milk and dairy products from Posilac-treated cows and to refrain from deterring rbST-free labeling. The analysis of this question raises issues of utilitarianism, rights, and justice.[49] Prior to engaging in these analyses, Monsanto has to satisfy itself that it has all of the relevant facts about the situation so that its analysis can be fully informed.

FACTS

An obvious factual issue concerns the scientific basis for concern about the safety of Posilac, both before and after it leaves the company. Monsanto may have to go no further than its own scientists to obtain answers to this question, but it would be prudent to consult independent experts who have additional insights and might be perceived as more credible. Independent scientists might emphasize that scientific findings are not static and that it could take a longer period of product use to arrive at firm safety conclusions. Also, farmer non-compliance or misuse of the product may be a source of unintended adverse effects that might harm both animals and humans. Therefore, one result of this safety investigation could lead the company to conclude that product safety could not be taken for granted, despite the extensive research already performed. This conclusion might prompt Monsanto to put into place a monitoring or alert system so that the company is always in possession of the current facts about the safety profile of the product. The company could also include those employees best placed to make the labeling decisions "in the loop" of the safety alert system. Decisions about whether to label may change over time, depending on the facts unearthed and on changes in scientific thinking about the probability of Posilac-related illness and injury. Therefore, an ongoing collection of facts would be appropriate.

Despite the close link between safety and the need to label foods, scientific evidence cannot be the sole labeling consideration. The values that people hold about something so personal as the food that they eat and feed to their children have led to the passage of labeling laws and regulations and have also influenced how companies approach product marketing.[50] The United States does not subscribe to a policy that says that consumers have only the right to know about scientifically credible food risks. As a matter of fact, many food risks are not included in labels, and many food labels carry information that has nothing or little to do with personal risk. Examples include labeling specifying that the food is kosher approved, vegetarian, or from free-range animals. Therefore, a second factual inquiry important to Monsanto would be into the reasons that foods are labeled in general. A pertinent trend to study is the shift away from *caveat emptor* for food products and the increased information contained on food labels that occurred over the past decades. Why did this trend occur? Was most food labeling based on safety concerns or was labeling also driven by consumer demand for other information? If based on consumer demand, what informational need did the labels fulfill, and why did companies feel the need to comply with these demands? Finally, were these reasons and trends applicable to the labeling of biotechnology foods or were biotechnology foods different in some relevant ways so as to justify excluding them from the trend?

Such a factual inquiry would reveal that in the past there have been very strident and widespread criticisms of such things as milk pasteurization and drinking water fluoridation, and, like Posilac, the criticisms were based on a mixture of scientific and nonscientific concerns. Unproved long-term safety was the primary scientific concern. Among the nonscientific concerns were freedom and choice. When it was publicized that tuna were being harvested in large nets that also caught and killed nonfood fish and animals, such as dolphin, many consumers ceased buying canned tuna because of the animal welfare and environmental concerns. Regardless of the nature of the concerns highlighted by these three examples, consumers knew what they were consuming, and those opposed to the technologies could usually avoid the objectionable products by buying nonpasteurized milk, bottled or filtered water, or tuna labeled "dolphin safe." Learning how the producers of these products handled these situations would be instructive to Monsanto in deciding how to manage Posilac labeling.[51] Monsanto also had the benefit of a growing body of commentary on the subject of labeling biotechnology foods, including books on the ethical and social implications of food labeling and the reasons (for example, safety, political, religious, esthetic, or scientific distrust) that people wanted information that would allow them to avoid rbST and other biotechnology-produced foods.[52] According to Paul Thompson, professor of applied ethics at Purdue University and the author of one of these books:

> Nothing would be more human than to adopt beliefs about the purity and authenticity of foods that would be difficult or impossible to support on scientific grounds. Is New York State Champagne an oxymoron? The French certainly think so. Avoiding impure or inauthentic foods may not be a safety issue in the narrow sense, but it can be extremely important to those who hold the relevant beliefs. Second, people routinely make consumer choices to express solidarity with other groups or political causes. This type of consideration overlaps with aesthetics to some extent, as the injunction to "buy American" echoes the French desire for authentic champagne. In the rBST case, however, solidarity may have more to do with loyalty to small dairy producers or animal well-being concerns. In either case, it may be important for some consumers to choose "non-BST" milk.
>
> Neither of these concerns relate to the probability of disease or injury that is associated with drinking rBST milk. They could be described as elements of food anxiety, rather than safety in a narrow sense. Ironically, controversy itself creates anxiety. As questions are raised about the technology, people naturally wonder who to believe. They may ultimately resolve the question by considering the costs of being fooled. If the critics of rBST are wrong, a consumer is losing several cents per gallon of milk purchased. Although this may add up to

significant social costs, even a family purchasing a hundred or more gallons of milk every year may find the three or four dollars a year cost a reasonable price to pay for avoiding the anxiety of a new and unfamiliar form of milk. If the scientists are wrong, after all, the cost would be measured in ill health, especially to children who drink more milk than adults. Even if one thinks it far more likely that the scientists are right, it may be rational to forego [*sic*] the marginal consumer price benefit in exchange for the familiarity of ordinary milk.[53]

Studying the history and the literature on food labeling and including these points of view into a factual investigation of the rbST labeling question could help Monsanto develop an understanding of the various points of view it must contend with. In addition, studying the labeling practices of other companies and industries could assist Monsanto in knowing whether its contemplated actions were outside the mainstream of business practice. Although being outside of standard practice can be considered innovative, especially if the practice has become questionable, it can also indicate that especially careful and reasoned justifications are needed for contrary practices.

Monsanto also needs to know who the rbST labeling proponents are, what their views are, what legitimacy there is for these views, how prevalent these views are, and to what extent they reflect the views of the general public. Monsanto need not look too far to discover the views of its vocal opponents but may wish to consult with more moderate but less vocal groups seeking labeling. Consumer polls are also useful in assessing public opinion. What the company will most probably learn in these endeavors is that groups and consumers who favor labels have no current scientifically credible evidence that Posilac is unsafe for humans and animals but that they fear that risks might exist. Their objections stem from this fear of the unknown combined with other nonsafety concerns. Further insights can be obtained from informational exchange sessions with company critics, in which corporate representatives could learn about the depth and breadth of concerns. In these sessions, Monsanto may learn that some of the safety fears arise from the suspicion that, by not labeling milk products from Posilac-treated cows, the company is trying to hide something and has reason to do so. Or Monsanto may hear that consumers feel helpless and controlled by the decisions of government agencies and large corporations who have been wrong before about the safety of technologies—the chemical and nuclear disasters at Bhopol and Love Canal come to mind. In such a climate, consumer trust is difficult to maintain, and as distrust grows, the company's motivations and actions are more heavily scrutinized and easily misconstrued.

If Monsanto comes to believe that mistrust was driving its critics and caus-ing market resistance more than scientifically assessed probabilities of risk, it may want to investigate how this came about. Some commentators and policy advisors had come to believe that antibiotechnology fears were, at least in part, driven by the public's unfamiliarity with the scientific process, which can easily lead to confusion and mistrust. This state of affairs is exacerbated by the fact that scientific findings are hardly ever conclusive since, by its nature, scientific understanding is continually evolving and growing. As with the claimed and then refuted anticancer effects of bran, antioxidant vitamins, and various types of fat, most consumers are left in a constant state of uncertainty about what foods do to the body. What is presented as "scientific fact" one day can be de-bunked a few years later. Also, scientists do not always agree on what constitutes credible scientific evidence. Stories about scientific feuds and the hazards of emerging technologies are increasingly found in lay publications. The press can contribute to public confusion and scientific skepticism if it fails to publish bal-anced reports. In addition to studying these issues, Monsanto could investigate if and how it had directly contributed to consumer confusion and mistrust.[54]

With such facts and conclusions as a guide, Monsanto could proceed to en-gage in an ethical analysis of the Posilac labeling question.

UTILITARIAN ANALYSIS

Under a utilitarian analysis of the labeling question, the company would at-tempt to act in such a way that the greatest good could be produced for the greatest number of people affected by the act. Such an outcome promotes hu-man welfare by minimizing harms and/or maximizing benefits on the whole and can then be defended as a morally correct action. The method used in a utilitarian analysis is usually described as follows:

1. Determine the alternative actions available

2. Estimate the costs and benefits that a given action would produce for each person or entity affected by the action

3. Choose the alternative that produces the greatest sum of utility and/or the least amount of disutility

Thus, Monsanto could consider the costs and benefits of two alternative actions—acquiesce to or deter rbST and rbST-free labeling. In each case, in order to arrive at an optimal utilitarian outcome, Monsanto must consider the impact of its actions on others and decide which entities are legitimate concerns of Monsanto when it makes a labeling decision. The entities for which the costs and benefits would be studied are listed below.

The Company

Monsanto could use financial projections to calculate the degree to which Posilac and rbST-free labeling could benefit the company by improving regulatory acceptance in other countries and preventing activist backlash, compared with the costs of labels, which include the potential for increased marketing and distribution costs, product stigmatization, and delay in the ability to recoup the huge Posilac R&D costs. These labeling consequences could be compared with the probable benefits of no labels, namely, lower marketing and distribution costs and quicker market penetration, compared with the costs of regulatory delay, activist boycotts and lawsuits, "no label" enforcement costs, damage to corporate reputation, and negative impacts on future product marketing. Projections could be made about how long it would take for labeling pressures to subside and, therefore, the length of time the costs of avoiding labels would persist. Another impact to consider is the difficulty of reversing a decision to label Posilac-derived foods. Once a standard was set that all biotechnology-derived products had to be labeled as such, the negative ramifications of that decision would last, perhaps longer than the time it would take for the antibiotechnology or biotechnology-shy groups to become comfortable consuming foods produced using biotechnology.

The Industry

The costs and benefits of Monsanto's labeling decisions would be magnified to the extent that they affect other companies in the same or related industries. If Monsanto's actions cause regulatory agencies to require labels, other companies that make similar products must label as well, the related costs for which can be similarly high. Posilac boycotts by school districts and grocery stores shrink not only Monsanto's markets but those of other businesses in the chain of distribution. In addition, mistrust of biotechnology foods or suspicions of consumers that Monsanto is trying to deprive them of information that they deem valuable could spill over to the biotechnology food industry in general. If the labeling issue causes an inability to make a market in biotechnology foods, financial institutions could lose confidence in other biotechnology-based foods, and funding for other products may be difficult to obtain. In contrast, other companies will benefit if the lack of Posilac labels coupled with a continued product safety record results in more rapid acceptance of biotechnology food products in general. And Monsanto's refusal to capitulate to demands to label safe biotechnology food products would inure to the benefit of other companies that would not have to fight the same battles as Monsanto. Moreover, the other companies would be spared the stigmatization that biotechnology food labels tend to generate.

Perhaps the two largest labeling costs for industry, however, are those related to compliance and product segregation. Because there was no test that could identify any milk product as having been derived from an rbST-treated cow, labeling compliance would have to come from on-site farm inspections, which are expensive, time consuming, and difficult. Also, given the common practice by dairies to pool all milk, it would be especially costly to duplicate milk processing methods so that milk from rbST-treated cows could be segregated and labeled separately. There may be infrastructure in place for organic milk processing, however, that can accommodate the rbST-free milk without any further restructuring costs. Financial impact projections could be done for these various scenarios.[55]

Farmer Customers

The economic and other interests of customers who benefit from using the product would be an important part of this utilitarian analysis. The efficiencies and profits gained with more productive cows versus the shrinking markets that labeling could cause and the costs of segregating treated from nontreated milk could all be included in the risk-benefit calculus. Monsanto might also want to consider other factors, such as the possibility that farmers using Posilac might be subject to protests and sabotage similar to those against farmers growing genetically modified crops.

Noncustomer Farmers and Dairy Producers

Monsanto might want to consider the impact of its labeling decisions on those farmers who do not contribute to Monsanto's market and some of whom actively undermine it by labeling milk products as rbST-free. Labels could allow such farmers to sell into a niche market and might increase their profits if they price their products high enough to offset the costs of verifying that Posilac is not used in their herds and the costs charged to segregate the product. If Monsanto successfully prevented these labels from being used, these milk producers could lose their market. Although these dairy producers figure importantly in the labeling issue, whether Monsanto wishes to include them in its calculation of "the greatest good for the greatest number" raises the "scope" question discussed in the preceding chapter.

Consumers

The increased prices charged for rbST-free milk products are an obvious outcome of the use of negative labels. Monsanto might legitimately believe that the higher price buys very little since the rbST-free product is no different from lower-cost milk products from Posilac-treated cows. Consumer health also could be affected by the use of labels. For instance, if all dairy products from rbST-treated cows were labeled and consumers who consistently ate these products developed a certain health problem, it would be much easier to implicate or rule out rbST as a cause of the health problem and this information could benefit the public health. Although it would probably be difficult to measure in any quantifiable way, it might also be worthwhile to attempt an analysis of whether the presence or absence of Posilac or rbST-free labels increases or decreases the well-being of consumers. Assuming that Monsanto is right about the safety of the product, many consumers may not care that milk products are generated with biotechnology processes, and the presence of labels could cause heightened and unnecessary confusion and anxiety. By contrast, parents may wish to take a conservative approach and make food choices for their children as risk-free as possible. The well-being of these people might be served with labels. Or Monsanto might conclude that, since labels falsely imply that milk products from rbST-treated cows are less safe than regular milk, all labels undermine consumer well-being by creating confusion about biotechnology food safety.

Activist Groups

Monsanto might consider that activist groups are a vehicle through which its labeling decisions have a wider impact. Labeling would obviously quell activist protests and their attempts to influence the regulatory and legislative processes, stop the lawsuits, and diminish the negative publicity against the company and the food biotechnology industry. The impact of the company labeling policy grows with the extent that activists' views are shared by the general public, so it behooves Monsanto to explore this issue. If the activists' views are not popular, there would be less reason for Monsanto to alter its business practices to comply with their demands.

Cows

Monsanto's labeling decisions could affect the dairy cows that are treated with Posilac. If labeling allowed milk to be traced to a particular Posilac-treated herd, any human harm caused by Posilac could be identified as having been caused by the drug itself, by improper use, or by problems with the animal or its care. Either way, the ability to identify and correct such problems could prevent future harm to both animals and humans.

Biotechnology

Many of the same impacts of labeling versus nonlabeling that apply to the industry as a whole also apply to biotechnology as an emerging technology. According to some, labeling of biotechnology foods encourages "reckless and irresponsible" criticism of biotechnology and "may do more to undermine the promise of food biotechnology than anything else."[56] However, labeling may allow the fears about biotechnology to abate. According to this view, the longer labeled biotechnology foods are on the market without producing adverse effects, the more they will be accepted as safe. As the public policy communications manager for the Grocery Manufacturers of America once said, the public will eventually accept the fact that "a tomato is a tomato is a tomato," regardless of whether it was produced conventionally or through biotechnology.[57]

Obviously, some of these listed impacts would be difficult if not impossible to quantify, but attempts should be made to factor them into the utilitarian risk-benefit calculus as meaningfully as possible. Also, this list of risks and benefits points out the utilitarian analysis problem that differences of opinion can tilt the risk-benefit balance one way or the other. Such differences of opinion include whether the product is safe, whether regulatory agencies can sufficiently protect the public safety, how long it may take for the product backlash to die out, whether it is relevant that demand for labeling is driven by a scientifically unfounded fear of technology, or the extent to which food labels help or undermine consumer well-being. These difficulties make a utilitarian analysis less than precise. However, the art of a utilitarian analysis comes from a recognition of the imperfections combined with an ability to objectively include all of the relevant considerations and to equitably account for those factors that cannot easily be measured.

Assuming that Posilac use and outcomes are monitored and that no reliable data surface to indicate that it poses a health risk to humans, the utilitarian outcome seems to indicate that the risk-benefit calculus would weigh in favor of not labeling Posilac-derived dairy products. Guessing on what Monsanto's numbers would reveal, the overall costs and risks of labeling are probably very large and wide-ranging—the huge collective costs to many companies and consumers of restructuring dairy production practices to segregate milk and enforce labels, the prolonged inability of Monsanto to recoup its R&D costs, the stigmatization of biotechnology leading to the inability to achieve broad market acceptance of beneficial food products, coupled with the probability that a decision to label would be very difficult to reverse, therefore prolonging all of the negative consequences of labeling.

The benefits of labeling are less tangible and may be more speculative; these include the possibility that regulatory acceptance may be easier to achieve in Europe (but only after safety concerns are satisfied), that product detractors will stand down (although, again, those who worry about long-term safety will persist), and that consumer well-being and confidence will improve if they are able to make choices about purchasing biotechnology foods. In comparison, the consequences of not labeling Posilac-derived foods seem to produce less disutility and smaller benefits. The regulatory and market reversals caused by product detractors would be most likely temporary and could abate as confidence in product safety grows. Also, the confusion that results from a label that implies that biotechnological processes produce different or inherently unsafe food seems to outweigh the more moderate benefit to a smaller number of people of promoting the peace of mind that comes from avoiding safe but otherwise objectionable food.

The calculus is different for the use of rbST-free labels. Although the use of these labels will undermine Monsanto's market and also stigmatize biotechnology and reduce the acceptance of biotechnology foods, these effects will likely be smaller than for Posilac labels, since not all farmers will use "free" labels and the effects will also likely diminish over time as confidence in product safety improves. In addition, the dairy industry costs of implementing rbST-free labels would be smaller than for Posilac labels if rbST-free milk producers can use the existing organic milk processing infrastructure. The decision to use rbST-free labels is also easier to reverse because dairy producers can easily stop using them whenever the market for the "free" products dwindles. The benefits of rbST-free labels include the ability of farmers and dairy producers to sell a specialty product to those who want to avoid biotechnology foods. In addition, the well-being of these consumers could improve with the choice provided by these labels. On the whole, compared to Posilac labels, the use of rbST-free labels seems to result in less overall cost but possibly close to the same benefits. In and of themselves, the rbST-free labels could be utilitarian if one concluded that these labels would also reduce the fear that the industry is forcing unwanted biotechnology foods on the public. Reducing distrust in the industry could lead to confidence, which could, in turn, lead to greater market acceptance of these products.

Monsanto's industry and market projections may or may not be consistent with what is presented here. However, this exercise is intended to show how a utilitarian analysis can lead to specific conclusions, in this case that Monsanto is justified in its position that, by taking the interests of all affected entities into account, the use of Posilac labels will produce more overall harm than good and Monsanto is justified in continuing to oppose them. In contrast, the question is much closer when it comes to whether rbST-free labels are utilitarian and whether Monsanto should refrain from opposing them. The conclusion about Posilac labels also highlights the principle limitation of a utilitarian analysis. What about those people who genuinely believe that Posilac may be dangerous and wish to avoid all foods derived from its use? What about dairy producers who seek to develop a market for these consumers? Their interests are better accounted for with a rights analysis, as described below.

RIGHTS ANALYSIS

Despite the fact that Monsanto and its U.S. regulators and many independent scientists did not believe that Posilac use endangered public health or the health of treated animals, there were people who demanded labels with rbST information. A rights analysis could help determine if Monsanto had a duty to respect those demands. According to a Kantian view, to qualify as a right, conditions of universality and reversibility must be satisfied and Monsanto must approach the question of rights and duties by treating individuals as ends and never solely as a means to an end, in this case, a sales end. A rights analysis can begin by asking: Who has rights? Are they claimed or granted? What are the bases for the claimed rights? What interests are the rights intended to promote? What actions can be taken to further those rights? Any limitations on these rights are then assessed in order to rank the claimed or granted rights in order of their importance and to take actions based on the priority of the rights identified.

Some potential rights can be eliminated from consideration at the start. For example, as a preliminary matter, if it appears that some consumers demand a right to food safety, Monsanto can justifiably conclude that it has no duty to honor that right since no food can ever be made risk free. But there is a right to reasonable safety for food products that is both legally granted and justifiably claimed. Given the scientific data and the expert and regulatory opinions about Posilac, Monsanto could reply that it is fulfilling its duty to consumers by providing a reasonably safe product, especially if ongoing monitoring continues to confirm this conclusion.

With regard to labeling, it may be more difficult to create a suitably circumscribed and unambiguous description of potential rights. Monsanto cannot claim an unfettered right to control the label of Posilac dairy foods since drug and food product labeling is closely regulated by government agencies. However, Monsanto can claim that it has a right to market a safe product unencumbered by labels that, for no good scientific reason, would undermine product acceptance. The FDA happened to agree with Monsanto's position and did not require Posilac labels on dairy products. In addition to being legal, the right not to be encumbered by detrimental labels has a moral basis in that it is universal and reversible (Monsanto, in claiming the right for itself, would agree that the right applies to all other similarly situated entities) and, given Monsanto's belief in the safety of Posilac, such a right would not be tantamount to viewing consumers solely as a means to sell products. The interest the right can be said to protect is a fair opportunity to engage in business. The action consistent with this right is to continue to resist efforts to label foods as Posilac-derived.

The company might also want the right to stop others from implying that Posilac-derived milk products are inferior to rbST-free products. If this claimed right is viewed generally as a right to stop others from implying that a company's safe product is unsafe, there are legal rights to sue for unfair competition and food disparagement that protect Monsanto's interests under law. The right would also seem to have a moral basis under a Kantian framework since it should be a universal and reversible rule that businesses should not be allowed to compete unfairly in this way. The interest that such a right protects is an interest in fair business competition. However, there are difficulties when attempting to apply this right to the rbST-free labels. FDA issued guidelines with suggested general language for rbST-free labels, and these guidelines are insufficient alone for Monsanto to stop all rbST-free labeling. To invoke the right to be free of unfair competition and food disparagement, Monsanto would have to use the law courts to convince a jury of its position that the wording of these labels improperly implies that its product is inferior to conventional milk products. The likely defense to this position is that these labels do not disparage Posilac or imply that it is unsafe but, instead, truthfully describe the product for interested consumers. For these reasons, Monsanto's claimed right is only possibly granted in law. The action consistent with this claimed right is to oppose the use of rbST-free labels that imply that Posilac-derived products are inferior. The sticky problem with this action is in having the parties agree on the content of such a label.

Farmers and dairy producers who do not use Posilac can claim a right to label their products truthfully as rbST-free. This is both a claimed right and legally (albeit ambiguously) granted by FDA regulation and some state laws. The problem with the FDA guideline is that the specification that the rbST-free labels be "truthful and not misleading" and the suggestion (but no requirement) that the labels include language to the effect that milk from rbST-treated cows was no different from, or not inferior to, milk from untreated cows, left dairy producers with uncertainties about how they could exercise their right to label. Some state laws were also vague. The right to label has moral status insofar as labeling a product to truthfully describe its character can be said to be universal and reversible and also respects consumers as ends by providing information that allows them to exercise choice. The interests the right protects include a business interest to develop a market by informing consumers about the nature of products, and a consumer interest in accurate food information. However, when applied to the rbST-free labels, there is again the problem of determining what else these labels imply, if anything, about Monsanto's Posilac. And should these dairy producers be forced to label their products with favorable messages about competing Posilac-derived products? Depending on how one viewed these labels and what exactly they said, Monsanto or these rbST-free dairy producers could be seen as infringing on each other's business rights.

Consumers and their advocates want label information so that they can choose whether to purchase milk products from rbST-treated cows. Consumers can claim a right to have Posilac-derived labels on dairy products. However, this claim lacks legal entitlement. Further, labels are forbidden unless approved by FDA. Regarding rbST-free labels, the right to these labels is granted to consumers by FDA guidelines and by some state laws since these labels were allowed partly for consumer benefit. The right to food label information seems to have a moral basis (everyone wants it, everyone would agree to provide it, and the information respects people as ends) depending on what information is requested. For example, information that would be too costly for the food producer to supply (maybe Posilac labels) would not meet the universal/reversible Kantian requirements. There can also be difficulties in agreeing that there is a consumer right to information to satisfy what can be viewed as idiosyncratic preferences. The interest protected by a right to have food labeled is consumer autonomy, that is, the ability of consumers to exercise free choice about the foods they eat. For the consumers who want Posilac labels, an interest served by such a right also includes an interest to be free of the concealment of relevant food information. The action consistent with these consumer rights is to label Posilac-derived and/or rbST-free dairy foods.

It is obvious that there are conflicts among these claimed and granted rights, leaving it unclear which rights should trump others. To resolve the conflicts or to decide which action to take in light of the conflicts, the rights at stake need to be prioritized. Claimed rights forbidden by law are ranked lowest. Therefore, consumer demand for Posilac labels can be ranked lowest. Clearly granted rights take precedence over ambiguously granted rights, and all granted rights take precedence over claimed rights. Once rights are sorted into granted and claimed groups, priority is then determined according to the importance of the interests the rights are intended to promote. For example, most people would probably agree that, in this society, consumers' right to food information, to choose the food they eat, and to be free of concealment of food information they consider important has higher priority than the rights of businesses to control label claims about their products.

Using this analysis, these rights and their various aspects would look like Table 3.1.

Prioritizing the various rights is a starting point in deciding what can reasonably be accomplished so that the rights of all can be respected as much as possible. It is clear that consumers do not have a legal right to know if milk products come from Posilac-treated cows, but consumers do have the right to information that will facilitate autonomous choices that promote their well-being and that of their families. Therefore, when feasible, consumers should have access to labels that allow them to avoid foods that they consider harmful or that they otherwise find objectionable. From this analysis, one could conclude that Monsanto should respect this right and cease attempts to prevent rbST-free labels so long as these labels do not misleadingly imply that Posilac-derived products are inferior. This suggests that in states where the laws are not clear about rbST label content, Monsanto should engage in negotiations with legislators and dairy producers to arrive at mutually acceptable label language. This solution would go some of the way in respecting Monsanto's right to fairly sell its product at the same time respecting the rights of dairy producers to make a business in the specialty rbST-free market without also forcing them to promote competing products made with Monsanto's hormone. These solutions do not, however, resolve the most direct conflict between those consumers who claim a right to Posilac labels and Monsanto's right to avoid them. Since the fundamental conflict stems from a disagree-

TABLE 3.1

Applied Rights Analysis: Monsanto and rbST Labeling

Rights	Claimed/Granted	Base	Interests the Right Protects	Priority	Actions Consistent with the Right
Monsanto: To sell a safe product unencumbered by harmful label	Claimed/granted	Moral/legal	Fair opportunity to engage in business	2	Resist Posilac labels
Monsanto: To be free of product disparagement	Claimed/possibly granted or prohibited in some states	Moral/legal	Fair business competition	4	Oppose disparaging labels
Dairy producers: To inform consumers about product characteristics	Claimed/ambiguous granted	Moral/legal	Fair opportunity to engage in business	3	Allow "rsBT free" labels
Consumers: Food information; Posilac labels	Claimed/prevented by law	Moral	Autonomy/free choice; freedom from concealment of relevant information	5	Posilac labels
Consumers: Food information; "rbST free" labels	Claimed/indirectly granted	Moral/legal	Autonomy/free choice	1	"rbST free" labels

ment about the safety of using Posilac, Monsanto could attempt to ameliorate some of this conflict with educational programs and meetings with consumer groups to supply safety information. Monsanto could also commit to actively monitor for health and safety problems and disclose any risks as soon as possible. In this way, Monsanto could fulfill a duty that respects consumers' right to know about the safety of the food they consume.

Paul Thompson, who authored a text on ethical issues in food biotechnology, agrees with some these conclusions. He views an aspect of consumers' right to choose the foods they eat as being one of informed consent:

> In most cases, consumers have a choice to select foods even if the food they
> want to avoid is not labeled (fluoridated water, pesticide treated veggies, etc).
> In each of these cases, the principle of informed consent is protected, but in
> none of them are the offensive products the object of mandatory labeling laws.
> Indeed, they are not labeled at all. The principle of consent is protected in
> each of these cases by the availability of alternatives. These alternative foods
> give food consumers the right of exit from a system of food transactions that
> they find objectionable. If there are identifiable alternatives to the products
> of biotechnology, then consumer sovereignty and the principles of consent
> are protected. There are several ways in which the principle of exit can be
> protected and the most obvious of them all involve labels that identify a
> product as "biotech free" [p. 77].[58]

JUSTICE

This case study raises issues about the fairness of allocating the burdens of society. This is a prototypical justice issue involving various free and equal persons or entities attempting to advance their own interests in conflict with others pursuing their self-interests. Monsanto seeks to avoid the burdens of labeling, and consumers do not want to bear the risk of Monsanto and the FDA being wrong about their assessments of Posilac safety. Without labels, there is no way to avoid the use of Posilac-derived milk products and any of their possible risks. Some material justice principles of allocations are relevant here. Monsanto may be seen as having been the largest contributor to the problem and therefore should be made to fix it. The company also has the financial and other resources and abilities to accomplish labeling via FDA and dairy producers. However, it does not seem fair to place two significant burdens on Monsanto (the costs of the labeling effort and the negative impact on the sale of Posilac and future products) since the company would incur these expenses for no good reason, believing as it does that labeling will not protect consumer health and well-being. Monsanto can also apply this reasoning to claim that it is unfair for it to be burdened by the labels of its rbST-free competitors. Consumers, in contrast, claim a need for Posilac information but have no ability to obtain it without labeling. There does not appear to be a way that the parties can bear these burdens equally.

Neither does Nozick's libertarian view that "if the process is fair, the outcome is fair" seem to work here. The processes here are regulated, which obliged Monsanto to comply with government requirements in the marketing and labeling of Posilac. Given that the FDA and other agency procedures were developed independently of the food and drug industry to protect the interests of consumers, Monsanto can claim that the marketing approval process was fair and that, if FDA required no label, that was a fair result. However, a common consumer advocacy complaint is that FDA is too heavily influenced by the companies it regulates. Consumers would argue that the agency made the label decision with more input from Monsanto and the biotechnology industry than from consumer interest groups and that consumer interests in Posilac labeling were not given equal consideration. However, FDA did seem to heed consumer views when it issued voluntary guidelines allowing rbST-free labels, which also allowed dairy producers to develop this market. If consumers and dairy producers felt that this was a fair process and a fair result, Monsanto may claim the opposite, perceiving that FDA had buckled to the vociferous antibiotechnology minority and had then abandoned their scientifically based position that there was no safety reason to label Posilac-derived products. Either way, one party or another could view the processes and outcomes to be unfair.

Rawls's approach, applying principles of equal liberty, difference, and fair equality of opportunity, may offer some assistance in arriving at a fair result. If no one knew who they would be in this situation, they may be able to freely and impartially arrive at a fair solution that maximizes the amount of freedom for everyone involved. Under considerations of equal liberty, Monsanto and the consumers have equal interests that must be protected from invasion by others. However, the conflicts here seem to prevent application of this principle; true equality cannot be achieved, which makes it clear that compromises regarding the inequalities are in order. Under the difference principle, the consumers seem the least advantaged since they have no rbST information and no way to get it unless it is disclosed. But Monsanto can argue that, since Posilac is safe, the added costs and the market inefficiencies of Posilac labels may make everyone worse off. Therefore, the difference principle is difficult to apply here. Under the equality of opportunity principle, the inequalities can be managed if there is a fair and equal opportunity to avoid the burdens in question. Application of this principle suggests that Monsanto should not be forced to accept Posilac labels and that consumers should be able to avoid Posilac foods. These goals can be accomplished by allowing rbST-free labels. This solution places the labeling, processing, and monitoring cost burdens on those who want to sell biotech-free products, and these costs can be passed on to consumers who want to avoid Posilac-derived food. In exchange, these two parties reap the benefits of selling product and having food information. Monsanto is left to cope with the smaller burden of the competing rbST-free labels and, again, can negotiate about the label language in an attempt to reduce the negative implications of these labels. This solution can be considered just since rational principles were used to allocate burdens among the parties involved.

ETHICAL REASONING CONCLUSIONS

The utilitarian analysis favored an outcome in which Monsanto could rightfully continue to resist Posilac labels but was equivocal about resisting rbST-free labels. This conclusion ignored the rights of consumers who wanted label information and ignored the rights of dairy producers seeking to develop biotech-free markets. The utilitarian outcome also created some unfairness for these two groups. The rights analysis gave a priority to the interests of the consumers for labeling information, and the justice imbalance was resolved by allowing the use of rbST-free labels. The ethical systems applied to this labeling question did not provide conclusive resolutions to the conflicting positions but would allow Monsanto to reason through the ethical implications of its labeling decisions and consider consequences to itself and to others affected by its decisions. *In toto*, this analysis favors the conclusion that Monsanto can continue to resist labels placed on dairy foods from rbST-treated cows, that Monsanto refrain from preventing the use of rbST-free labels, and that it continue to carefully monitor for safety problems, promote safe use, and educate the interested public and address its concerns about biotechnology foods. Such a solution allows Monsanto to maintain its highest priority for Posilac, that being establishing the scientific evidence that the product is efficacious and safe, and also allows competitors to develop their markets and prevents consumers from being forced to eat something they believe to be harmful. While compromises are needed on all sides, this solution tends to preserve the utility of Posilac while respecting the rights and needs of others affected by the use and sale of this product.

Notes

1. This abbreviated case study was developed from information contained in the following sources: Monsanto Web site at www.Monsanto.com, and www.monsanto.com/dairy/Default.htm and Monsanto financial reports; Walters DK. Stores won't stock milk of cows treated with hormone. *Los Angeles Times* 1994 Feb 5; Sect. D:1; Day K. Where did the milk come from? Tracking dairy hormone may prove impossible. *Washington Post* 1994 Feb 13; Sect. A:1; Steyer R. ABC's of BST; answering key questions on Monsanto's new milk drug. *St. Louis Post-Dispatch* 1994 Mar 3; Sect. C:5; Mason M. Milk? It may not do a body good; a furor over hormones, labeling and health. *Washington Post* 1994 Mar 7; Sect. C:5; Schneider K. Lines drawn in a war over a milk hormone. *New York Times* 1994 Mar 9; Sect. A:12; Steyer R. BST is Monsanto's splice of life; a behind-the-scenes look at drug that raises production of cow's milk. *St. Louis Post Dispatch* 1994 Apr 25; Sect. Business:12; O'Neill M. The debate over milk and an artificial hormone; move over, Elsie: Recasting the cow as a political animal. *New York Times* 1994 May 18; Sect. C:1; Feder B. Monsanto has its wonder hormone: Can it sell it? *New York Times* 1995 Mar 12; Sect. 3:8; Steyer R. Monsanto wins case against challenging BST. *St. Louis Post-Dispatch* 1995 Aug 8; Sect. C:11; Steyer R. Backers and critics both wrong on BST; a small number of farmers are using the product. *St. Louis Post-Dispatch* 1996 Aug 11; Sect. E:1; Steyer R. BST milk drug turns 3 with little fanfare; protests fade, but product lags expectations. *St. Louis Post-Dispatch* 1997 Mar 16; Sect. E:1; and Schmickle S. BST has blended into the dairy case; only a few oppose growth hormone. *Minneapolis Star Tribune* 1999 Jan 22; Sect. A:1. Dr. Paul B. Thompson, professor of applied ethics, Purdue University, kindly reviewed the Monsanto case study included in this chapter and gave helpful suggestions and background information. His advice and input is appreciated.

2. The recombinant DNA technique involved isolating the gene for the growth hormone and splicing it into a self-replicating DNA molecule called a vector. This "recombined" product was then inserted into bacteria or yeast, which were thus programmed to produce growth hormone.

3. Walters DK. Stores won't stock milk of cows treated with hormone. *Los Angeles Times* 1994 Feb 5; Sect. D:1; Schmickle S. BST has blended into the dairy case; only a few oppose growth hormone. *Minneapolis Star Tribune* 1999 Jan 22; Sect. A:1.

4. Daughaday W, Barbano D. Bovine somatotropin supplementation of dairy cows: Is the milk safe? *Journal of the American Medical Association* 1990; 264:1003–5.

5. Juskevich J, Guyer C. Bovine growth hormone: human food safety evaluation. *Science* 1990; 264:875–84.

6. These research recommendations were: continue the study of long-term effects of rbST on cows, including reproduction; evaluate more thoroughly both clinical and subclinical mastitis in rbST-treated cows and their relationship to milk production; define and characterize "stress" in dairy cows; determine the mechanisms underlying the galactopoietic effects of growth hormone; determine the concentrations of IGF-I in human saliva as a function of age; and determine the acute and chronic local actions of IGF-I, if any, in the upper human gastrointestinal tract.

7. Office of Medical Applications of Research. *Bovine somatotropin*. Technology Assessment Conference Statement. Bethesda, MD: National Institutes of Health; 1990. Available at www.monsanto.com/dairy/documents/NIHTASSESSMENT.htm.

8. Steyer R. ABC's of BST; answering key questions on Monsanto's new milk drug. *St. Louis Post-Dispatch* 1994 Mar 3; Sect. C:5.

9. Day K. Where did the milk come from? Tracking dairy hormone may prove impossible. *Washington Post* 1994 Feb 13; Sect. A:1.

10. Steyer R. New age for milk industry; cow drug on market after years of study. *St. Louis Post-Dispatch* 1994 Feb 4; Sect. A:1.

11. Schneider K. Lines drawn in a war over a milk hormone. *New York Times* 1994 Mar 9; Sect. A:12; see also Note 10, Steyer.

12. This was not the first time that Dr. Shalala had been involved in the rbST controversy. When farmers criticized the University of Wisconsin in the late 1980s for proposing to study rbST, Shalala was the university's chancellor and she became known as a defender of the hormone.

13. Mason M. Milk? It may not do a body good; a furor over hormones, labeling and health. *Washington Post* 1994 Mar 7; Sect. C:5.

14. The labeling questions about rbST occurred at a time when Monsanto and other bio-agriculture companies were also facing widespread opposition, especially in Europe and India, about the development and marketing of genetically modified crops, such as Monsanto's RoundUp Ready soybean, genetically engineered to contain a gene that conferred resistance to the herbicide of the same name. Because there were no apparent differences between genetically modified and conventional soybeans, no labels indicated that some soybeans were grown from the RoundUp Ready technology. Also, the genetically modified soybeans were mixed with natural soybeans so that consumers could not tell if the genetically modified product was in their food. Protesters wanted the product banned or, failing that, labeled. The forms of protest included lobbying government agencies, filing lawsuits, publishing articles, picketing company headquarters, organizing boycotts, bomb threats, burning and destroying crops in the fields in a "Cremate Monsanto" campaign, and otherwise trying to sabotage Monsanto's marketing efforts for its genetically modified seeds and foods.

15. See Note 8.

16. Steyer R. Monsanto wins case against challenging BST. *St. Louis Post-Dispatch* 1995 Aug 8; Sect. C:11.

17. Feder B. Monsanto has its wonder hormone: Can it sell it? *New York Times* 1995 Mar 12; Sect. 3:8.

18. See Note 11, Schneider.
19. See Note 13.
20. See Note 11, Schneider.
21. Ibid.

22. Associated Press, Steyer R. Court OK's Vermont's law requiring BST milk label. *St. Louis Post-Dispatch* 1995 Sept 6; Sect. C:1; Associated Press, Steyer R. Court rejects milk hormone label law. *St. Louis Post-Dispatch* 1996 Aug 9; Sect. D:13.

23. Steyer R. Ben & Jerry's caught in middle of BST label confusion. *St. Louis Post-Dispatch* 1997 Mar 16; Sect. E:9; see also Note 3, Schmickle.

24. Steyer R. Europe may order a permanent ban on Monsanto milk drug. *St. Louis Post-Dispatch* 1999 Oct 31; Sect. E:7.

25. See Note 23, Steyer.

26. International Food Information Council, U.S. consumer attitudes toward food biotechnology. Wirthlin Group Quorum Surveys; 1997. Available at www.ific.org.

27. See Note 17.

28. DeGregori TR. Genetically modified nonsense. Institute of Economic Affairs; 2000. Available at www.biotechknowledge.com/showlib_us.php3?2769.

29. Advisory Group, Harvard School of Public Health, and International Food Information Council Foundation. Improving public understanding: Guidelines for communicating emerging science on nutrition, food safety, and health for journalists and all other communicators. *Journal of the National Cancer Institute* 1998; 90:194–99.

30. According to one 1999 media study of 1,260 food news stories conducted by the International Food Information Council Foundation and the Center for Media and Public Affairs, stories devoted to the harms of biotechnology-developed foods outnumbered the stories about the benefits by 70 percent to 30 percent. See "Food for Thought III," available at www.ific.org.

31. Pollan M. Playing God in the garden. *New York Times Magazine* 1998 Oct 25; 44–51, 62–63, 82–92.

32. IGF-1 is a BST intermediary compound, which occurs naturally in both untreated cattle and humans unexposed to foods from rbST-treated cows.

33. Walsh J. Milk hormone may be dangerous, study finds; researcher says longer life for cancer cells could result. *Minneapolis Star Tribune* 1995 Aug 9; Sect. B:6.

34. See Notes 8 and 13.

35. Groves M. Canada rejects hormone that boosts cow's milk output; agriculture decision comes on report that the substance could harm animals; Monsanto said it will continue to pursue approval. *St. Louis Post-Dispatch* 1999 Jan 15; Sect. C:1.

36. See Note 3, Schmickle.

37. Weiss R. British report: Label gene-modified food; call by U.K. doctors group adds to trade tensions with U.S., brings strong reaction on Hill. *Washington Post* 1999 May 18; Sect. A:2.

38. Greenberg D. The right to know what we eat. *Washington Post* 1999 Jul 7; Sect. A:19.

39. See Note 17.

40. Ibid.; Steyer R. Backers and critics both wrong on BST; a small number of farmers are using the product. *St. Louis Post-Dispatch* 1996 Aug 11; Sect. E:1; Steyer R.

BST milk drug turns 3 with little fanfare; protests fade, but product lags expectations. *St. Louis Post-Dispatch* 1997 Mar 16; Sect. E:1.

41. Monsanto. Status update regarding Posilac bovine somatotropin. St. Louis, MO; 2000 Jul 14. Available at www.monsanto.com/monsanto/biotechnology/background_information/oojul14_posilac.html.

42. Posilac was also being sold in sixteen other countries, including South Africa, Brazil, Mexico, Israel, and Turkey.

43. See Note 23, Steyer.

44. See Note 17.

45. See Note 31.

46. The gene in question made a toxin lethal to caterpillars such as the corn borer, an insect that fed on corn causing roughly $1 billion in damage annually.

Kilman, S. Modified corn seed is found to poison monarch butterfly. *Wall Street Journal* 1999 May 20; Sect. B:2.

47. Weiss R. Biotech vs. "Bambi" of insects? Gene-altered corn may kill monarchs. *Washington Post* 1999 May 20; Sect. A:3. See also, Kaufman M. Consumers want engineered food labeled; shoppers express "outrage" that product choices aren't clear, FDA reports. *Washington Post* 2001 Feb 12; Sect. A9.

48. Steyer R. Backers and critics both wrong on BST; a small number of farmers are using the product. *St. Louis Post-Dispatch* 1996 Aug 11; Sect. E:1.

49. The analysis presented here is a simulated example of how the labeling question can be approached, not to suggest that Monsanto did or did not manage this situation appropriately.

50. Thompson PB. What is happening to food? In *Food biotechnology in ethical perspective.* London: Blackie Academic & Professional; 1997. pp. 1–13, p. 11.

51. Thompson PB. Food safety and the ethics of consent. In *Food biotechnology in ethical perspective.* London: Blackie Academic & Professional; 1997. pp. 57–80, p. 77.

52. MacDonald JF. *Agricultural biotechnology at the crossroads: Biological, social, and institutional concerns.* Ithaca, NY: National Agricultural Biotechnology Council; 1991; Thompson PB. *Food biotechnology in ethical perspective.* London: Blackie Academic & Professional; 1997; Thompson PB. Food biotechnology's challenge to cultural integrity and individual consent. *Hastings Center Report* 1997; 27:34–38.

53. Thompson PB. Biotechnology policy and the problem of unintended consequences. In Thompson PB, editor, *Food biotechnology in ethical perspective.* London: Blackie Academic & Professional; 1997. p. 46.

54. See Note 29.

55. See Note 51.

56. See Note 50.

57. Kay, J. Genetic engineering v. labeling laws: A new frontier. *San Francisco Examiner* 1999 Jul 11; Sect. A:1.

58. See Note 51.

Research Ethics

Of all of the activities of medical product research and development, human and animal research have raised the most complex and potentially troublesome ethical and social issues, principally because of past histories of research abuses. Questions about the ethical conduct of clinical research persist, especially when the research is sponsored by commercial entities. Not uncommonly, regulatory enforcement and litigation follow allegations of research ethics abuse. This chapter describes the history and background of the development of modern human and animal research ethics and the various contexts within which ethical and social issues arise. Because pharmaceutical and medical device companies sponsor and pay for most animal research and nearly three-quarters of all human clinical research performed in the United States every year (spending about $3 billion on human research alone), companies must understand the ethical and social aspects of clinical research since they will undoubtedly confront these issues at one time or another.[1]

HUMAN RESEARCH

Modern History of Ethics Codes for Human Research

World War II and the Nuremberg Code

Current ethical standards for clinical research have their roots in the research atrocities that took place during World War II, carried out by physicians under orders from the Third Reich. Examples of the abuses that took place included biological warfare experiments where healthy concentration camp inmates were involuntarily infected with yellow fever, smallpox, typhus, cholera, and diphtheria germs, which caused the death of hundreds of people. In other camps Nazi doctors conducted experiments to test the consequences of exposure to high altitude, malaria, freezing, mustard gas, bone transplantation, ingested sea water, and incendiary bombs. Methods were also tested to determine the fastest way to sterilize as many people as possible in order to meet the demands of the mandatory sterilization laws directed toward Jews, homosexuals, Gypsies, and those with birth defects or genetic disorders. The postwar Nuremberg Trials that disclosed these research practices resulted in the issuance of the Nuremberg Code, the first major set of modern research ethics guidelines, which continues to inform current research standards.[2] The Nuremberg Code contains a set of basic principles to guide the conduct of medical experimentation on human subjects. The ethical foundations for the code lie in the values of respect for the autonomy and liberty interests of subjects and of the need to consider the consequences of the research on the subjects involved. To implement these values, the code specifies that informed and voluntary consent be obtained from all subjects, that the degree of risk should never exceed the importance of the problem to be solved (implying that some research is too risky to be performed even if subjects would consent), that the risks of research harm be minimized, that medical research be conducted only by qualified physicians, that subjects be free to withdraw from the research project, and that the research should be terminated if continuation poses unacceptable risks to subjects.[3]

Declaration of Helsinki

The principles of the Nuremberg Code were used to generate a more extensive moral code of conduct for medical researchers when the Declaration of Heısinki was adopted by the Eighteenth World Medical Association General Assembly at Helsinki, Finland, in 1964.[4] The Declaration of Helsinki was promulgated following a growing recognition that research abuses had occurred before Nazi Germany and were still continuing to occur in many countries, including the United States. In 1963, reports surfaced that medical researchers had injected live cancer cells into twenty-two patients in the Jewish Chronic Disease Hospital in Brooklyn, New York. This research was done without the knowledge of the patients involved and was intended to study the role of the immune system in fighting cancer. About the same time, mentally impaired children in the Willowbrook State School in New York were infected with live hepatitis A virus in an attempt to reduce the spread of fecal borne infections. The parents were not fully informed about the nature of this research. Many more studies came to light that used equally problematical methods. Despite the general postwar standard that it was unethical to sacrifice individuals to the greater good of expanded medical knowledge, it was clear that the zeal that drove researchers to answer important medical questions sometimes led them to ignore the interests of the human subjects. These revelations highlighted the need for more specific research standards and a heightened awareness of the ethical obligations of researchers.[5]

The Declaration of Helsinki contains the same basic requirements as the Nuremberg Code—human subject rights to autonomy and free choice should be respected and the benefits of research should not be outweighed by the risk to subjects. The Declaration of Helsinki also contains more specific provisions about how these rights should be preserved, and many of these have been topics for continuing debate in the medical research community. One important problem that the Declaration of Helsinki addresses is when the need to obtain scientific information is given priority over the interests of human subjects. To prevent this from happening, the declaration provides that it is the duty of the physician researcher to remain the protector of the life and health of human subjects, and not to allow scientific or societal interests to ever take precedence over the well-being of the subject. While most medical researchers do not dispute that the interest of human subjects should remain paramount, disagreements about what amount of risk is reasonable to impose in the interests of science remain controversial.

Another contentious provision of the Declaration of Helsinki states that medical research is justified only if there is a reasonable likelihood that subjects stand to benefit from the results of the research. This provision conflicts with the widely held notion that research should be conducted solely to obtain scientific data. Providing benefit is the province of medical treatment. No benefit can be expected, for instance, in Phase I drug trials, in which healthy volunteers are recruited to obtain information on a drug's adverse effects. In addition, this declaration requirement conflicts with the need to use placebo or no-treatment controls in drug trials. If investigators have a reasonable belief in advance that the drug will prove to be better than placebo or no treatment, such a study could be considered unethical under the standards of the Declaration of Helsinki.

This declaration standard also confused those who believed that humans should not be subjected to randomized controlled studies unless the investigator is substantially uncertain about which of the comparative interventions (for example, the drug or placebo) is better. Called the uncertainty principle, proponents often adhere to the notion that the proper degree of uncertainty exists when the investigator is in a state of equipoise—equally uncertain about which investigational intervention is better. Under any formulation of this principle, however, it is agreed that, without uncertainty, it would be unethical to deny the treatment to the control group. The pharmaceutical industry has come under periodic criticism for failure to abide by this uncertainty principle. Because so many company-sponsored drug trials result in positive results, some medical commentators have wondered whether industry trials are biased in that direction. In other words, did industry sponsors conduct only those trials in which their product was compared to a control such that the outcome was likely to contribute positively to their FDA application and marketing efforts? This skepticism is often misplaced because company drug studies *only* continue if the past data are encouraging and the company believes that it is worthwhile to continue. That belief, however, is often shattered, as evidenced by the high number of drug trial failures (only one out of every five experimental drugs tested in humans is eventually approved for marketing), thereby underlining that uncertainty (if not equipoise) is always an aspect of industry research. Pharmaceutical companies would be placed in a bind if the statistical certainty provided by the use of placebo controls were deemed unethical by a strict interpretation of the uncertainty principle.[6]

Another related and troublesome aspect of the Declaration of Helsinki is that it has been interpreted to condone combining medical treatment with medical research. It is always problematical to blur the distinction between medical treatment (where the physician is solely devoted to the well-being of patients) and research (where the physician has two goals: to collect data to advance medical knowledge and to protect the interests of their human subjects). Many researchers have deplored the lack of a distinct line in this process because physicians must be clear in what they are doing in order to obtain valid consent from patients and subjects. The distinction between treatment and research is not only an issue for physician researchers. Questions about the propriety of therapeutic research become most difficult when experimental treatments are given to dying patients or patients suffering from great pain or distress. Despite attempts to convince these patients that they may receive no benefit from the experimental intervention, their desperate situation convinces them that any chance of therapeutic benefit is worth taking, a situation that is sometimes called the "therapeutic misconception." Medical ethicists debate whether such patients are too easily exploited and whether they can give genuine and informed consent.[7]

An even more controversial issue arose in 2000 when the Fifty-Second World Medical Association General Assembly adopted the provision that the use of placebos in medical research is always unethical if treatment is available for the condition in question. According to the revised declaration, placebos may be used only when there are no other therapies available for comparison with a test procedure. The revision was intended to prevent the risk that placebo treatment would worsen the medical condition of research subjects. Given FDA's and many researchers' belief that the use of placebo controls in specific trials provides the most efficient and the highest level of scientific certainty in medical treatment research, debates are ongoing about whether this provision will become widely adopted in the United States. It was feared that bioscience companies attempting to eliminate roadblocks to product approval would be forced to choose between providing data acceptable to FDA and violating an international research ethics standard. Publications of placebo-controlled research data have also been affected by the revisions because the "Uniform Requirements for Manuscripts Submitted to Biomedical Journals," which are followed by more than five hundred medical journals, dictates adherence to the standards set forth in the Declaration of Helsinki.[8] The Genzyme case study in Chapter 7 contains further information about the use of placebo controls in human medical research.

Belmont Report

Despite knowledge about the reasons that the Nuremberg Code and the Declaration of Helsinki were written, American physicians did not universally heed their requirements. It was only after revelations of unethical U.S. research conduct were publicized that formal safeguards were introduced into American laws and regulations. In 1966, Henry K. Beecher, an anesthesiologist at Harvard Medical School who had closely studied the Nuremberg Trials documents, published an article in the *New England Journal of Medicine*, listing eighteen cases of nonconsensual and otherwise unethical research conduct. These studies took place at some of the country's most prestigious medical centers, and the results had been published in the most influential medical journals. Among examples described by Beecher were the Willowbrook study, studies where effective antibiotics were withheld to prove that a form of penicillin prevented rheumatic fever, and a study in which invasive and unwarranted cardiac tests were performed. Beecher deplored these abuses regardless of the usefulness of the data collected, and he concluded that "an experiment is ethical or not at its inception; it does not become ethical post hoc—ends do not justify means. There is no ethical distinction between ends and means."[9] The article created a firestorm of commentary and was widely reported in the newspapers, which also published editorials and letters to the editors expressing outrage that American physicians were ignoring ethical codes of conduct and praising Beecher for speaking out. The medical community expressed similar sentiments, but some research physicians also denied that such abuses had taken place and were highly critical of what they viewed as Beecher's indiscretion.[10] Public awareness of research problems was kept alive by Beecher's continued publications and also the writings of the influential German philosopher Hans Jonas (1903–93), who worried that modern technology disturbed the balance between humanity and nature and created "freedom without values." Applying his views to human medical research, he wrote about the conflicts between a physician's duty to the welfare of patients and society's interests in scientific progress. He wrote that "the physician is obligated to the patient and to no one else. He is not the agent of society, nor of the interests of medical science." Jonas was willing to sacrifice the speed of medical progress to preserve what he believed were more important fundamental moral values dedicated to preventing the exploitation of humans in research.[11]

Research abuse issues rose to national prominence again in the 1970s with the disclosure of the infamous Tuskegee syphilis study. In 1933, in Macon County, Alabama, the Public Health Service had begun a study to document the effects of syphilis in four hundred African American men. By the 1940s, it was clear to investigators that the men infected with syphilis were dying at twice the rate of the control group, and it was also known that penicillin was effective in treating the disease. Despite this knowledge, none of the men in the study received penicillin and the study continued until 1973. By that time, twenty-eight men had died from the direct effects of the disease, and one hundred more from complications of syphilis. Moreover, more than forty wives and nineteen children had also contracted the disease. Investigations revealed that the men had not been given information that would have allowed them to provide genuine informed consent, and some of the information given was intended to mislead them about the nature of the study.

The combination of Beecher's and Jonas's publications and the outrage that followed the Tuskegee reports led to the appointment of a U.S. national commission to clarify ethical guidelines for protecting human subjects.[12] The National Commission for the Protection of Human Subjects of Biomedical and

Behavioral Research was created by the National Research Act of 1974 and operated until 1978.[13] The commission was directed to consider the following: (1) the boundaries between biomedical and behavioral *research* and the accepted and routine *practice* of medicine, (2) the role of assessment of risk-benefit criteria in the determination of the appropriateness of research involving human subjects, (3) appropriate guidelines for the selection of human subjects for participation in such research, and (4) the nature and definition of informed consent in various research settings. Because the commission met at the Belmont Conference Center of the Smithsonian Institution, the report that contained the outcome of its deliberations was called the Belmont Report.[14] The Belmont Report identifies three basic ethical principles related to human medical research: (1) respect for persons, (2) beneficence, and (3) justice.

Respect for persons requires that individuals should be treated as autonomous agents and also that persons with diminished ability to exercise their autonomy are entitled to protection. Beneficence is defined as an obligation to "do no harm" to subjects and to maximize possible benefits and minimize the possible harms of research.[15] The justice aspect addresses the question of who ought to receive the benefits of research and bear its burdens. The Belmont Report gave recognition to the notion that human medical research can be unethical if its benefits and burdens are unfairly distributed, especially if the burdens fall disproportionately on vulnerable or disadvantaged people. Applying these ethical principles meant that, to respect persons, investigators must obtain informed and voluntary consent from all human subjects. Autonomy has come to mean a form of personal liberty, where a person is free to make individual decisions free from deceit, coercion, duress, or constraint. Autonomous decision making is also furthered when adequate information is provided to allow someone to fully understand the consequences of research participation. Beneficence requires a careful assessment of the risks and benefits of a clinical trial and a proper trial design to maximize the benefits and minimize and justify the risks. Application of justice principles requires that subjects be selected in a fair manner (individual justice) and also that vulnerable subjects such as children, prisoners, and the mentally incapacitated are protected (social justice).

While it was more comprehensive than most other research ethics documents, the Belmont Report did not prioritize the importance of the three ethical principles, leaving for others to determine how to balance the various imperatives and how to apply them. Some general guidance was offered; for example, that brutal or inhumane treatment of human subjects is never morally justified, that a higher level of justification is needed for recruiting vulnerable subjects like children, and that the "relevant" risks and benefits must be thoroughly presented in the informed consent process. Investigators who wished to comply with the ethical guidance of the Belmont Report would have to engage in a risk-benefit analysis to determine what specific human subject protections to employ to meet ethical obligations. Later, federal laws and regulations based on the Belmont Report put more flesh on the bones and listed detailed requirements, such as specific consent provisions, the need for institutional review board (IRB) review of research protocols, and the prompt reporting of adverse effects.[16]

Despite the specifications of ethical principles and the regulatory requirements that govern human medical research in the United States, reports of research abuses have persisted, resulting in sanctions and further regulatory restrictions. In the recent past, FDA and the United States Office for Protection from Research Risks (OPRR), which had responsibility for administering regulations regarding the protection of human subjects in research sponsored by the federal government, were required to restrict or suspend research activities at numerous institutions because of ethically and legally inappropriate practices. Medical and lay press reports during the 1980s and 1990s of OPRR's and FDA's enforcement work kept the public informed about studies in which, for instance, subject consent was obtained after the fact or not at all, subjects' signatures on informed-consent forms were forged, subjects were enrolled in studies they did not qualify for, studies were unacceptably risky for the subjects selected, data were fabricated, adverse reactions were not adequately monitored, subject deaths were not reported, study protocols were not followed, and investigators had significant conflicts of interest with the funder of the research.[17] Government agency investigations and audits led to the closure of research programs at medical centers including those at Duke University, University of Colorado Health Sciences Center, the West Los Angeles Veterans Affairs Medical Center, and the University of Arizona. The failures were attributed to multiple causes, including lack of investigator awareness of research requirements, overzealous researchers who ignored human subject protection requirements that impeded research, an inability to determine if an adverse effect was caused by the experimental drug or the subject's disease, and sheer incompetence. IRB review was also often seen as inadequate especially in high-volume research centers where IRB members were just too overburdened to give each protocol a careful review.[18]

In 1995, the National Bioethics Advisory Commission (NBAC) was instituted and charged by President Clinton to review the U.S. federal protections pertaining to human subject research.[19] Continuing reports of recent research problems resulted in the movement of OPRR to a location higher in the Department of Health and Human Services hierarchy. The new Office for Human Research Protections (OHRP) is required to further strengthen protections for human research subjects in clinical trials.

Council for International Organizations of Medical Sciences

International entities continued to strengthen and augment the guidelines of the Nuremberg Code and the Declaration of Helsinki. The most notable effort has been made by the Council for International Organizations of Medical Sciences (CIOMS), which in collaboration with the World Health Organization (WHO) developed the International Ethical Guidelines for Biomedical Research Involving Human Subjects.[20] Among the goals of these guidelines was to eliminate the disparities in the way that human research was conducted among countries and to discourage researchers from using foreign subjects to conduct research that would be unacceptable in their home country. The guidelines were considered necessary because of abusive practices in countries, especially in the third world, with inadequate regulations, ineffective enforcement, and few ethical standards to protect human subjects. The CIOMS guidelines stemmed from the belief that there are fundamental values that cross cultures and that should be upheld no matter where the research is performed.

The CIOMS work addressed concepts of cultural relativism (*for example,* "when in Rome, do as the Romans," "no culture's ethics are better than others'"). This morally blind approach contrasts with what is known sometimes as ethical imperialism, which directs people to do everything exactly as they do at home or, put another way, counsels that moral behavior should not change as it travels. Both approaches have their advantages and their inadequacies. Cultural relativism fails when reliance on local standards causes great harm to the local people. Conversely, insisting on the imposition of home country standards can ignore a country's need to uphold its own values and prevents emerging countries from accepting expedient conditions in order to make any progress against devastating local conditions.[21]

The difficulty of these issues, particularly if a company attempts to abide by American standards, is exemplified by an African study conducted by Pfizer, Inc. In this study, the company's experimental antibiotic (Trovan®) was used during an outbreak of deadly meningitis in which fifteen thousand people had died.[22] After obtaining FDA and Nigerian government approval for the trial in 1996, the study was done in Kano, Nigeria, using two hundred children age 1 to 13, half of whom got Pfizer's drug and half an approved drug but, according to allegations, in less than the usual recommended dose. In this study, eleven of the children from both treated and control groups died, and others became paralyzed or deaf. In 2001, thirty Nigerian families sued Pfizer alleging that the company violated international laws and guidelines (including the Nuremberg Code) by failing to obtain informed consent, failing to provide a proven therapy for children who failed to respond to Pfizer's drug, and giving the control group less-than-effective doses of the control drug. The suit, which was the first of its kind based on the Alien Tort Claims Act, contained the allegation that "Pfizer took the opportunity presented by the chaos caused by the civil and medical crises in Kano to accomplish what the company could not do elsewhere—to quickly conduct on young children a test of [a] potentially dangerous antibiotic." Pfizer denied all of the allegations and asserted that informed consent had been obtained and that the study was conducted in the belief that the drug would be helpful in the afflicted population. Further, the fatality rates in the Kano study, approximately 6 percent for both Trovan and the control drug, were lower than published results for other forms of treatment in this epidemic. However, the circumstances guaranteed that the conflicting issues would be difficult to resolve.[23] Clearly, there are some situations where different research standards can be justified. However, some will undoubtedly believe that third world research conducted by first world companies too easily results in the same exploitation that was considered morally unacceptable when the American regulations were written.[24] For more on this subject, see the introduction to the VaxGen case study in Chapter 9.

Miscellaneous Guidelines That Govern Human Research Practices

Conflicts of Interest

Industry-sponsored clinical trials have raised continuous concerns about the conflicts of interest they can engender. The basic worry is that, if outside investigators are too closely allied with the company that sponsors the research, the investigator can lose objectivity, mislead subjects, or bias the research in the company's favor. "Rigging" a study design to produce favorable results also undermines the integrity of all subsequent research derived from the study and compromises the safety of patients who are treated according to the research findings. The primary source of biasing influence is, of course, money. Financial arrangements between industry and investigators can include:

- Payments for clinical research services (that can be fixed or "capitated," in which the investigator receives a specified amount for each subject enrolled in a study)
- Equity in the company (seen more often in smaller, newer companies that lack cash and in entrepreneurial medical schools where faculty found companies)
- Consulting fees
- Patent ownership (in which the company pays a royalty on drug sales to the investigator who holds the drug patent)
- Honoraria given to researchers to present the findings of research

Other connections, such as board positions, speaking engagements, authorship on research papers, and funding for future research can also potentially bias the investigator. These arrangements can involve small or large amounts of money. One reporter estimated that some medical researchers can be paid up to one million dollars a year for performing clinical research.[25]

For the most part, there has been only anecdotal evidence that financial conflicts of interest between bioscience companies and their investigators bias research results. Recently, however, empirical data have been collected suggesting that financial ties to drug companies can affect the outcome of drug research. One notable study from the University of Toronto compared the source of research authors' funding to the authors' conclusions about the safety of cardiac drugs called calcium channel antagonists.[26] The study data showed that 96 percent of authors who were supportive of the antagonists had financial relationships with the drug's manufacturer, compared with 60 percent who were neutral, and 37 percent who were critical. Harvard University health policy researcher David Blumenthal, commenting on this research, stated that "this kind of evidence supports what one expects of human nature—that personal connection, financial or other, [tends] to create a favorable inclination for the group or individuals to which you have a connection."[27] While few in the medical community believe that true financial conflicts of interest are widespread, most agree that awareness of the potential problem, management of conflicts, and disclosure of financial relationships are all warranted.

Most academic medical centers have internal conflict-of-interest policies and monitoring programs to prevent true and perceived conflicts of interest.

These policies vary considerably but most require disclosure of relationships and limit the amount of equity that a faculty researcher can hold in a company that funds his or her research. FDA does not restrict financial relationships between investigators and their research funders but does require that they be disclosed.[28] Bioscience companies either have conflict-of-interest policies or are becoming increasingly aware of the need to manage relationships with outside investigators to avoid creating situations where researchers are inclined to produce results agreeable to the company. Companies also monitor their investigators to ensure that no investigator practices bias the study data. For more on conflict of interest issues, see the introduction to the Novartis case study in Chapter 6.

Academic Freedom Guidelines

Because medical school faculty frequently perform research for bioscience companies, policies have been developed to guide these relationships to avoid negative impacts on academic freedom. Faculty codes of conduct encourage openness in research, collaboration, data sharing, and unfettered ability to publish. Industry, however, often needs to control these aspects of research to maintain patent positions, protect trade secrets, or to otherwise preserve competitive advantages.[29] Given these differences, it is not surprising that some industry-faculty relationships generate conflict. Faculty allegations have included that companies attempt to exert undue control over research results by misinterpreting data, preventing disclosure of negative findings, and prohibiting publication of results.[30] At times, disputes about publications have led investigators to air their grievances in medical journals, such as when seven researchers published an announcement that they had withdrawn their names from a publication of an industry-sponsored study because the sponsor had attempted to wield undue influence on the nature of the final paper. They wrote that "this effort was so oppressive that we felt it inhibited academic freedom and led to substantial differences within the [study] group with regard to the ultimate presentation and interpretation of the results."[31]

One of the most widely known instances of alleged industry heavy-handedness involved a study conducted by University of California, San Francisco, clinical pharmacist Betty J. Dong. Beginning in 1988, Dr. Dong conducted a study to compare four formulations of levothyroxine (a form of thyroid) tablets, one by Boots Pharmaceuticals on its product Synthroid® and three less expensive competing generic thyroid tablets. This study was supported in part by a grant from Boots Pharmaceuticals Inc., which had an 84 percent market share for levothyroxine. The study was done because, although fifteen million levo-thyroxine prescriptions were filled annually, there were no data to show whether the more expensive Synthroid was therapeutically superior to the cheaper ge-neric products. Based on some prior publications by Dong that it was risky to switch patients from Synthroid to generic tablets, the company expected that the Synthroid data would be superior. However, the data instead indicated that all four products were essentially equivalent. According to Dong, the company then wrongfully attempted to discredit the study and the conduct of the re-searchers. A university investigation followed that exonerated Dong's research, finding only minor and insignificant flaws in her research methods and conclu-sions. Boots countered that there were major flaws in the study, making publi-cation of the results scientifically irresponsible since it would encourage physi-cians to prescribe generic levothyroxine, which would put patients at risk.[32] After years of wrangling over the data, Dong prepared a paper reporting her findings that was accepted for publication in the *Journal of the American Medical Association* (JAMA). The company threatened to sue Dong based on a research contract she signed that gave the company control over publication. Dong then withdrew the paper one week before it was scheduled to be published. The company, which had sent letters to the editors of several medical journals advis-ing them that the Dong study was flawed, then published its own paper in which Dong's data were critiqued and reanalyzed to show that Synthroid was better than the other formulations. The Boots-approved paper was published in a new journal called the *American Journal of Therapeutics*, where the senior au-thor, also a Boots medical-services director, was an associate editor.[33]

Eventually, the company (which had by then been purchased by the parent of Knoll Pharmaceuticals), the university, and Dong came to an agreement that Dong's study could be published. JAMA published the paper unchanged seven years after Boots had first raised objections about the data and over two years after the paper had first been slated for publication.[34] In this paper, Dong and her colleagues asserted that health-care costs could be cut by $356 million a year if Synthroid were replaced by the cheaper but equally effective levothy-roxine drugs. In the meantime, FDA's Division of Drug Marketing, Advertis-ing and Communication, after its own investigation, found that the Boots/ Knoll paper, to the extent that it was being disseminated by the company, amounted to misleading labeling about Synthroid. In addition, a large class-action lawsuit followed the publication of Dong's paper, alleging on behalf of all Synthroid users that Knoll had defrauded them of hundreds of millions of dollars in inflated costs. The company offered to settle for up to $135 million.[35]

Although the Dong incident was extraordinary, academic-industry research conflicts were frequent enough to prompt most research universities to implement academic freedom policies that govern relationships with industry sponsors of research. The primary intent of these policies is to prevent the loss of control over the conduct and publication of faculty research. This topic is discussed further in the Novartis case study in Chapter 6.

ANIMAL RESEARCH

Prior to the time that products can be tested in humans, they are tested in animals. The purpose of animal research is to determine as much as possible that the drug or device is safe and effective for the target patient group. Animals are used to develop a pharmacokinetic profile to determine how a drug is absorbed, distributed, metabolized, and eliminated from the body. These studies also monitor for side effects. Animals are used to determine the minimum doses that produce toxicity and to compare this dose with the amount that produces the desired effect. If the toxic and effective doses are too close together (that is, the drug has a "narrow therapeutic window"), the drug is often abandoned as too unsafe to give to humans. Animal research is important because it provides research data that are more predictive of the human condition than lab data, spares humans from being exposed to unacceptably toxic drugs, and, for devices, allows physicians to perfect techniques before attempting them in humans. Often, if the disease the drug is intended to treat is chronic, animal tests may be required to last for up to two years to assure regulators that the drug is sufficiently effective and safe to administer to the first human subjects.

Research animals are purchased from facilities that breed, raise, and sell them for research purposes. Many of these animals are bred for specific types of research, such as mice prone to tumor development, dogs that have sleep disorders, surgically altered animals (such as those with the thyroid gland removed), or transgenic mice implanted with human genes to study human gene function. Supplying research animals is a big business. One of the largest mouse research and supply facilities, the Jackson Laboratory of Bar Harbor, Maine, with over $88 million in 2000 revenue, each year supplies approximately two million mice from over 2,700 stocks and strains to universities, medical schools, and research laboratories.[36] Raising and selling these animals requires rigorous quality controls to ensure the standardization, health, and genetic purity required for scientific research.

In addition, these facilities must adhere to the Animal Welfare Act and other federal and state animal welfare laws and the regulations of the U.S. Department of Agriculture (USDA), Department of Health and Human Services (DHHS), and animal health authorities that control the conditions under which animals are transported, housed, and used in clinical research.[37] Research oversight committees at animal research facilities are also responsible for adherence to these laws and regulations.[38] As with human research, the U.S. laws and the requirements for oversight committees were developed primarily in response to disclosures about the abuse and misuse of animals in research settings. To avoid problems and to assure as much as possible the humane treatment of laboratory animals, more than 630 animal research facilities have voluntarily become accredited by the nonprofit American Association for the Accreditation of Laboratory Animal Care-International (AAALAC-I), which sets standards for responsible animal care above and beyond the state and federal legal requirements.

FDA does not specifically regulate industry animal research, but, along with drug development laboratory data, the agency must be satisfied that the investigational product is sufficiently safe and effective to justify the first human experiments. Therefore, the company's regulatory affairs group often gets involved in these early laboratory and animal research stages to ensure that the company knows what FDA considers necessary for a successful application to commence human trials. FDA generally asks the company sponsor to provide animal data showing: (1) a pharmacological profile of the drug, (2) acute toxicity in at least two species of animals, and (3) short-term toxicity.

Although animal testing is a necessary prerequisite to testing drugs in humans, there are often questions about the extent to which animal data can be extrapolated to humans. Because of intra- and interspecies differences, false positive and false negative test results are common. Two examples of false negative results occurred when animal testing failed to predict two potentially lethal side effects in humans—blood clots with oral contraceptives and aplastic anemia with the antibiotic chloramphenicol. It is also commonly believed that the conservative approach to animal tests for carcinogenicity often produce false positive results since these tests always expose the animal to doses of the drug far in excess of what humans will take. However, out of caution, drugs rarely make it beyond the animal test stage when animals develop cancer even if the researchers believe that the result is a false positive. Because of the limited ability of animal research data to predict drug effects in humans, constant efforts are being made to develop animal models that more closely mimic human diseases and drug effects.

One such effort is notable in its achievement. At the beginning of the AIDS epidemic, it was discovered that there were no good animal models for this disease. The only animals susceptible to experimental HIV-1 infection were chimpanzees, gibbon apes, and rabbits, but AIDS-like disease did not develop in these species. This difference made it impossible to use animals to test the efficacy of anti-AIDS drugs or vaccines beyond looking at what the product did to blood virus levels, which was only an indirect indicator of efficacy at best.[39] Without a good animal model, preliminary research on potential AIDS cures was severely restricted. An important advance came with the creation of a mouse bred for research on severe combined immunodeficiency (SCID), called the SCID-hu mouse. The progenitor to this mouse was the SCID mouse, which was bred with SCID. These mice had no functioning immune system and, therefore, no natural means of fighting disease. What was valuable about this mouse was that it would also not immunologically fight (or reject) the transplantation of tissues from other species.

The initial research that led to the creation of the SCID-hu was performed at Stanford University by J. Michael McCune and his associates, including Irving Weissman, who were looking for better animal models for the testing of AIDS drugs and vaccines. They came upon the idea of transplanting a human immune system into a mouse, and the existence of the SCID research mouse made this attempt plausible since the SCID mouse would not reject the implantation of the foreign human tissue. In order to create the new mouse, researchers painstakingly transplanted human fetal thymus gland and lymph nodes into the adult SCID mouse, then injected them with embryonic human immune cells.[40] Some of these cells traveled to the implanted human thymus, where they matured into various types of immune cells called T cells, B cells, and macrophages. A second group of researchers implanted mature human T cells in the SCID mouse. In September 1988, Stanford University announced that a mouse with a human immune system had been created, thus the name SCID-hu, the "hu" for human. This mouse allowed for predictive studies on the effects of drugs and vaccines on viruses, including HIV. Working with NIH funding and in specially secure laboratory facilities, the researchers then went on to demonstrate that these mice could become infected with AIDS and, later, that the anti-AIDS drug AZT inhibited the proliferation of the virus. This chimeric mouse thereafter became an invaluable model for testing the efficacy of anti-AIDS drug candidates, for the testing of compounds against other human pathogens, and for the study of the human immune system. Stanford obtained a patent on the mouse, and, with start-up funding and a license from

Stanford, McCune and Weissman formed a company called SyStemix, Inc., to commercialize this highly useful research animal.[41]

Despite such success stories and the high utility of many animals to the drug development process, most companies must deal with the growing concern about animal cruelty. Several aspects of animal use are considered cruel by animal rights groups. Developing and breeding animals with diseases or other medical conditions can make life miserable for the animal. Many research techniques are also painful and subject animals to a high level of distress. The laboratory conditions (cages, lack of access to the outdoors, abnormal social conditions, and so on) especially for larger, more socially complex animals have also been criticized. Modern concern for animal welfare has been a social issue going back to 1789 when the English jurisprudence professor and philosopher Jeremy Bentham, eschewing the Biblical notion that man had complete domain over all other creatures, asked in his book, *An Introduction to the Principles of Morals & Legislation*, what "insuperable line" prevented humans from extending moral regard to animals: "The question is not, Can they reason? nor, Can they talk? but, Can they suffer?" The point that the degree of suffering, not the species of the sufferer, is what should count in deciding how to use animals is still a widely held notion in animal research.

Based on this notion, antivivisectionist leagues and other animal rights groups have continuously questioned the need to use animals in anatomy laboratories and as research specimens. However, the animal rights movement became a real force in 1975 following the publication of the book *Animal Liberation* by the Australian philosopher Peter Singer. Singer believed that if experiments would cause unacceptable suffering in a human, the experiment should not be done on an animal that would suffer as much. This book struck a chord within a vigilant movement of animal rights activists adamantly opposed to the use of animals in research, and some of these activists have periodically used violence to promote their point of view. Over the past twenty years, most animal research workers in university, industry, and private laboratories have become used to the frequent protest campaigns of the animal rights activists and increasingly have had to defend themselves from bomb threats, vandalism, and break-ins to free the animals. Therefore, security at these facilities must be vigilant and high-profile animal researchers occasionally have reason to fear for their personal safety. Although most people's views on animal research are more balanced, public perceptions of animals have become increasingly protectionist. In 1985, one survey showed that 63 percent of American respondents agreed that "scientists should be allowed to do research that causes pain and injury to animals like dogs and chimpanzees IF it produces new information about human health problems." In 1995, only 53 percent agreed with this statement.[42]

Scientists have responded to animal welfare concerns and are frequently engaged in efforts to improve laboratory conditions and treatment of animals and to spare animals from euthanasia after the research is completed. AAALAC accreditation helps keep researchers up to date on the best animal treatment practices. Others work on reducing the numbers of animals used in research, or attempt to use lower species of animals. For instance, it is common in drug studies to produce a statistic called the LD50, the dose of a drug that kills half of the animals in the study. These studies once required the use of up to two hundred rats, dogs, or other animals, but it is now common to use up to one-tenth that number of animals to produce an LD50 measurement. Some of these animal protection changes are difficult to make since they can reduce the scientific value of the experiment. Therefore, scientists have also worked on devising alternative methods to obtain the data traditionally collected on animals. While this activity is more common in Europe, where animal welfare is a stronger concern, several U.S. governmental agencies have started to fund studies to discover laboratory tests that can substitute for animal studies. A number of companies have also participated in this work by funding the Center for Alternatives to Animal Testing (CAAT) at Johns Hopkins University. However, since the mechanisms of drug toxicity are still not understood well enough to forgo the use of animals, controversy about animal research issues likely will remain a feature of drug development.[43]

CONCLUSION

Responsible management of human and animal research will ensure the continued viability of this important corporate work. Fundamental to this endeavor is an understanding of the applicable ethical guidelines and concepts. Therefore, business managers responsible for corporate research should obtain copies of the codes of ethics described earlier and, especially when legal requirements are absent or unclear, use these ethical standards to guide research decisions.

Notes

1. Brody BA. Troubling ethical issues in the conduct of clinical trials. In *Ethical issues in drug testing, approval, and pricing*. New York: Oxford University Press; 1995. pp. 99–157; Malone RE. Ethical issues in industry-sponsored research. *Journal of Emergency Nursing* 1998; 24:193–96; *Institutional review boards: Promising results*. Washington, DC: Office of Inspector General, U.S. Department of Health and Human Services; 1998. Report No. OEI-01-97-00191. Available at www.dhhs.gov/progorg/oei/reports/9274.pdf.

2. Ironically, before the ascendancy of the Third Reich, Germany was one of few countries with legal guidelines that protected the interests of human subjects of research. Requirements included that "clear and unmistakable" and bona fide consent to research must be obtained, subjects must be provided information about the research, research design must be careful, and vulnerable subjects must be protected. These laws were ignored under the Nazi regime and provided no protection against the medical experiments that were carried out by force and without consent on German citizens before and during the war.

Lock S. Research ethics: A brief historical review to 1965. *Journal of Internal Medicine* 1995; 238:513–20; The Nuremberg Code, from trials of war criminals before the Nuremberg Military Tribunals under Control Council Law No. 10. U.S. Government Printing Office. 1946–49. Available at www.ushmm.org/research/doctros/Nuremberg_Code.htm; Ernst, E. Killing in the name of healing: The active role of the German medical profession during the Third Reich. *American Journal of Medicine* 1996; 100:579–81.

3. Brody BA. Troubling ethical issues in the conduct of clinical trials. In *Ethical issues in drug testing, approval, and pricing*. New York: Oxford University Press; 1995. pp. 99–157; Baram, M. Making clinical trials safer for human subjects. *American Journal of Law and Medicine* 2001; 27:253–82.

4. World Medical Association. Declaration of Helsinki. *Journal of the American Medical Association* 1997; 277:909–14.

5. Lock S. Research ethics: A brief historical review to 1965. *Journal of Internal Medicine* 1995; 238:513–20.

6. Djulbegovic B, Lacevic M, Cantor A, et al. The uncertainty principle and industry-sponsored research. Lancet 2000; 356:635–38.

7. Levine RJ. Research and practice. In *Ethics and regulation of clinical research*. New Haven, CT: Yale University Press; 1988. pp. 3–4; Annas GJ. *Some choice: Law, medicine, and the market*. New York: Oxford University Press; 1998; Miller FG, Rosenstein DL,

DeRenzo EG. Professional integrity in clinical research. *Journal of the American Medical Association* 1998; 280:1449–54.

8. Enserink M. Helsinki's new clinical rules: Fewer placebos, more disclosure. *Science* 2000; 290:418–19; see also Note 3, Brody; Baram.

9. Beecher HK. Ethics and clinical research. *New England Journal of Medicine* 1966; 274:1354–60; Beecher's medical paper was based on a 1965 presentation at the Brook Lodge Symposium for Science Writers, sponsored by the Upjohn Company.

10. Kopp VJ. Henry Knowles Beecher and the development of informed consent in anesthesia research. *Anesthesiology* 1999; 90:1756–65.

11. Jonas H. Philosophical reflections on experimenting with human subjects. *Daedalus* 1969; 98:219–47.

12. National Commission for the Protection of Human Subjects of Biomedical and Behavioral Research. *The Belmont report: Ethical principles and guidelines for the protection of human subjects of research.* Report No. GPO 887-809. Washington, DC: Department of Health, Education and Welfare; 1979. Available at www.nih.gov:80/grants/oprr/humansubjects/guidance/belmont.htm.

13. National Research Act of 1974, Public Law No. 93-348.

14. National Commission for the Protection of Human Subjects of Biomedical and Behavioral Research. *The Belmont report: Ethical principles and guidelines for the protection of human subjects of research.* Report No. GPO 887-809. Washington, DC: Department of Health, Education and Welfare; 1979. Available at www.nih.gov:80/grants/oprr/humansubjects/guidance/belmont.htm.

15. Some medical ethicists divide this principle into beneficence (the obligation to do the good that can be done) and nonmaleficence (the duty to avoid causing harm).

16. An IRB, or institutional review board, is a multidisciplinary review board that must approve all human research protocols at an institution. The IRB review is intended to ensure: that subjects are selected equitably; the risks of the research to subjects is minimized to the extent possible and are in relation to the benefits to subjects, if any, and the importance of the knowledge to be gained; that subjects are informed in advance of the risks or discomforts and the anticipated benefits of a study; that a study has adequate monitoring provisions; that privacy of subjects is provided for; and that safeguards are in place to protect vulnerable subjects. These requirements for IRB review for federal research are codified in 45 *Code of Federal Regulations* Part 46 and are further described in the IRB Guidebook, available from http://ohrp.osophs.dhhs.gov/irb/irb_guidebook.htm.

45 *Code of Federal Regulations* Part 46. These federal "Protection of Human Subjects" regulations apply to research conducted or supported by seventeen federal departments or agencies. The FDA human subject regulations (21 *Code of Federal Regulations* parts 50, 56, 312, and 812) govern research that involves the use of investigational drugs and devices. These two sets of regulations are generally consistent with each other. Most states also have laws that protect the human subjects of research.

17. Reporters at *U.S. News and World Report* became so interested in the subject that they obtained FDA research audit records under a Freedom of Information re-

quest that revealed the following citations from about one thousand FDA spot-checks of all types of trials from January 1996 through June 1999: 213 researchers failed to obtain proper consent from subjects, 364 failed to stick to their approved research plan, and 140 did not report adverse reactions from test drugs.

Kaplan, S, Brownlee, S. Dying for a cure. *U.S. News and World Report* 1999 Oct 11; 34–43.

18. Bell J, Whiton J, Connelly S. *Final report: Evaluation of NIH implementation of Section 491 of the Public Health Service Act: Mandating a program of protection for research subjects.* Office for Protection from Research Risks, National Institutes of Health; 1998 June 15. Available at http://grants.nih.gov/grants/oprr/hsp_report/hsp_final_rpt.pdf; Monmaney T. VA not alone in ethical shortcomings. *Los Angeles Times* 1999 Mar 29; 1. Weiss R. U.S. halts research on humans at Duke. *Washington Post* 1999 May 12; Sect. A:01; see also Note 17, Kaplan.

19. Executive Order Number 12975, Protection of human research subjects and creation of National Bioethics Advisory Commission. 60 *Federal Register* 52,063; 1995 Oct 3. See www.bioethics.gov.

20. *International ethical guidelines for biomedical research involving human subjects.* Council for International Organizations of Medical Sciences. Geneva; 1982, rev. 1993. Available at www.codex.uu.se/texts/international.html.

21. Donaldson T. Values in tension: Ethics away from home. *Harvard Business Review* 1996 Sept–Oct:48–62; Woodward B. Challenges to human subject protections in U.S. medical research. *Journal of the American Medical Association* 1999; 282:1947–52.

22. Pfizer's drug had been approved for use in adults for other infections, but FDA approvals were restricted in 1999 after it was discovered that the drug was toxic to the liver.

23. Malakoff D. Nigerian families sue Pfizer, testing the reach of U.S. law. *Science* 2001; 293:1742; Pfizer, Inc. Pfizer statement re Trovan suit. Press release. 2001 Aug 30. Available at www.pfizer.com/pfizerinc/about/press/trovansuit.html.

24. Jost TS. The globalization of health law: The case of permissibility of placebo-based research. *American Journal of Law and Medicine* 2000; 26:175–86.

25. American Medical Association. Report by the Council on Scientific Affairs and Council on Ethical and Judicial Affairs. *Journal of the American Medical Association* 1990; 263:2790–93; Eichenwald K, Kolata G. Drug trials hide conflicts for doctors. *New York Times* 1999 May 16; Sect. A:34; Lo B. Conflict-of-interest policies for investigators in clinical trials. *New England Journal of Medicine* 2000; 343:1616–19.

26. Stelfox HT, Chua G, O'Rourke K, et al. Conflict of interest in the debate over calcium-channel antagonists. *New England Journal of Medicine* 1998; 338:101–6.

27. Kreeger KY. Studies prompt closer scrutiny of conflict of interest policies. *Journal of the National Cancer Institute* 2001; 93:895–97.

28. The FDA regulation "is intended to ensure that financial interests and arrangements of clinical investigators that could affect reliability of data submitted to FDA in support of product marketing are identified and disclosed by the sponsor of any drug, biological product, or device marketing application." 63 *Federal Register* 5233, 1998 Feb 2.

29. Reasons for secrecy or publication delays include the need to file patent applications, protect proprietary findings, negotiate licensing agreements, or allow time to resolve disputes over intellectual property. Competitive needs have led companies to control the release of study data for more controversial reasons, e.g., to promote stock prices, ensure a lead against competitors, or slow dissemination of undesired results.

30. Freeman RA. Minimizing bias in industry-sponsored research. *Medical Interface* 1994; 7:130–34; Fox JL. Industry-linked groups, geneticists, hoard data. *Nature Biotechnology* 1997; 15:504–5; Blumenthal D, Campbell EG, Anderson MS, et al. Withholding research results in academic life science; evidence from a national survey of faculty. *Journal of the American Medical Association* 1997; 277:1224–28.

31. Applegate W, Furberg K, Byungton R, et al. The multicenter isradipine diuretic atherosclerosis study (MIDAS). *Journal of the American Medical Association* 1996; 277: 297–98.

32. Knoll made the following points to support their conclusion during an FDA meeting: Dong's assay used to establish pharmaceutical equivalence was inaccurate; some patients enrolled in the study did not meet protocol entry specifications; food consumption in subjects in relationship to blood tests was not controlled; tablet counts showed that study subjects were noncompliant; and reports of thyroid-related symptoms were inadequate.
Synthroid Meeting Minutes. Center for Drug Evaluation and Research, Food and Drug Administration. 1997 Jan 8. Available at www.fda.gov/cder/foi/special/97/synthroidspectop.pdf.

33. Mayor GH, Orlando T, Kurtz NM. Limitations of levothyroxine bioequivalence evaluation: Analysis of an attempted study. *American Journal of Therapeutics* 1995; 2:417–32; King RT. Bitter pill: How a drug firm paid for university study, then undermined it. *Wall Street Journal* 1996 Apr 25; Sect. A:1.

34. Dong BJ. Bioequivalence of generic and brand-name levothyroxine products in the treatment of hypothyroidism. *Journal of the American Medical Association* 1997; 277:1205–13.

35. Rennie D. Thyroid storm. *Journal of the American Medical Association* 1997; 277:1238–43; Synthroid Meeting Minutes. Center for Drug Evaluation and Research, Food and Drug Administration. 1997 Jan 8. Available at www.fda.gov/cder/foi/special/97/synthroidspectop.pdf.; Vogel G. Long-suppressed study finally sees light of day. *Science* 1997; 276:523–25; Richards B. Knoll will make payments to settle claims over drug. *Wall Street Journal* 1997 Aug 12; Sect. B:4.

36. Facts about the Jackson Laboratory, a nonprofit institution. The Jackson Laboratory. 2001. Available at www.jax.org/about/jax_facts.html.

37. The Animal Welfare Act is at 7 United States Code, sections 2131–56 and the USDA regulations are at 9 Code of Federal Regulations, Chapter 1, Subchapter A. Further information about the federal animal welfare laws and regulations are available at www.nal.usda.gov/awic/legislat/usdaleg1.htm#L1.

38. These are called institutional animal care and use committees (IACUC) and are composed of veterinarians, scientists, and lay people unaffiliated with the research

facility. IACUCs exist to review and approve research protocols and monitor the care and use of the research animals.

39. Cohen J. Animal illogic. In *Shots in the dark*. New York: W.W. Norton; 2001. pp. 78–101.

40. Human immune tissue from aborted fetal tissue donated for research was chosen to implant into SCID mice since early fetal tissue would likewise not reject the mouse tissue as would human adult immune system tissue.

41. National Cancer Institute. *Understanding the immune system; the SCID mouse.* 2001. Available at http://rex.nci.nih.gov/PATIENTS/INFO_TEACHER/bookshelf/NIH_immune/html/imm31.html; McCune JM, Namikawa R, Kaneshima H, et al. The SCID-hu mouse: Murine model for the analysis of human hematolymphoid differentiation and function. *Science* 1988; 241:1632–39; Namikawa R, Kaneshima H, Lieberman M, et al. Infection of the SCID-hu mouse by HIV-1. *Science* 1988; 242:1684–86; McCune JM, Kaneshima H, Lieberman M, et al. The SCID-hu mouse: Current status and potential applications. *Current Topics in Microbiology and Immunology* 1989; 152:183–93.

42. Hoge W. British researchers on animal rights death list. *New York Times* 1999 Jan 10; Sect. 1:10; Sorkin AR. Behind biggest drug merger, quest for research pipeline. *New York Times* 2000 Jan 18; Sect. C:1; Hodgson J. UK keen to mimic German venture scheme. *Nature Biotechnology* 2001; 19:495.

43. Mukerjee M. Trends in animal research. *Scientific American* 1997 Mar. Available at www.sciam.com/0297issue/0297trends.html.

5

Industry Regulation and the Product Approval Process

The pharmaceutical and biotechnology industry markets are huge. Every year, Americans spend $117 billion to have three billion prescriptions filled. Because these medical products have great potential for good as well as harm, they are closely regulated by the Food and Drug Administration. According to FDA, as of the year 2000, it regulated over $1 trillion worth of products (food, drugs, biologics including blood products, insulin and vaccines, cosmetics, medical devices, radiation-emitting products, and animal feed and drugs). There were 95,000 firms on their list of regulated companies. The agency considers its core public health protection function as the assessment of the risks of the products over which it has jurisdiction—and for drugs, biologics, and medical devices, weighing the risks against the potential benefits and approving or disallowing the marketing of new products. To perform this work, FDA has approximately 9,000 employees (2,100 scientists, 900 chemists, 300 microbiologists, and 1,100 investigators and inspectors), who review product marketing applications and monitor the manufacture, import, transport, storage, and sale of these products. FDA personnel inspect and investigate over 15,000 facilities a year for manufacturing and labeling compliance and, in the process, collect about 80,000 domestic and imported product samples for examination.

If the agency uncovers violations, it typically issues warning letters asking the company to correct problems voluntarily. FDA also can require the company to send out "Dear Doctor" letters to immediately notify the medical community of product safety concerns or to correct some unjustified claim or promotional information that the company has made. Further, if need be, the agency can exercise its authority to revoke facility licenses, recall any product, force a company to stop selling, and order items seized and destroyed. About three thousand products a year are found to be unfit for consumers and are withdrawn from the market, either by voluntary recall or by court-ordered seizure. Reasons for drug recalls include an unacceptably high incidence of adverse reactions; failures in good manufacturing procedures; discrepancies in company filings; deficiencies in product stability, uniformity, potency, purity, and sterility; and labeling errors.

Most FDA notices of discrepancies or violations are resolved informally and voluntarily. However, if regulatory violations are alleged by FDA and disputed by the company, the agency can institute enforcement proceedings to require the company to correct problems. This process often results in a consent decree. A consent decree, which is a court-supervised, mutually agreed-upon corrective action, is one step short of FDA initiating criminal charges against the company. Usually in a consent decree, the company agrees to punitive measures and pays for all of FDA's expenses for the investigation. Courts must oversee any consent decree to ensure, among other things, that FDA is not being too lenient on the company. When warranted, FDA can ask the Justice Department to bring criminal charges against a company or its employees. Under FDA laws, company employees can technically be charged for wrongdoing that occurs under their command even without their knowledge. Penalties include fines and prison sentences. FDA can also institute debarment procedures, usually against clinical researchers, to prevent anyone from participating further in FDA-regulated activities.

STRIKING A BALANCE BETWEEN SPEED AND SAFETY

According to the Tufts University Center for the Study of Drug Development, in 2001 it was taking twelve years and costing up to $800 million for a company to develop and market a new drug.[1] This includes the cost of failure. For every five thousand chemical entities tested, only five make it to human trials, and of these only one is eventually approved by the FDA for marketing. Naturally, given the time and costs, companies are anxious to avoid any delay and obtain marketing approval as soon as possible. However, drugs and other medical products are expensive and can cause serious adverse reactions and death. Therefore, both the FDA and regulated companies need to strike the right balance between rapidly approving drugs (which can overlook problems) and instituting more rigid safety requirements (which adds cost and can diminish company sales revenues and delay public access to important new drugs).

Because FDA has the ultimate control over whether a company's product is approved or rejected, it is not surprising that the relationship between a company and FDA can range from cooperative to adversarial, depending on the company, the product, the people involved, and FDA's timing and decisions. The adversarial nature can come from perceptions by FDA regulators that pharmaceutical companies, especially the large ones that qualify as Big Pharma, can be exceptionally strong and powerful and that they try to use that power to bend regulatory procedures to suit their needs, even to push the boundaries of permitted conduct. FDA also encounters problems with small or new companies that lack regulatory experience because they can be prone to make mistakes or are unaware of requirements. These difficulties cause regulators to believe that companies must be closely scrutinized and controlled. The utmost caution is required to prevent problem drugs from reaching the market. An oft-cited example involved the 2001 withdrawal from the market of Bayer's drug Baycol®, which after less than three years on the market, had been linked to fifty-two drug-associated deaths.

On the company side, managers can view FDA regulators as insufficiently expert to review their product submissions and unnecessarily bureaucratic and demanding in their requirements for more data. In addition, the lengthy FDA review times have always been an issue of contention, one that is not easily resolved given the nature of the science, data requirements, and the need to address public safety. Companies like to say that, for a product with a $350 million market, each day of FDA delay in product approval costs the company $1 million. Ultimately, however, companies have a vested interest in working cooperatively with the FDA and ensuring that only safe and effective products reach the market. Baycol, for example, was Bayer's third-largest drug with 2000 sales of $554 million and on track to top $800 million in 2001 sales. Bayer reported that the Baycol withdrawal cost about $575 million in 2001, and, to recover from the loss, the company planned to eliminate eighteen hundred jobs and close fifteen manufacturing plants. In addition, the company started to receive notices of lawsuits from injured patients and families.[2]

STAGES OF FDA PRODUCT REVIEW[3]

Investigational New Drug Exemption

After preclinical (that is, lab and animal) research has been completed, the company sponsor can submit an Investigational New Drug Exemption Application (referred to as the IND), which is technically needed to exempt the sponsor from the law that prohibits the interstate transport of unapproved materials.[4] The main purpose of the IND is to compile the evidence demonstrating that it is reasonable to begin testing the drug in humans. The IND includes: (1) information on the composition and source of the drug; (2) data from laboratory and animal studies; (3) clinical study plans and protocols, including the numbers of human subjects to be studied, where the studies will take place, how the data will be analyzed, and how adverse reactions will be identified and reported; (4) names and credentials of physicians and clinical investigators who will conduct the clinical trials; (5) submission of brochures and consent forms for investigators and patients, including relevant disclaimers on product safety; and (6) some basic manufacturing information for the study drug and any comparative products, including the placebo. The IND, which can be two thousand pages long, is reviewed by numerous departments at FDA. If the agency does not issue an objection within thirty days after IND submission, the sponsor can proceed with the first clinical trials.

In the process of preparing the IND and prior to going "into man" or "into the clinics" with clinical trials, the company must often make difficult decisions about how the research should be conducted. The most obvious tasks are to ensure as much as possible that the candidate product to be studied in humans is pure and has the lowest toxicity and maximum potential for efficacy. This decision can involve vigorous debates about whether further laboratory work and manipulation can improve the candidate in question. Some company scientists will want to "get on with it" while others believe that going into clinical trials with less than the optimal compound or with incomplete understanding of how the compound works is too risky for subjects and a potential waste of money if the product washes out. The frequent lack of correlation between animal and human responses to drugs exacerbates the difficulty of this decision. When drug compounds have more than one possible use, choosing which of these to pursue can also be difficult, and there might be disagreements about whether the choice should be driven by medical need or commercial promise. The type of clinical data that should be collected is another question. Deciding whether clinical signs and symptoms are sufficient (for example, reducing blood pressure) or whether outcomes are needed (for example, fewer heart attacks, reduced death rates) will significantly influence the determination of the number of subjects needed and the time required to complete the studies, and therefore the cost of the trial.

Clinical Trial Design Issues

Clinical trials are designed by company scientists and physicians with the aid of statisticians who attempt to ensure that no statistical errors will be made and that the studies are designed to detect true product effects. One way to do this is to compare the effects of the study product with an inert look-alike called a placebo. The experimental product can also can be compared with no treatment, a similar product, the standard treatment for the disease, or the past experience of other patients treated for the same disease. Using these comparison groups is a way to "control" a study.[5] The use of control groups helps to prove that the study product caused the disease to improve because investigators can say "the drug was better than a blank pill" or "the drug was better than another treatment." Without a comparative control group, there is no way to know if the disease improved on its own or because of some other factor, including mere chance. Control comparisons allow researchers to obtain a quantitative assessment of a drug's effect, and the placebo control is often believed to provide the most reliable benchmark. For more on the use of placebo controls in the design of clinical trials, see the introduction to the Genzyme case study in Chapter 7.

Statisticians must also collaborate with company physicians to avoid problems such as when statistically significant results are not clinically significant. Statisticians must also account for variability and bias in the study. For instance, by predicting variability in the likely responses to the product, statisticians determine such things as how many subjects are needed to produce reliable data and how long the study must last. Sources of bias must also be eliminated as much as possible, such as when the study design causes the therapeutic benefit of a drug to be overestimated. This can occur when the test drug is compared with another treatment of inferior quality or where study subjects have a predilection to respond favorably to the test product.[6]

Because research often reveals surprises—when, for instance, animals don't respond to drugs the same way humans do or because a disease process is not fully understood—it is often difficult to design a reliable study. If there is little confidence in the predictability of outcome of a major trial, several small pilot trials may be needed in order, for example, to eliminate certain types of patients from the study or to predict the most promising trial design. Deciding how much data can be collected per trial is another issue for companies that want to maximize the data-producing potential of their studies. Asking too many questions in a study, however, can muddy the conclusions and undermine the usefulness of the data. To respond to this problem, small discrete studies are performed in addition to the major trials. Examples include separate trials to evaluate specific drug interactions or studies in select patient populations that are of special concern (for example, patients with a limited ability to excrete the drug).

The choice of investigator and the setting and location for clinical trials are also important factors. For instance, a tightly run private contract research organization (CRO) may have a track record for efficient and careful research processes but may have little medical credibility compared with an academic center run by a nationally renowned physician. The status of the investigator will not help the company, however, if his or her research work is sloppy. Clinical research also needs to be done in centers where there is a sufficient patient population for recruitment. Medical centers in "retirement" states like Florida or Arizona are good places to locate studies for drugs that will be used in geriatrics. Anti-AIDS drugs are studied at centers with ready access to populations of intravenous drug abusers or gay men. Conversely, a drug company would not want to conduct a study of an experimental laser device unless the medical centers had sufficient numbers of physicians trained in the use of laser interventions. Oftentimes, studies need to be run in several centers in order to recruit enough patients to meet study criteria. These multicenter trials are obviously more difficult to manage and also make it difficult to ensure consistency in the way that study subjects are treated.

Studies will also fail if not enough patients are enrolled. Competition for human subjects has become a relatively recent problem, with nearly three million Americans recruited annually to participate in fifty thousand to sixty thousand ongoing clinical trials sponsored by government, academia, and industry.[7] According to industry analysts, close to 80 percent of clinical trials fail to enroll the required number of patients in the time promised by the investigators. This problem either compromises the integrity of the data as a whole or prolongs the study until the full complement of subjects can be enrolled. The scarcity of human subjects is most acute in the late-stage trials, which often require thousands of subjects. The problem will be exacerbated by the increasing numbers of drugs expected to be coming through company pipelines from genetic discoveries. Moreover, well-known research centers often have many drug trials in progress at one time and can be plagued by internal competition for subjects.

Pharmaceutical companies also compete for subjects with the government, such as with the National Cancer Institute, whose late-stage studies can require as many as ten thousand subjects and last up to seven years. This challenge cannot be addressed by reenrolling patients since often once a patient has participated in a drug study, he or she is ineligible for enrollment in studies of similar drugs.[8] Not only do companies need to recruit sufficient numbers of subjects, they also need to be careful not to overburden subjects with study requirements, such as by asking them to travel to a clinic for daily blood tests. Requiring too much from subjects means either that few will volunteer or, if they do, they may fail to comply with study requirements or even drop out of the study. Companies also need to be aware of the cultures and values that exist in the intended study population since beliefs or practices in different groups can influence subject behavior, which can influence study data. Such a problem can occur, for instance, when contraception product research is performed using women who come from a culture where it is common for husbands to attempt to control the use of female contraception.

To remedy some of the problems associated with conducting drug studies, many companies are doing research in foreign countries. An increased supply of potential subjects, less stringent regulatory requirements, lower costs, and faster local approval times are among the benefits. Clinical trial data are also most often accepted more readily in the country in which the studies are done. Some of the large companies can afford to conduct trials in several countries at once, and by combining data they can seek regulatory approvals simultaneously in several countries. Drawbacks to doing offshore research include the difficulty of proving that the foreign population is sufficiently similar to the patients in the country where regulatory approval is sought. Japan, for instance, will only accept clinical drug data collected in Japanese people. The qualifications of the investigators must also be carefully assessed. Some foreign medical centers in economically emerging countries actively compete for American drug trials since these can be important sources of income. Companies need to ensure that financial need does not prompt investigators to take shortcuts and that procedures followed in such centers are as careful as those in the United States.[9]

As in any complex endeavor, trade-offs are inevitable in the clinical trials process. Statisticians lobby for reliable study design, which can conflict with medical and logistical realities. Investigators may be at top-tier medical centers but be overcommitted with other work. The patients with the target disease, such as those with some psychiatric disorders, may be noncompliant study subjects. On top of problems such as this, clinical trial designers are always under pressure to make the research processes as efficient as possible because the cost of delay is always huge. Medical staff, statisticians, the regulatory affairs groups, and even marketing must work together to find acceptable solutions to these disparate needs. And at the end of the clinical trial design process, the study plans need to be acceptable to FDA regulators.

FDA Regulation of Clinical Trials[10]

The need to conduct clinical trials is based on the fact that it is impossible to know whether a potential new drug with promising effects in the laboratory and in animals will prove to be safe and effective in humans. Because of the unknowns, testing new drugs in humans necessarily places human subjects at risk, which is the primary reason that clinical studies are very closely regulated by FDA.[11] FDA requires that the company show that the trials they intend to conduct will be reasonably safe, that they will exercise care in choosing subjects, and that they will secure their fully informed consent. The company is also required to monitor subjects' responses to the tests involved and alter or stop experiments when new information indicates that subjects are endangered or harmed. Although the risks to human subjects are largely unknown before the first trial commences, the FDA requirements attempt to reduce uncertainties at the beginning and, by requiring timely reporting and investigation of all adverse experiences, manage subsequent risks thereafter.[12] Many of these regulations are grouped under what are called good clinical practice (GCP) standards.[13] In addition to internal clinical research review and to ensure that GCP standards are followed, FDA inspects and audits the conduct and reporting of clinical trials. This program of inspections and audits, known as the Bioresearch Monitoring (BIMO) program, covers all of the parties involved in regulated clinical trials, including clinical investigators, institutional review boards (IRBs), sponsors, monitors, and contract research organizations. FDA conducts more than one thousand inspections annually under this program. Together, the reviews and regulatory standards are intended to assure that the clinical study data and reported results are credible and accurate and that the rights, safety, and well-being of clinical trial subjects are protected.

The clinical trial process is the most expensive aspect of research and development of a medical product. Because of the expense, these studies must be carefully designed and monitored to be as efficient as possible. The clinical studies are run and supervised by the company medical department, whose personnel must work closely with the company regulatory affairs department to guarantee that what is intended will meet FDA criteria. At each stage of the clinical research work, the regulatory affairs groups of most pharmaceutical companies actively coordinate with FDA to eliminate surprises in the review process. Meetings and formal conferences between FDA officials and drug sponsors can often minimize wasted effort and expense from poorly designed clinical trials and inadequately prepared drug application submissions. Coordination with FDA also helps to anticipate and resolve scientific and medical disputes.[14]

Institutional Review Board Review

Once FDA has allowed human studies to begin, companies must also obtain approval by the IRB at every site where the research will take place.[15] IRBs are FDA-mandated research oversight committees that review each study protocol, authorize approval with or without changes, and exercise continuing oversight of all approved research. The main goal of the IRB is to protect the rights and welfare of human research subjects recruited to participate in human studies. To ensure that the members of the IRB are competent to assess compliance with research protection requirements and are reasonably free of any conflict of interest, regulations require that members of the IRB are a mix of scientists and nonscientists and at least one member must not to be affiliated with the institution where the research is conducted. During the time that the study takes place, investigators must promptly report all moderate or severe unanticipated adverse events to the IRB and the drug sponsor.

Beyond these federal requirements, companies often take additional steps to ensure that the risks to human subjects are minimized. For example, they may use independent data safety monitoring boards (DSMBs) to monitor specific areas of concern so that, if a significant problem arises, a trial can be terminated at the earliest possible time. DSMBs can also determine if a study needs to be terminated prematurely because the drug has proved so effective that it would be unethical to continue to deny the drug to the control group subjects. Decisions such as this need to be coordinated with FDA.

CLINICAL TRIALS PROCESS

FDA divides the major clinical trials process for new drugs (also called new chemical entities or NCEs) into four phases. The first three of these phases must be complete before the company can submit its marketing application to FDA. The studies are generally carried out by physicians in medical centers and are most often managed by the medical department of the company sponsor. However, an outside contract research organization (CRO) may also be used to handle the entire clinical trials management process.[16]

Phase I Trials

In Phase I clinical research, drugs are evaluated for safety in healthy volunteers. These are small trials, the first of which is conducted with a single dose of the drug that is believed to be well below the toxicity threshold. If the drug produces no problems, multiple and larger doses of the product are evaluated for safety in larger numbers of subjects. With these subsequent trials, the safe dosing range of the drug can be established. In other words, the company attempts to learn what side effects are caused by the drug and what dose of the drug is toxic. Blood tests are also performed to learn the drug's pharmacokinetic profile, that is, how the drug is absorbed, distributed, metabolized, and excreted from the body and how often the drug must be taken to maintain desired blood levels. These trials are conducted usually on less than one hundred healthy volunteers, who presumably can tolerate any side effects better than sick patients. Phase I trials take about one year to complete. Phase I study volunteers are often paid to participate but not enough to induce participation for the money. If the drug is toxic but potentially effective for a serious disease (for example, cancer chemotherapeutic agents), Phase I subjects can be patients with the disease. The problem with using sick patients is that it can be difficult to sort out whether adverse effects were caused by the study product, the disease, or other drugs taken by the subjects. In all Phase I studies, both the patient and the investigator know what is being administered; that is, the study is open and nonblinded. About 35 to 40 percent of clinical research failures of NCEs occur in Phase I.

Phase II Trials

If the drug is successful in Phase I trials, Phase II trials can commence. The primary goal of Phase II clinical trials is to evaluate both the safety and efficacy of a drug in patients with the target disease or condition. As with all subsequent studies, the study population must be carefully selected to eliminate those with other complicating diseases or treatments so that the drug effect can be clearly studied. For the same reason, subjects should also be sick enough but not too sick to qualify for these studies. However, these studies often select patients with advanced stages of disease who have fewer treatment options and less to lose if the drug fails to benefit. Testing a drug in such a severely ill patient population can stack the deck against the drug but is done also to spare patients with milder forms of the disease from the unknown risks of side effects. Regardless of what group of subjects is used, Phase II trials begin to answer the question "Is the desired therapeutic effect observed at doses that can be tolerated by sick patients?" Phase II trials are usually conducted on one hundred to three hundred subjects and last an average of two years. These studies also incorporate a control element, and, if placebo is the control, the studies are generally single-blind, meaning that the investigators, but not the subjects, know who is receiving the drug and who is receiving the placebo. More than half of clinical research failures of NCEs occur in Phase II studies.

Phase III Trials

These "late stage" trials evaluate safety and efficacy in larger and more varied groups of patients with the target disease, including the elderly, various racial and ethnic groups, patients with other diseases, those who take other drugs, and patients whose organs are impaired. In this way, these trials attempt to simulate actual drug use conditions. The product is also tested in its final formulation and packaging. Phase III trials usually involve one thousand to five thousand subjects recruited at a variety of research centers, and then take an average of three years to complete. In these studies, certain less frequent side effects may first become apparent, especially those caused by immunologic processes such as allergic reactions. The larger number of subjects involved provide a basis for extrapolating the results to the general population. The trials usually contain the most rigorous study designs. The design of Phase III trials is usually set after a meeting with FDA to discuss whether the intended protocol, trial design, and statistical analysis will be acceptable. Based on this meeting, and the results from Phase I and II results, an amendment is submitted to the IND. This amendment also includes information on longer-term animal studies and any revised manufacturing specifications that have occurred in the interim. After this point, it is not easy to change product specifications without further Phase II trials. About 20 percent of clinical research failures of NCEs occur in Phase III.[17]

Clinical Trial Monitoring

During all clinical trials, companies must carefully supervise the investigators to ensure that the protocols are carefully followed and all required data are collected, that no shortcuts are taken, that all significant product side effects and injuries are immediately reported, and that publications of results are timed appropriately and coincide with Securities and Exchange Commission and media disclosures. When a company gets into trouble with any clinical trial, it is many times attributable to inadequate trial supervision.

New Drug Application

If Phase III trial results meet expectations, the new drug application (NDA) will be filed with FDA. This application constitutes a request for approval to market the drug for a particular use. These applications are typically one hundred thousand pages long and contain an integrated analysis of all the clinical trial data, which can come from as many as seventy clinical trials involving over four thousand to five thousand patients, each of whom produces one hundred or more pieces of data (for example, blood tests, symptom scores) to assess the safety and efficacy of the investigational product. For certain drug applications, FDA will assign the application to an advisory committee, which reviews the submission and produces a nonbinding approval recommendation (yea or nay) to the agency. Generally, sponsors will also meet with FDA officials before they file the NDA and throughout the review process to make sure the appropriate information has been included and easily correctable deficiencies are addressed. At this point, manufacturing procedures must be final and applicable to full-capacity production, and, before approval, the sponsor must be able to produce three consecutive lots of drug with no failures. Manufacturing site inspections are also conducted. Labeling review is also performed at this point, work that FDA considers fundamental to the marketing approval process to ensure that the product is not misbranded. The labeling includes not only what is physically affixed to the product but also the accompanying information about product approved use(s), doses, pharmacology, contraindications and warnings, precautions about drug interactions, cancer, birth defect and fertility risks, adverse reactions, and drug abuse potential, all of which must conform to the study data. This extended information is contained in the package insert, which is shipped with the product. FDA must also approve the product marketing and advertising material, a subject that is explored in the Zeneca case study material in Chapter 12.

Prior to 1992, it took FDA close to a median time of thirty months to complete an NDA review. After that, FDA was allowed to assess prescription drug user fees of $225,000 per product application. With this money, FDA hired extra reviewers, and the NDA review time decreased to ten to eighteen months unless the drug was for a life-threatening illness and designated for expedited review. The Merck case study material in Chapter 11 contains information on FDA programs to speed the review and approval of products that fill serious unmet health-care needs. Despite the shortening of FDA review times over the past decade, the percentage of applications rejected by FDA (10 to 15 percent) has remained essentially the same.

Postmarketing Safety Surveillance and Product Recalls

Postmarketing studies (for drugs, these are called Phase IV studies) are often required as a condition of medical product approval. The purpose of these studies is to monitor for product safety. FDA often specifies the nature of the studies to be performed. In addition, drug manufacturers are required to report to FDA within fifteen days all serious and unexpected adverse reactions associated with their products and to report less serious adverse reactions at regular intervals. FDA also runs the MedWatch program, under which health professionals can submit serious adverse reaction reports about FDA-regulated products.[18] However, because the MedWatch reports are anecdotal and uncontrolled, FDA considers postmarketing surveillance studies to be a more reliable means to detect product problems that did not surface in premarketing studies. If an adverse event occurs in one in five thousand or even one in one thousand users, it could be missed in clinical trials. But such a low-incidence effect could pose a serious safety problem when the drug is used by many times that number of patients. Also, once a medical product is marketed, FDA does not regulate the way that physicians use the product and a drug can be (and often is) used for other diseases and conditions, thereby increasing the number of patients exposed to product risks.

Physicians, guided by the product labeling information, are responsible for using professional judgment in prescribing the dose and dosing regimen for drugs, for deciding what other drugs can be used concomitantly, and for determining the types of patients who can benefit from a drug or other medical product. The wider postmarketing use can introduce new safety problems for any approved medical product. An FDA study of postapproval drug risks during 1976–85 led to the conclusion that over 50 percent of all drugs had serious risks that remained undiscovered until after marketing. These adverse events led to hospitalizations, increases in the length of hospital stays, severe or permanent disabilities, and deaths. Among drugs approved in less than four years, those that had serious postapproval risks had generally been approved in a shorter time than those without such risks. Studies such as these lead some experts to conclude that the risk of adverse drug events cannot be predicted without systematic research.[19]

Regardless of whether FDA requires postmarketing surveillance studies, many companies believe that it is prudent to systematically monitor for adverse events in order to institute warnings and prevent subsequent patient injury and liability. Many of the large pharmaceutical companies establish global systems to track, investigate, evaluate, and report adverse drug reactions. Postmarketing safety surveillance can provide assurance of product safety or uncover problems that, on the company's own initiative or mandated by FDA, can be corrected (for example, by issuing new warnings, changing dose recommendations). At some point, there may be enough evidence of adverse effects that the company or FDA is prompted to recall the product from the market. Obviously, the sooner this happens, the better it is for patients, who are spared future risk. But those patients who had a real need for the drug and have no equivalent therapies available will feel the loss. Also, the timing of the recall determines whether the company has been able to recoup R&D costs. Balanced against this economic impact is the cost of lawsuits that may result from public knowledge of the recall and the reasons for it.[20] In addition to the Baycol example above, the recall experience with the drug Rezulin® is described in the introduction material to the OncorMed/Myriad case study in Chapter 10.

Other Postmarketing Studies

Postmarket research also can be done purely for marketing purposes to eliminate packaging inconveniences, determine whether a line extension product (for example, for pediatrics) would be useful, remove other barriers to use, or compare the company's drug with competitors. Companies, monitoring the extent to which physicians are using the drug for unapproved purposes, may also want to conduct studies to support FDA approvals for new product indications.

Another important area of product research, which can be conducted before or after product approval, is in the field of pharmacoeconomics. This research attempts to provide information about the cost-benefit of the product. Pharmacoeconomic data are considered necessary because drug prices have escalated while health-care budgets have declined, making it ever more difficult to convince hospitals and HMOs to place particular drugs on formulary lists or persuade third-party payers (for example, insurers, Medicaid) to reimburse the cost of drug treatment.[21]

Without widespread formulary approvals and third-party payer reimbursements, the market for most new drugs will probably be too small to pursue. Some pharmacoeconomic research seeks to prove that a drug is cost effective since using it will lower the total cost of medical care by eliminating such things as surgery, hospitalization, other therapies, physician visits, and nursing care. For instance, the total cost of care for adults with HIV infection has declined since the introduction of effective antiretroviral drugs. One study showed a 43 percent drop in hospital inpatient care for HIV-infected patients during the sixteen months after availability of antiretroviral drugs.[22] According to Samuel A. Bozzette, a physician with the Veterans Affairs San Diego Healthcare System who headed the study, "The drugs are almost a perfect substitute for hospital care. We can afford them because, in fact, we are already spending the money on HIV care in the form of hospitalization."[23] All told, full access to new AIDS drugs helped realize a net savings of $18 million in the cost of care for this group of patients in 1997.[24] Other economic research looks at the wider costs of illness and the impact of drug treatment on such things as worker productivity, absenteeism from work, or lost home care services. Because of the stakes involved for the company and because of the continued emphasis on controlling health-care costs, pharmacoeconomic data increasingly are used to justify pricing decisions and to obtain competitive advantages in the medical product marketplace.[25]

Likewise, quality-of-life data are becoming an important competitive tool. Quality-of-life studies attempt to determine the degree to which the drug contributes to patients' psychological or physical well-being—are patients more comfortable, calm, mobile, self-sufficient, or better able to interact with family? A medicine that reduces arthritis pain but produces continuous nausea will not only be considered more toxic than others but will score lower on a quality-of-life scale. And although it is difficult to quantify quality-of-life findings, companies are becoming more innovative in their attempts to demonstrate that their drugs produce a higher quality of life than competitive products.

MEDICAL DEVICE REGULATION

Medical device regulation, which is controlled by the Medical Device Amendments of 1976, differs markedly from that of drugs and biologics. Devices on the market prior to the 1976 law are allowed to remain on the market until FDA promulgates regulations requiring market applications. New devices, regardless of how risky, that are substantially the same as those already on the market prior to the 1976 law can be marketed after the submission of a premarket notification, commonly referred to as a 510(k) after the applicable section of the FDA law.[26] If FDA concludes that the device is substantially equivalent to a pre-existing device, it can be marketed without further regulatory review. New devices that are not substantially the same as a pre-1976 device must undergo more extensive FDA review and approval prior to marketing.

The device legislation established three risk classes for all medical devices, Classes I, II, III.[27] Class I (for example, stethoscopes, crutches, cold packs) are those that present no unreasonable risk of illness or injury and are subject only to minimal regulation. Class II devices (for example, hearing aids, powered wheelchairs, many lab tests) are potentially more harmful and may be marketed without advance approval but are subject to more rigorous controls. Class III devices (for example, infant breathing monitors, replacement heart valves, bone cement) are those that either "present a potential unreasonable risk of illness or injury" or which are "purported or represented to be for a use in supporting or sustaining human life or for a use which is of substantial importance in preventing impairment of human health." New Class III devices must obtain FDA approval through a rigorous premarket application (PMA) process before marketing the device.[28] In a PMA, the device manufacturer must provide FDA with a reasonable assurance that the device is both safe and effective, a process somewhat akin to an NDA submission.

Eventually, FDA was to generate specific marketing requirements for all types of devices, both new devices and those on the market prior to 1976. However, many medical devices on the market today have not received premarket approval because FDA has lacked financial and other resources to both handle the increasing number of PMA submissions and to promulgate new PMA requirements. As a result, the 510(k) premarket notification process is still often the means by which new medical devices, including Class III devices, are approved for the market. Most device manufacturers do not complain about this situation since, compared to the PMA, the 510(k) notification process takes much less time to prepare, requires much less information, gets processed very quickly, and has a low rejection rate.

CONCLUSION

The regulation and oversight of drugs and devices is justified by the need to protect the public health. The regulatory system has evolved over time, continuously responding to simultaneous pressures to protect safety in a timely manner while not stalling the introduction of valuable new medical products to patient populations. A stringent system of clinical trials aims to produce data in an incremental way to inform companies of the value of their investment while meeting regulatory requirements about the safety and efficacy of the experimental agent. Because different product profiles and health needs are always at play, regulatory mechanisms are frequently being modified to respond in a flexible way to health-care and industry needs. There remains, however, a tension between the views of regulators and industry about the best way to proceed in such a highly regulated and complex environment.

Notes

1. See http://csdd.tufts.edu/.

2. Kolata G. Anticholesterol drug pulled after link with 31 deaths. *New York Times* 2001 Aug 9; Sect. A:12; Financial news; Groups sue Claritin's maker. *Washington Post* 2001 Aug 10; Sect. E:2; Fuhrmans V. Bayer reports a loss of $16.2 million, plans Glaxo-SmithKline marketing deal. *Wall Street Journal* 2001 Nov 15; Sect. B:5.

3. Further information about the aspects of FDA drug approval regulation can be obtained from the Agency's Center for Drug Evaluation and Research Handbook, available from www.fda.gov/cder/handbook/.

4. For information on the regulation of animal research, see the section in Chapter 4 dealing with animal research ethics.

5. A control in a biomedical research study provides a mechanism by which to compare results from subjects taking an experimental intervention to results from a group that is not receiving the treatment being studied.

6. Moher D, Cook JJ, Jadad AR, et al. Assessing the quality of reports of randomized trials; implications for meta-analysis. *Health Technology Assessments* 1999; 3:19–24; Malone, RE. Ethical issues in industry-sponsored research. *Journal of Emergency Nursing* 1998; 24:193–6.

7. Washburn J. Informed consent. *Washington Post* 2001 Dec 30; Sect. W:16.

8. Alger A. Trials and tribulations; the drug revolution could run into a brick wall: Not enough guinea pigs. *Forbes Magazine* 1999 May 17. Available from www.forbes.com/forbes/1999/0517/6310316a.html?_requestid=40573.

9. Ibid.

10. Human clinical research unrelated to the approval of drugs and medical devices is governed by the Department of Health and Human Services (DHHS) if the research is funded by the NIH or another DHHS division whether in their own facilities or at other institutions. See 45 *Code of Federal Regulations* Part 46.

11. 21 *Code of Federal Regulations* 312 et seq.

12. Greenberg MD. AIDS experimental drug approval, and the FDA new drug screening process. *New York University Journal of Legislation and Public Policy* 1999–2000; 3:295–350; Baram, M. Making clinical trials safer for human subjects. *American Journal of Law and Medicine* 2001; 27:253–82.

13. A list of the regulations that contain GCP requirements for FDA-regulated clinical trials can be found at www.fda.gov/oc/gcp/regulations.html.

14. DiMasi JA, Manocchia M, Lasagna L. Initiatives to speed new drug development and regulatory review: The impact of FDA-sponsor conferences: PIII-13. *Clinical Pharmacology and Therapeutics* 1996; 59:191.

15. 21 *Code of Federal Regulations* 56. These committees are referred to sometimes as committees for the protection of human subjects and in other countries can be called research ethics committees.

16. DiMasi JA. Risks in new drug development: Approval success rates for investigational drugs. *Clinical Pharmacology and Therapeutics* 2001; 69:297–307.

17. Ibid.

18. MedWatch is FDA's voluntary adverse event reporting system that allows the agency to monitor for adverse events, issue product safety alerts, and initiate any other enforcement action needed to protect consumers from harm caused by regulated products. See www.fda.gov/medwatch/safety.htm.

Ropp KL. MedWatch, on lookout for medical product problems. *FDA Consumer Magazine* 1995 Jan. Available at www.fda.gov/fdac/special/newdrug/medwatch.html.

19. *FDA drug review: Postapproval risks 1976–85.* Pub. No. GAO/PEMID-90-15. Washington, DC: U.S. General Accounting Office; 1990; *Adverse drug events; the magnitude of healthy risks is uncertain because of limited incidence data.* Pub. No. GAO/HEHS-00-21. Washington, DC: U.S. General Accounting Office, Health, Education and Human Services Division; 2000. Available at www.gao.gov/new.items/he00021.pdf.

20. Bunney WE, Azarnoff DL, Brown BW, et al. Report of the Institute of Medicine Committee on the efficacy and safety of Halcion. *Archives of General Psychiatry* 1999; 56:349–52; Noah, BA. Adverse drug reactions: Harnessing experiential date to promote patient welfare. *Catholic University Law Review* 2000; 49:449–504.

21. Some countries (not the United States) also require pharmacoeconomic data as a condition of approval.

22. Bozzette SA, Joyce G, McCaffrey GF, et al. Expenditures for the care of HIV-infected patients in the era of highly active antiretroviral therapy. *New England Journal of Medicine* 2001; 344:817–23; Steinbrook R. Providing antiretroviral therapy for HIV infection. *New England Journal of Medicine* 2001; 344:844–46.

23. Pharmaceutical Research and Manufacturers of America. *Pharmaceutical industry profile 2001.* Washington, DC: Pharmaceutical Research and Manufacturers of America; 2001. Available at www.phrma.org/publications/publications/profile01/.

24. Rahman A, Deyton LR, Goetz MB, et al. Inversion of inpatient/outpatient HIV service utilization: Impact of improved therapies, clinical education and case management in the U.S. Department of Veterans Affairs. International Conference on AIDS 1998. Abstract No. 443/42429; 12:859.

25. DiMasi JA, Caglarcan E, Wood-Armany M. Emerging role of pharmacoeconomics in the research and development decision-making process. *Pharmacoeconomics* 2001; 19:753–66.

26. Food Drug and Cosmetic Act 510(k); 513(i), codified at 21 *United States Code* § 360(k), 360c(i).

27. 21 *United States Code* § 360c(a)(1)(A), (B), and (C).

28. 21 *United States Code* § 360e(a).

PART III   CASE STUDIES

6

Research Collaborations Between Academia and Industry

Biomedical and agricultural companies frequently draw on academic scientists and clinicians to conduct company research, and often license discoveries that result from university-based research. A 1989 survey of seventy-six major U.S. manufacturing companies found that the pharmaceutical industry obtained 44 percent of its new products and 37 percent of its processes from university-based research.[1] The number and extent of research collaborations between industry and academia have escalated with the rapid advances in genetic science. Much of this research activity is mutually beneficial and also benefits society, since it helps to produce needed medical products and get them to market. However, because academia and industry exist for such different purposes and operate under very different principles, research collaborations between the two entities can often result in conflict.

Traditionally, academia exists to teach students, to expand knowledge through scholarly endeavors and research (both of which should result in publications), and to train new academics. In order to achieve these goals, faculty require autonomy and academic freedom to research any question, and are encouraged to collaborate and share research results. In contrast, medical and agricultural companies exist to develop and market products in such a way as to maximize profits. Whether companies fund particular research or collaborate or share research data depends on whether these activities promote corporate goals. There are many circumstances, therefore, that prompt companies to control the research agenda and protect the secrecy of research data. Although these are the general differences that can lead to conflict, modern relationships between corporations and universities are much more complicated and nuanced, and have led to debates about the overall impact of these research collaborations on the institutions themselves, on the people who use the products that result from this research, and on society in general. As research collaborations have grown in number and size, commentary about industry-academia conflicts of interest has proliferated among academics, economists, legislators, regulators, and executives in the bioscience industry, and the lay press has also begun to present these debates to the public.[2] As a result, companies that make use of academic faculty to conduct industrial research are increasingly under the spotlight and often are critiqued on how they structure these relationships.

BENEFITS AND RISKS OF COLLABORATION

There are many reasons that research collaborations between industry and academia exist.[3] Bioscience companies seek academic researchers to gain special technology or expertise not available in-house. Some development companies, almost entirely dependent on obtaining access to outside discoveries, have always sought academic collaborations to keep the discovery "pipeline" supplied. The earlier the access, the higher the chance of obtaining valuable but inexpensive intellectual property rights and a jump start on competitors. Sometimes the reputation of a faculty researcher alone is deemed valuable enough for a company to seek the establishment of a long-term research relationship with that individual. Data published by top scientists are automatically more credible at the regulatory agencies and are persuasive in physician marketing programs. Companies can also be kept informed of discoveries as they come off the bench. For clinical research, such as human drug studies, access to patients at university hospitals can be a primary motivator for collaborative research.

Universities, however, can be difficult places to conduct corporate research. Experience has shown that it often takes more time and money to sponsor academic research than to conduct it in-house, and the company has less control in the academic setting. According to a 1994 survey[4] of 210 life science companies, conducted by health policy researcher David Blumenthal and colleagues at Harvard University, about half of the companies reported that university bureaucracies and regulations prevented contracting or interfered with contract negotiations. Disputes over intellectual property rights were also disruptive for 34 percent of companies. One-third of companies complained that faculty researchers had changed the direction of the research or created conflicts of interest by establishing additional relationships with competing companies. Some companies (12 percent) also disclosed that academic researchers had engaged in questionable scientific practices and misconduct that rendered the research worthless. Other complaints involved the timeliness of the university research. The teaching, research, and patient care responsibilities of faculty slowed their ability to conduct specific projects, which while not vexing to the university, could seriously increase the cost to the corporate sponsor. Given the fact, for instance, that some drugs can command markets in excess of $300 million, even a one-day delay in getting FDA approval could cost the company close to $1 million in sales revenue.[5]

These drawbacks to working with academic researchers have led some companies to turn to for-profit contract research companies for clinical drug research. Unfettered by conflicting academic responsibilities, these outfits (called contract research organizations or CROs) can often produce data more cheaply and quickly. In recent years, large amounts of corporate research money has shifted to these new entities.[6] Regretting the loss of income, some academic medical centers have made concerted efforts to compete with the CROs to win back clinical drug trial work, claiming that academic research is conducted with more rigor and objectivity than that performed by commercial research houses. Skeptics also wondered whether CROs would be more likely to bias research results since drug companies were their only source of revenue.[7]

From the university perspective, working with industry also has its benefits and risks. There is no doubt that in the medical and agricultural sciences, universities have benefited from research collaborations with industry, especially in times when government research funding was declining or uncertain. Increased funding allows universities to expand other research programs, attract new faculty, build facilities and purchase equipment, and enhance the reputation of the school. Faculty are able to perform higher levels of research using industry resources and keep abreast of the latest industry developments, which creates a synergy beneficial to research and the training of students and young scientists. Patients at university medical centers can potentially benefit from access to experimental new drugs and products not otherwise available. Individual faculty members can benefit directly by obtaining additional consulting fees and royalties on inventions licensed to industry. Faculty can also benefit financially from these collaborations when companies offer executive positions and consultation work to faculty performing foundational research. For companies that are young and cash-poor, faculty scientists are frequently paid for their work with potentially valuable stock options.

By contrast, several drawbacks to university involvement with industry research have been identified. University officers and faculty chairs worry about constraints on academic freedom and the conflict between commercial trade secrecy requirements and traditional academic openness. Corporate research diverts faculty from teaching and other academic service activities, and other faculty can become irritated when they have to pick up the slack. There is potential for exploitation of graduate students and junior faculty if they feel compelled to work on commercial research directed by the department chair. Industry funding often creates unequal faculty camps of "haves" and "have nots"; corporations tend to fund medical and engineering but not other faculty, which makes some faculty unhappy and the university budget allocation process more difficult. Conducting corporate research that is too routine can also get nonprofit universities in trouble with the Internal Revenue Service, which could take the position that mundane laboratory work performed for a for-profit entity does not qualify as research under the tax-exempt charter of the academic institution. In addition, university administrators are increasingly worried that antibiotechnology industry activists might include the companies' academic research partners in their protests, acts of civil disobedience, and terrorist acts.[8]

Another prime concern centers on the differences between basic and applied science and the relative roles of the public and private sector in supporting them.[9] Basic science is the quest for fundamental knowledge, primarily conducted in public laboratories and in universities and funded with tax dollars. As such, these research efforts are generally considered to be in the public interest. Fundamental to the concept of academic freedom and inherent in basic research is the ability to research any idea without regard for immediate utility or commercial promise. In contrast, applied science is more often performed by or for private industry and thus benefits private interests, at least initially. Applied science is often conducted with short-term product objectives in mind, contrasted with basic science, which tends to be more long term, fundamental, or novel. It follows then that if the universities are diverted by corporate funding to engage in research geared more toward commercial applications, they will not engage in other more fundamental research areas that have the potential to open up vast new areas of scientific understanding. Critics point out that it is inevitable that large amounts of private money will ultimately influence the direction of research and that universities, because of insufficient public support, might be too willing to engage in market-driven science.[10]

With the increase in the numbers of university-industry research collaborations, some critics are concerned that academic researchers will compromise scientific or academic goals to accommodate industry objectives or to keep corporate partners interested in continual funding. Some went so far as to suggest that data could be skewed (consciously or not) to favor the industry patron. Traditional university values such as openness of communication among scholars are also at risk when companies insist on data confidentiality. All of these concerns fuel a fear that even society could be harmed by the increasing numbers of commercially connected academic scientists. According to one academic commentator, "These conflicts of interest threaten the objectivity of science, the integrity of scientists and institutions, and the safety of medical products."[11]

One of the most widely publicized situations where these issues were raised involved the first death of a human subject enrolled in a gene therapy trial. The trial was conducted in 1999 at the University of Pennsylvania's nationally prominent Institute for Human Gene Therapy, directed by Dr. James Wilson. The human subject who died was eighteen years old. His death was followed by a lawsuit where the subject's family lawyer accused the physicians involved of acting like entrepreneurs, because of Wilson's ties to a biotech company. Wilson had founded and owned 30 percent of the stock in a company called Genovo, which had exclusive rights to commercialize the gene therapy discoveries that Wilson and his colleagues had shown to be beneficial in clinical trials. The university's conflict-of-interest rules had been altered to permit this amount of faculty ownership and the institute obtained 20 percent of its budget income from Genovo. The university also received money from the relationship. Genovo had, in turn, obtained $37 million from Cambridge, Massachusetts-based Biogen, Inc., and another investment from Genzyme, Inc., for rights to Genovo's products. These investments were to be renewed contingent upon Genovo having made progress in transforming the gene therapy discoveries into viable commercial products. There was no evidence to support the view that Wilson's corporate ties had influenced his scientific and medical judgments regarding the gene therapy trial. He had disclosed his connection to Genovo in the consent form signed by all trial participants and had given direct control over the trials to other physicians at the institute. "To suggest that I acted or was influenced by money is really offensive to me," he told a reporter. "I don't think about how my doing this work is going to make me rich. It's about leadership and notoriety and accomplishment. Publishing in first-rate journals. That's what turns us on. You've got to be on the cutting edge and take risks if you're going to stay on top."[12] Still, the appearance of conflict made the tragic situation more difficult to handle for all involved parties.[13]

Based on comments like this, supporters of academic-industry alliances assert that universities should look at other motivations before attributing all conflicts of interest to corporate influence. According to two M.D.-M.B.A. faculty members at the University of Pittsburgh Medical Center:

> Conflicts of interest from consulting fees or stock options can be trivial in comparison to the potential bias caused by desires for academic productivity, a faculty promotion, a large clinical-referral base, a grant from the National Institutes of Health, fame, or the Nobel prize. These sources of bias, unrelated to relationships with industry, have not been seen as black marks on research requiring public disclosure, despite their remarkable ability to lead to unethical behavior.[14]

These faculty suggested that no company benefits from obtaining biased research data that could undermine the development of beneficial and safe medical products.

ASSESSING THE IMPACT OF UNIVERSITY-INDUSTRY RESEARCH RELATIONSHIPS

Concerns and debates like this led Harvard's Blumenthal to attempt to assess the impact of industry collaborations on university faculty. With wide-ranging faculty surveys conducted from October 1994 to April 1995, Blumenthal's group collected survey data from 2,052 faculty members from the fifty U.S. universities receiving the most research funding from NIH, the principal biomedical research funding agency in the federal government.[15] From these surveys Blumenthal learned that 28 percent of responding faculty received research funding from industry and that overall, industry accounted for about 9 percent of the research funds given to academic life science researchers. The good news: "Faculty members receiving industrial funds had more peer-reviewed articles published in the previous three years, participated in more administrative activities in their institutions or disciplines, and were more commercially active [meaning they had more projects and money from industry] than faculty members without such funding." These variables were highest for faculty members who received one-third or less of their total research budget from industry. The bad news: faculty productivity and university "citizenship" activities tended to decline as the proportion of research funds from industry increased. Faculty who received more than two-thirds of their research support from industry were less productive academically and their articles were less influential than articles published by researchers with no industrial support.[16] Also, faculty with corporate support were significantly more likely than those without to report that they were required to keep information secret to protect its proprietary value to the company. Furthermore, these faculty members were significantly more likely to report that they had refused requests from other academic scientists to share research results or biomaterials. As well, faculty members with industry funding were also significantly more likely to report that their choice of research topics had been affected somewhat or greatly by the likelihood that the data would have a commercial application—thereby increasing the likelihood that the faculty member would share in the royalties obtained when the research was licensed.

Given academic sensibilities, withholding of data is always a significant issue in these types of alliances. While faculty believe that unfettered freedom in the timing of the publication of data is the best way to advance scientific knowledge, it is accepted practice for companies to require that faculty keep data confidential to allow time for the filing of a patent application. Although NIH guidelines state that thirty to sixty days is reasonable, in the past many companies have reported that patent filing can take as long as six months, and it was not uncommon for the period of confidentiality to last longer. In the Blumenthal industry survey, 56 percent of companies reported that in practice, the results of university research they supported often or sometimes were kept confidential to protect their proprietary value beyond the time required to file a patent.

In another Blumenthal survey of 2,167 faculty conducted in 1993, data-withholding behaviors among academic faculty were studied. This survey evaluated whether faculty delayed publication of their research results for more than six months and whether they had refused to share research results with other university scientists in the past three years. Almost 20 percent of the responders reported that their research publications had been delayed by more than six months at least once in the past three years to allow for patent application, to protect their scientific lead, to slow the dissemination of undesired results, to allow time to negotiate a patent, or to resolve disputes over the ownership of intellectual property. Also, 9 percent of responders reported refusing to share research results with other university scientists in the last three years.

The authors concluded that "participation in an academic-industry research relationship and engagement in the commercialization of university research were significantly associated with delays in publication."[17]

Other studies suggested (but did not prove) that receipt of industry funding or stock options could compromise the objectivity of the researcher. These studies showed that faculty researchers paid by industry were more likely to report research results favorable to the corporate sponsor compared with scientists without corporate support.[18]

Occasionally, there were reports of conflicts between companies and faculty about the content in publications of industry-sponsored research results. Studies resulting in disappointing data were an obvious problem since companies did not need (and many times did not want) to publish these data, while academics sometimes did, believing that the insights to be gained would advance scientific understanding. Disagreements also arose when the parties could not agree on data interpretation. One scientist at the Wake Forest School of Medicine, who had years of experience in industry-funded drug trials, stated, "Companies can play hardball, and many investigators can't play hardball back. You send the paper to the company for comments, and that's the danger. Can you handle the changes the company wants? Will you give in a little, a little more, then capitulate? It's tricky for those who need money for more studies."[19] One pertinent example involved Sandoz, a large Swiss-based pharmaceutical company that had not yet merged with Ciba-Geigy to form Novartis. The conflict involved Sandoz's study of the cardiac effects of one of its blood pressure drugs compared to another common drug. Some of the faculty researchers alleged that Sandoz had wielded undue influence in controlling what was said in the publication about the research results. For this reason, these faculty researchers refused to have their names included as authors on the publication.[20]

The scope of industry-academic relationships has also become an issue for universities and the companies that sponsor their research. Traditionally, these relationships tend to be limited in scope and targeted in nature. Comparing survey data from 1984 and 1994, the Harvard researchers found that about 75 percent of life sciences companies sponsored projects under $100,000 per year and that 80 percent contracted for collaborations that lasted two years or less. These statistics indicated that the companies had short-term, focused goals and were seeking specific data. Only 6 percent or fewer of the companies sponsored yearly projects costing $500,000 or more or projects lasting more than three years—figures that suggested that the company had sponsored more basic research with longer-term goals.[21]

CHANGES IN INDUSTRY-ACADEMIC RELATIONSHIPS
AND THE FEDERAL RESPONSE

Recent history, especially with biotechnology companies, shows a trend toward larger and more long-term academic research agreements. One notable example again involved Sandoz, and its proposed agreement with the Scripps Research Institute in 1992.[22] Scripps was the largest nonprofit independent biomedical research institution in the United States at the time, and its research projects were heavily subsidized with federal funds. Of Scripps's $120 million annual budget, $70 million came from NIH and other federal sources. The original Sandoz proposal was that it pay Scripps $300 million over a period of ten years, in exchange for which Sandoz would obtain first rights to all Scripps medical discoveries. The agreement could last sixteen years if options were exercised. Sandoz also would have the right to vote on the selection of research to be conducted, to halt Scripps projects, and to place Sandoz researchers in the Scripps facilities. Sandoz would oversee all other Scripps consulting arrangements and could preview all of Scripps's scientific publications. Finally, Scripps's officers would share in the profits of private research collaborations. This proposal led to forceful criticism from NIH, resulting in congressional investigations into whether the arrangement gave Sandoz excessive control over the federally funded institute. Congressman Ron Wyden, who investigated the arrangement based on an NIH complaint, found the deal unacceptable, calling it a corporate takeover of one of the country's biomedical research crown jewels. In addition, one of the goals of NIH funding was to assist small businesses in obtaining access to new technologies, and the Sandoz deal seemed to preclude that possibility at Scripps.[23]

Under this pressure, the agreement was revised so that Sandoz would pay $100 million over five years for first rights to only 47 percent of Scripps's discoveries. The agreement could be extended for an additional five years. Sandoz also agreed to give up its vote on the Scripps research selection committee, reduce its representation on the Scripps board, and give up its rights to oversee Scripps consulting, preview Scripps publications, and pull other projects. Small businesses had more access to Scripps's research discoveries. The Scripps officers gave up their profit-sharing rights. Even though the scope of the Sandoz-Scripps agreement was significantly diminished, criticisms persisted. "The perception of scientists and science is blackened when the public feels that the scientific community is not simply seeking truth but seeking to profit," said professor Sheldon Krimsky of Tufts University.[24]

As a result of this and other problematic industry-university contracts, NIH published guidelines on the parameters that should be followed when NIH-sponsored academic institutions contracted with commercial entities to conduct research. The guidelines explicitly recognized the potential for conflict in these relationships by stating that faculty "should be aware that their interest in the scientific endeavor covered by a sponsored research agreement and the interest of the industrial sponsor may not be totally consonant."[25] These guidelines were intended to preserve academic freedom, promote rapid dissemination of research results, and prevent undue influence by industry while at the same time fostering open commercial access to federally funded research activities and technology (especially for small businesses), speedy commercialization of technology, and fair access to the intellectual property rights of the discoveries resulting from federally funded research. The view was that broad-based funding by one company of the general research program of a federally funded institute or university department could potentially stifle these goals. Therefore, these guidelines called for heightened scrutiny by the university of the proposed relationship if any of the following criteria applied: (1) funding of $5 million per year or $50 million total, (2) the proportion of the funding exceeds 20 percent of the department's total research funding, (3) corporate prospective licensing rights cover all or a substantial proportion of the department's intellectual property output, and (4) duration of five years or more. Furthermore, the guidelines stated that NIH-funded institutions "should avoid any other unusual practice or stipulation that might generate public concern or undermine rather than serve the public interest."

As one medical faculty researcher put it, "Companies translate biologic advances into useable products for patients. They do it for a profit motive, but they do it, and it needs to be done."[26] While the NIH guidelines did provide suggested boundaries for the academic role in this endeavor, it was still up to the individual parties to determine optimal working relationships, since neither NIH nor the regulatory agencies controlled most aspects of these research relationships. This situation guaranteed that commentary and study would continue on the most appropriate manner in which to conduct collaborative research so as preserve the benefits to industry and academia and to generate reliable data that could be translated into useful and safe products, all the while preserving the public's trust in the institutions that generate these products.

Case Study

Novartis–UC Berkeley
Research Collaboration[27]

In November 1998, Steven Briggs was the newly appointed CEO of the Novartis Agricultural Discovery Institute, Inc. (NADII), a new research institute created under the corporate umbrella of Novartis AG. NADII had a mandate to jump start Novartis's basic research program in plant genomics, and Briggs was considering the latest research proposal terms offered by the University of California, Berkeley (UC Berkeley). Novartis was the finalist in an auction launched by the university in April 1998 to find a corporate partner with whom it could establish a broad plant genomics research alliance.[28] Since May, Novartis had been negotiating with UC Berkeley to finalize the proposal. The arrangement was unprecedented and required a great deal of trust on the part of Novartis—trust that the Berkeley faculty could produce useful discoveries for the company's fledgling plant genomics initiative. On the surface it appeared that recent advances in the cost-intensive field of life sciences, combined with heated competition in industry for leadership in biotechnology, had aligned the interests of the university and Novartis. Briggs was ready to approve the proposal before him (see Appendix 6.1). Before putting pen to paper, however, he considered the forces that had led to the historic agreement between Novartis and UC Berkeley, the funding of research, his firm's strategic choices, and academia's contribution to new discoveries.

STEVEN BRIGGS AND NOVARTIS

Novartis was a major international player in the life sciences group of companies that combined three primary businesses—pharmaceutics (in which it was the world's second largest company), agrochemicals (in which it was the world's largest and more than twice the size of its nearest rival), and foods/nutrition (it was among the top five companies worldwide).[29] Novartis and its competitors all recognized the need to enter the fields of biotechnology and genomics to become more competitive in these three business fields.

Briggs was relatively new at Novartis, having started with the company in April 1998, eight months earlier. Previously he had worked for a competitor, Pioneer Hi-Bred. His mandate at Novartis was to initiate and accelerate the company's basic research efforts in plant genomics, an area in which Briggs believed Novartis to be at least four years behind its major competitors (notably Pioneer Hi-Bred, Monsanto, and DuPont). On his recommendation, Novartis had just formed NADII to accomplish this mission. As CEO of NADII, he was to decide how NADII would obtain basic research discoveries to funnel into Novartis's R&D laboratories for future commercialization. One promising avenue was UC Berkeley's proposal for a research alliance. The proposal, which came from the Department of Plant and Microbial Biology, had many potential benefits but—judging from the reaction it had received so far, both within Novartis and at Berkeley—was risky and controversial. The basic provisions consisted of the following: (1) NADII would give the UC Berkeley department $25 million over five years to conduct plant genomics research, (2) virtually all of the faculty in the department would participate in this research program, (3) the faculty, not NADII, would control the selection of the projects NADII would fund, (4) NADII would make its proprietary genomics data bases and other research tools available to the department faculty to facilitate the research, and (5) NADII would get first crack at negotiating rights to a percentage of the discoveries resulting from the research.

After UC Berkeley had decided to make the proposal public, there had been a vociferous campus and public debate about the propriety of the arrangement. The gist of the criticism focused on the unprecedented scope of the collaboration and revolved around the notion that an entire department of a public university was "selling itself to industry," thereby jeopardizing some fundamental academic priorities—freedom to research any question regardless of the commercial potential, freedom to publish research results without regard to corporate need for secrecy, responsibility for conducting public interest research that resulted in socially optimal technologies, and overall independence, objectivity, and impartiality.

At Novartis, executives had keen concerns about the usefulness of the arrangement, primarily because the company could not specify the kinds of research to be performed. In the end, it came down to Briggs to make the decision. He had to assess the commercial benefits to Novartis of the Berkeley offer. Novartis had given Briggs no target number of discoveries to obtain, and Briggs had the freedom to choose NADII's research partners and the circumstances under which these partnerships would exist. Should Briggs decide to sign, there were questions that had yet to be resolved relating to the responsibilities of a company that would become a major patron of a publicly funded university research department. The corporate and academic cultures were very different, and the size of this relationship forced the parties to consider closely whether they had struck the right balance between their own needs and those of their partner.

Briggs knew his reputation was very much on the line with this university alliance and with the others that NADII would form: "Five years from now, I may be begging on the streets or washing windshields. This is definitely an experiment." Briggs knew of some other industry-university research collaborations that were larger than this one but none where all of the department faculty were involved and none where the direction of the research was controlled by the faculty. As far as he knew, this was the first arrangement of its kind.

PROMISE OF PLANT BIOTECHNOLOGY

Agricultural biotechnology research focuses on identifying and understanding the role of plant and plant pest genes. Once this is accomplished, scientists can develop techniques to alter, manipulate, and transfer specific genes into plants to improve their characteristics. Seeds are the delivery vehicles for these genetic enhancements. Such genetically altered seed products hold the promise of transforming the crop protection and seeds industries since plant traits can be altered more precisely and with greater specificity and speed with genetics than with traditional plant breeding or cell culture techniques.

Research in the late 1990s focused on developing seeds that made plants resistant to disease, pests, and environmental insult. Plants that were resistant to these insults required fewer chemicals for crop protection. Plant genomics research was also leading to discoveries that would make crops produce nutritional substances, medicines, vaccines, and even plastics. Genetic technology was also being developed for the use of plants in environmental cleanup, such as for oil spills. The results of these research efforts promised to make plant genomics science the major pathway to increasing crop productivity and quality and also a significant contributor to environmental protection. This innovation was needed in a world challenged by more people to feed, less land on which to grow crops, third world hunger, disease and poor nutrition, and environmental degradation.

CONSUMER AND ENVIRONMENTAL ACTIVISTS

Although many looked to plant biotechnology to improve human life, others feared that genetically altered crops and foods had entered the marketplace without a full understanding of their safety and ecological consequences. Monsanto, for instance, had suffered severe criticism, picketing, boycotts, lawsuits, and regulatory reversals, especially in Europe, as a result of decisions made about its genetically modified (GM) foods, the most controversial of which was the decision not to label Roundup Ready® soya as a GM food.[30] Any company entering the plant genomics business had to expect that they would encounter the scrutiny and criticism of these activists.

INVESTING IN GENOMICS

Despite the criticism, however, the market for such genetically engineered plant products was growing. Analysts estimated that the global market for genetically enhanced seeds for crop protection alone was close to $50 billion a year.[31] Although the markets for new products were estimated to be quite large, so were the costs of research. The president of BIO had said that the biotechnology industry was "one of the most capital intensive and research intensive industries in the history of civilian manufacturing."[32] Companies were spending an average of $59,000 in research expenditures per employee, while the corporate average in the United States was $7,106. The top five biotechnology companies were spending an average of $121,400 per employee on R&D compared to an average of $31,200 per employee for the top five pharmaceutical companies.[33] The accounting and consulting firm Ernst & Young reported that biotechnology firms spent $6.17 billion on research in 1998, a 21 percent increase over the prior year.[34]

Because of the promise of biotechnology and its impact on the use of farm and other chemicals, large chemical companies had been vertically integrating into the seed and biotechnology industries. This integration had created several companies considered to be dominant in plant biotechnology: DuPont ($62.7 billion), Monsanto ($29.6 billion), Pioneer Hi-Bred ($8.4 billion), and Novartis ($128.4 billion).[35] These companies saw the benefits of investing in genomics and began a race to acquire plant genomics information and technology in 1995 and 1996. That this race was important was highlighted by the success of one of the first genetically modified seeds (Roundup® herbicide-resistant crop seed), developed and licensed by Pioneer.[36] This product was so successful that in its first year it accounted for 17 percent of the company's total sales.[37]

Pioneer's success prompted the large agricultural companies to go on what one writer called a "seed and biotechnology company buying spree."[38] These active merger and acquisition activities coincided with the formation of the large life sciences companies. Monsanto (which had already acquired the pharmaceutical company Searle) led the industry with aggressive merger and acquisition activity.[39] In an eighteen-month period over 1997 and 1998 alone, Monsanto merged with or acquired DeKalb Genetics Corporation (agricultural genetics and biotechnology), 94 percent of Calgene (agricultural biotechnology), Plant Breeding International (plant breeding), Cargill's international seeds business, and Delta and Pine Land Co. (breeder, producer, and marketer of cotton seed).[40] By the end of the third quarter of 1998, Monsanto had acquired eighteen companies.[41] DuPont followed suit, purchasing a 20 percent stake in Pioneer for $1.7 billion. From 1997 to 1998, DuPont spent $3 billion buying seed and crop protection companies, crop patents, and biotechnology companies and had formed joint ventures with many more companies.[42]

Very large pharmaceutical companies were also engaged in similar mergers to create life science companies to translate biological knowledge into human, plant, and animal products, as Novartis had done. In 1998, Zeneca started to focus on its agricultural business and then merged with Astra AB, creating a company with a market capitalization of $35 billion and sales of $3.8 billion. At about the same time, Hoechst and Rhone-Poulenc Rorer merged their pharmaceutical and agricultural chemical businesses to create a new company called Aventis, which then became the largest of the new life sciences companies.[43] These companies were setting themselves up to become contenders in the plant genomics markets. Smaller agricultural companies without the ability to develop a biotechnology business were easy targets for big companies. The big companies were also divesting themselves of other more traditional agricultural/chemical businesses to focus more on biotech and plant genomics, as did Monsanto in 1997 and DuPont in 1998.[44]

FUNDING OF AGRICULTURAL RESEARCH

While the corporate race to acquire plant genomic information and technology was on, trend studies had been showing that federal government funding for agricultural research was dwindling in comparison to corporate spending. The fraction of the U.S. research budget spent on agriculture had declined from 40 percent in 1940 to less than 2 percent by the 1990s. During the 1980s and early 1990s, federal and state funding of agricultural research had remained fairly flat. In contrast, between 1960 and 1992, industry spending for food and agricultural research tripled in real terms. By 1996, public sector expenditures were $3.15 billion, about $800 million less than industry expenditures. Specifically, corporate plant genomics research spending had increased so much that in 1996 research in this area alone was approximately equivalent to the total agriculture industry R&D expenditures in 1992.[45]

The U.S. government had started funding plant genomics research with the National Plant Genome Initiative in 1998, which supported plant genome sequencing. But this program was dwarfed by the amounts spent by private industry. Prevalent estimates at UC Berkeley were that DuPont, Pioneer, Monsanto, and Novartis together must have spent at least $1.5 billion in plant genome sequencing in contrast to $40 million spent by the federal government.[46] Because industry had a head start with this research, the public program, which would be a natural source of funds for academic research, could not produce results with the same speed at which industry was advancing the science. For instance, Novartis's highly important rice genome project was on target for completion by June 2000, which was far in advance of government projections for the same project.[47] As another example, industry was expected to produce a DNA chip for *Arabidopsis thaliana*, a member of the mustard family composed of ten thousand genes, in the same time as publicly funded universities were able to produce a chip containing only one thousand genes.[48]

The consolidation within the industry and the rapid advance of the science resulting from the heavy corporate investment in research and development created a troubling situation: companies could not make use of all the data they acquired, and academic researchers could not compete in the cost- and technology-intensive race to conduct research. Companies without large cadres of molecular geneticists began to look outside for those skilled in this discipline, particularly to academe. Corporations were interested in assembling teams of industry and academic scientists to engage in scientific discovery and to move existing discoveries closer to new products. As a consequence, industry funding of academic research increased.

Academic researchers were ready for the resources and attention. Industry spending and acquisition in plant biotechnology had left university faculty researchers feeling as if they were at the back of the pack. Universities could not compete with industry in acquiring the expensive equipment and technology needed to conduct cutting-edge research. Their work was further complicated by the fact that industry now owned the rights to many plant genes and research tools, making it prohibitively expensive and time-consuming to conduct academic research. As a result, frustrated faculty either left academia to take jobs in industry or increasingly sought industry money to fund their research programs and give them access to advanced technology.

BAYH-DOLE ACT

Collaborative activity between the two sectors was not new to the life science academic community. For well over fifteen years it had collaborated with industry to transfer academic discoveries to industry for development into useful products. Moreover, the federal government endorsed and encouraged these arrangements. The Bayh-Dole University and Small Business Patent Procedure Act of 1980 (the Bayh-Dole Act) granted universities permission to retain the intellectual property rights to inventions resulting from federally supported research and to license these inventions to private industry for eventual commercialization.[49] Prior to this act, the federal government owned the rights to the inventions that resulted from its sponsored research, and private industry was forced to contend with slow and complex federal procedures in order to license rights to these inventions. As a result, commercialization of inventions was deterred, and many potentially useful discoveries languished on the shelf, thus fueling congressional concern about a reduction in the country's productivity. The Bayh-Dole Act was the federal government's recognition that the money it spent on research was ultimately valuable to the public only if beneficial products and services resulted (for example, computer chips, lasers, seeds, medicines). In return, the Bayh-Dole Act required the research institutions to make good-faith efforts to seek patents on discoveries and to secure licensees for those patents. Universities were to give preference to small businesses that agreed to manufacture in the United States any products resulting from the license. The Bayh-Dole Act also required universities to share royalties from the patents with the scientists responsible for the inventions. Researchers, in turn, were motivated to develop inventions and perform diligent work that would professionally and financially benefit the university and themselves.

The mutual benefits of these arrangements have been summarized as follows:

Universities are thus motivated by potential profits to transfer technology into the marketplace while acting in ways that will benefit American business. At the same time, American businesses are motivated to invest in university research by the legally imposed assurance that those companies that invest will be given preference when the university licenses its patents. Ultimately, both industry and universities benefit from promoting the welfare of each other.[50]

Another motivation for industry to invest in academic research involved R&D tax credits. For instance, in 1996 California sought to promote business investments in state university research when it raised the tax credit for such research from 12 to 24 percent. Similar federal tax credits were being proposed.

The Bayh-Dole Act and the other incentives prompted recognition of universities and colleges as sources of commercially valuable knowledge. A rapid increase in industry-sponsored academic research followed. According to a National Science Foundation study, between 1991 and 1997, industry funding of basic and applied research performed at universities and colleges rose by about 20 percent in constant dollars. Industrial funds accounted for an estimated 6.5 percent of all academic basic research expenditures and 9.1 percent of all academic applied research expenditures, amounting to $1.05 billion and $545 million, respectively.[51] Another study by the Association of University Technology Managers (AUTM) placed the 1998 industry spending on academic research at $2.4 billion.[52]

The impressive impact of academic technology licensing was summarized in the 1999 AUTM licensing survey.[53] According to this survey, the licensees of academic institutions introduced at least 417 new products that year, including health-care products, software programs, and agricultural products as well as research reagents and tools used by industry and academia for various research, development, and commercial purposes. AUTM estimated that these licenses generated $40.9 billion in economic activity and supported 270,900 jobs that year. Of the total 3,914 new licenses/options granted to companies, 62 percent went to companies with fewer that five hundred employees. Of the licenses to small companies, 344 were new companies created specifically to develop and commercialize the results of academic research. For the first time, the AUTM survey was also able to calculate the number of products currently on the market due to AUTM-member licensing activities. Of the 4,269 licenses that were generating so-called running royalties (obtained when the licensee has sold a product covered by the intellectual property in the license), about 2,000 were exclusive licenses. Since an exclusive license is a key catalyst in the development of products covered by that license, AUTM estimated that there were therefore about two thousand products that would not be presently available if not for AUTM-member licensing activities. Some of these products had produced tremendous revenues for the licensee companies. For instance, in 1987, Michigan State University licensed the anticancer drug cisplatin (Platinol®) to Bristol-Myers. Ten years later, this drug had an annual world market exceeding $100 million.[54]

All of these trends and events converged to make it highly likely that corporations and academic departments would increasingly become research partners. The most common arrangement involved a bioscience company funding various research projects of individual academic scientists. Such arrangements usually involved a research contract that specified the work to be done, under what circumstances the work was confidential, who owned the results of the work, and who had rights to license the work results. What Berkeley and Novartis were contemplating was taking such partnerships to the next level.

NOVARTIS AND NOVARTIS AGRICULTURAL DISCOVERY INSTITUTE, INC.

Novartis was formed in 1996 as a result of the merger of the two large Swiss companies, Ciba-Geigy and Sandoz, a deal worth $27 billion. This corporate merger was the biggest ever recorded, and afterwards the company quickly pared down to three divisions of health care, agribusiness, and foods/nutrition.[55] Its products included chemicals, pharmaceuticals, agricultural products (including seeds, crop protection chemicals, and veterinary products), and nutritional products and supplements. Because of this particular fusion of businesses, Novartis called itself a "life sciences" company and planned not only to develop these businesses individually but also to create new products out of the synergies that could be achieved among them. In November 1998, Novartis had a total market capitalization of $128 billion and yearly sales of $22 billion, 26 percent of which came from its agricultural businesses.[56] It was one of the top three seed companies in the world, with sales of close to $1.8 billion.

Novartis's plan was to focus on biotechnology as a means to innovate within and across its businesses individually and, eventually, synergistically. Within its agricultural division, plant genomics became a target for discovery, knowledge and technology acquisition, and growth. In 1998, however, most of what had been achieved in the area of commercial plant genomics was still in the R&D phase, and much of it had been accomplished by smaller companies. To set itself up competitively, Novartis had to decide how the company would go about obtaining access to genomics research and technology.

Briggs had a Ph.D. in plant pathology, a distinguished twenty-year career in plant pathology and genetic research, and, for a number of years, had been the director of research at Pioneer Hi-Bred. Initially, Novartis had proposed that Briggs operate out of the company's in-house R&D division in South Carolina, Novartis Agribusiness Biotech Research, Inc. (NABRI). Soon after his arrival at Novartis, however, the company asked Briggs to rethink assumptions that had been made about the best way to conduct the new basic research effort. Briggs, along with managers at Novartis, considered how their competitors had ramped up in this effort—by buying technology and companies or by hiring scientists and building in-house programs—and thought these approaches would be too slow for Novartis.

Briggs recommended that gene discovery and functional genomics work would be more likely accomplished by amassing a network of outside scientists to collaborate with Novartis scientists. Briggs felt that Novartis's research discovery efforts should be performed separately from NABRI, where the focus was on capturing the value of research discoveries and developing them into products rather than on discovery. In addition, Briggs knew that profitability was more difficult to achieve in the agribusiness division of Novartis since, in contrast with the pharmaceutical division, both markets and margins in agrochemical products were smaller. Briggs believed his unit would be less subject to corporate cutbacks in the event of a downturn in the market if his unit were separate from the main company. Finally, to facilitate work with outside scientists, Briggs wanted to establish an entity that was less corporately directed, and more focused on basic research, and for these reasons more likely to attract good researchers from strong academic programs. Briggs anticipated that academic scientists would more readily collaborate with an institute devoted to basic research than with a more commercially oriented entity. Although Novartis's upper management had reservations that the company would not be able to exert enough control over the research conducted at such an affiliated entity, they gave Briggs the green light and NADII was born.

NOVARTIS AGRICULTURAL DISCOVERY INSTITUTE, INC.

On July 21, 1998, NADII was created as the first phase of a ten-year, $600 million investment by Novartis to conduct agricultural genomics research and development. The money came from the Novartis Research Foundation, and the investment was one of the largest single research endeavors dedicated to this purpose.[57] Briggs set up NADII in San Diego, California, and staffed the institute with about 180 researchers.[58] NADII was given $250 million to establish and operate its new facilities. In addition to spearheading Novartis's basic biotechnology research, NADII was charged with maximizing the company's cross-sector cooperation with Novartis's Crop Protection and Seeds and working in tandem with NABRI and with the numerous Novartis research stations worldwide. The close proximity of NADII to the recently announced Novartis pharmaceuticals genomics institute (Novartis Institute for Functional Genomics), which was being built in La Jolla, California, was intended to optimize cross-business synergies in genomics research in both agribusiness and in pharmaceuticals.[59] The Novartis Research Foundation that funded NADII was to own the intellectual property developed at NADII.

According to Briggs, NADII's success would be based on the number and value of useful inventions that came from its own research and the research of its partners. One facility that Briggs immediately targeted as a research partner was the well-regarded Department of Plant and Microbial Biology at UC Berkeley, headed by his friend and colleague Willhelm "Willi" Gruissem.

UC BERKELEY AND THE COLLEGE OF NATURAL RESOURCES

According to the official history of UC Berkeley, "the roots of the University of California go back to the gold rush days of 1849, when the drafters of the State Constitution, required the legislature to 'encourage by all suitable means the promotion of intellectual, scientific, moral and agricultural improvement' of the people of California."[60] The university that was created nearly twenty years later was the product of a merger between the College of California (a private institution) and the Agricultural, Mining, and Mechanical Arts College. This latter college was a public land grant institution formed in 1866 under the auspices of the federal Morrill Land Grant Act of 1862. According to the UC Berkeley administrators, this act was intended to encourage cooperation between the agricultural industry and state and private universities. Land grant colleges often formed cooperative relationships with the government and various industries to disseminate research, provide extension programs, and improve agricultural productivity.

In 1974, the College of Agriculture and the School of Forestry and Conservation merged to become the College of Natural Resources. The College of Natural Resources (along with UC Davis and UC Riverside) was a California

Agricultural Experiment Station, which received state funds that supported part of the college's research program. In 1998, the College of Natural Resources had a $75 million budget and received about $50 million in grants. There were approximately 120 faculty members in the college who taught and conducted research in agricultural and resource economics; environmental science, policy, and management; plant and microbial biology; and nutritional sciences and toxicology. The mission of the college was to assist in meeting the societal demands for environmental quality, sustainability of natural resources, food safety, nutrition, and economic development.[61]

According to the dean of the College of Natural Resources, Gordon Rausser, "One of the reasons U.S. agriculture was the most efficient in the world was that the land grant university system recognized and capitalized on the complementarities between scientific and practical knowledge."[62] He recognized that in order to achieve these complementarities, it was necessary to incorporate a commercial component into the work of the college. This appreciation for the financial aspects of the college's mission came naturally to the dean. By training, Rausser was an economist with varied experiences that included measuring the economic returns of agricultural research.[63]

Just before Rausser's appointment as dean of the College of Natural Resources in 1994, the university chancellor, Chang-Lin Tien, had become concerned that the university was losing good faculty to the biotechnology industry. To preserve these faculty, the chancellor felt that the university needed to increase its support for biotechnology research, and that forging closer relationships with the biotechnology industry was one way to do this. It was believed that funds and access to new technologies would both improve the biotechnology research programs at the university and keep the faculty on campus. To assist in this endeavor, the chancellor formed a Biotechnology Advisory Board and invited faculty members to participate. As a result of the initiative, the departments of Microbial and Cell Biology and Plant and Microbial Biology began to work on proposals that would connect faculty scientists to scientists in industry. The chair of the Department of Plant and Microbial Biology, Willi Gruissem, was a plant biologist with a well-respected research program. Gruissem took the initiative to develop a strategy that would connect his department to the companies engaged in plant genomics research.

The Department of Plant and Microbial Biology was a key research and training program of the Agricultural Experiment Station in the California Division of Agriculture and Natural Resources, with 32 faculty members, 110 postdoctoral researchers, and 70 graduate students. The research efforts of the program were focused on contemporary basic plant research and the design of biotechnologies. The total annual budget for the department was about $15 million, and funding for research came from both public and private sources. About 80 percent of the funding came from public sources (for example, National Science Foundation, National Institutes of Health, and the state) and 20 percent came from private sources (for example, Monsanto, Pioneer, DuPont). Gruissem had been struggling with the problem of dwindling support from the public sector and was looking for ways to identify more stable sources of funding. At the same time, he recognized that the ability of his faculty to engage in research that would advance the field of agricultural biotechnology was hindered by the fact that many corporations owned most the useful plant and seed genes and many of the necessary research tools.[64] This made it both cumbersome and expensive for the department to acquire research-enabling knowledge and materials and technology, since these acquisitions would often require negotiating with multiple companies to collect what was necessary. Lack or difficulty of access had put the department far behind industry in terms of the sophistication of their research and also in the speed with which research results could be achieved. Under the circumstances, Gruissem believed that faculty flight to industry was a risk.

Gruissem believed that the best way to keep faculty engaged in useful contemporary research and get access to new tools and technologies was to seek industry-funded projects from companies with larger, better-financed, and more-advanced research programs. There were both good and bad consequences to seeking out and participating in these industry projects. On the positive side, necessary research funds were generated from the initial funding and from royalties obtained through technology transfer.[65] Conducting research for corporations meant that faculty frequently (but not always) could obtain access to useful advanced proprietary corporate data. On the negative side, competition among the companies funding the department required that faculty maintain confidentiality of company information, meaning they often could not confer with their colleagues about their research. Confidentiality requirements often extended after the data were ready for publication. These delays were frustrating and made it difficult for graduate students to participate in industry-funded research since students needed to publish their research quickly in order to successfully compete for their first job out of graduate school.

In 1993, with these benefits and risks in mind, Gruissem set up a Biotechnology Advisory Board for his department composed of industry scientists.

Gruissem hoped that advisory board members would not only provide private funding for the department's teaching and research programs but also guidance and training for students interested in industry careers. At first, faculty members were uneasy about inviting so many corporate scientists into the department. But the meetings became useful discussions about the science, and both groups of scientists came to see value in each other's work. Over the next two years, the board grew to include sixteen representatives from private industry, including Monsanto, Pioneer, CalGene, DNA Applied Technology, Ciba-Geigy, DuPont, and some U.K. companies. In formal written requests and in meetings, Gruissem attempted to get these companies interested in funding student research—but without success. Undaunted, Gruissem made attempts to increase formal research collaborations with faculty, but responses from industry were again not forthcoming. In 1997, a Monsanto scientist informally suggested to Gruissem that the department consider an exclusive research relationship with the company. This suggestion made Gruissem wonder if other companies might be willing to compete for an exclusive affiliation with the department, and he discussed this idea with Dean Rausser.

Rausser had studied aspects of university-industry partnerships and concluded that corporate research agreements had increasingly diverted universities from conducting important public benefit agricultural research.[66] He had written that "public/private partnerships cannot be allowed to leverage universities resources and divert research from public good outposts not produced elsewhere."[67] He had not concluded that such relationships should be discouraged; rather, he believed that university-corporate collaborations were beneficial but that the universities had to carefully negotiate these deals to preserve the academic public mission. He believed that mutually beneficial relationships were possible. One reason for this optimism was Rausser's belief that in some respects the cultures of academia and industry were not as separate as they once were. He commented, "As some private firms have restructured themselves as life science companies, their culture and values have become a bit more like those of a research university. Similarly, as research universities have responded to the Bayh-Doyle Act of 1980, expanding their technology transfer activities, they too have become a bit more like private companies."[68] As Rausser saw it, the newer life sciences companies were developing more long-term basic research programs similar to those at universities, and both companies and universities were interested in capturing the economic value of their discoveries. In addition, the fact that universities did not have the resources or infrastructure to commercialize their discoveries made industry-university alliances a natural development. With Rausser's blessing, Gruissem investigated exclusive collaborative possibilities for the college and the Department of Plant and Microbial Biology.

In the summer of 1997, Gruissem, faculty members Peggy Lemaux and Bob Buchanan, and Dean Rausser actively worked on plans to form a research alliance with a single company. Through contacts with company scientists, they became convinced that access to company research resources would markedly improve the sophistication, quality, and speed of the department's research. Gruissem also came to realize how unfair it was to ask the students to spend weeks or months performing research that could be accomplished in days with access to corporate research data bases. As the benefits of a partnership became apparent, department faculty members were asked to consider what would be useful and acceptable aspects of such an industry collaboration.

During the same year, Gruissem had discussed an affiliation proposal with Steven Briggs, then head of research at Pioneer. Pioneer was the first company to have developed a plant genomics program and had an extensive collection of gene maps and functional genomics tools, but, similar to its competitors, the company lacked the capability to fully exploit on its own the value of the data base and tools. Briggs believed that by collaborating with academia, Pioneer could increase the utility of the data. Briggs held the UC Berkeley plant scientists in high repute for the quantity and quality of their research work. The department was considered to be one of, if not the, best academic departments in this field. Briggs also knew that Berkeley had a reasonable technology transfer operation that would not create significant delays in negotiating licenses to discoveries that resulted from the research.

At the same time, Dean Rausser was expanding his investigation by studying targeted companies' plant genomics strategic foci and their alliances. He made visits to business development directors at these corporations to discuss how best to create a viable corporate relationship for the department. He learned that companies would value functional genomics research work and knew that the UC Berkeley department could deliver this work. He was fairly certain that several companies would want access to this type of research and might be willing to compete for it. In November 1997, as a consequence of an initial lack of response from the companies and based on his own research findings, Rausser proposed to Gruissem to change tactics and suggested that the department engage in an "auction," inviting companies to bid for access to faculty research.

This novel approach reversed the usual university-industry research proposal process, which typically involved individual faculty responding to re-search funding announcements either from public or private sources, with the scope of work specified by the sponsor. In the department's new proposal, however, UC Berkeley would specify the terms of the agreement and invite companies to compete for access to the department's research. Gruissem and Rausser believed UC Berkeley could achieve more control over the negotia-tions and be better able to preserve what elements of the relationship were ac-ademically valuable; namely, faculty autonomy, access to genomic information and tools, avoidance of oppressive restrictions on the publication of informa-tion, and the ability to obtain funds for student research.

Department faculty reaction was immediately negative because such ag-gressive courting of industry support seemed improper. Gruissem managed to assuage the faculty by asking them to assist with others on campus in setting the principles and guidelines that would govern the relationship so that aca-demic integrity would be maintained. By January 1998, the principles were in place and approved by the UC Berkeley administration. The principles in-cluded freedom of the faculty to choose their own research (to preserve aca-demic freedom), inclusion of as many faculty as possible (to promote faculty collaborations), access to proprietary company data, technology, and tools, and absence of oppressive restrictions on publication. Gruissem then sent letters to nine companies indicating that a large group of faculty were interested in a substantial strategic industry relationship and inviting the companies to send in proposals commensurate with the principles laid out by the department. Proposals were due by April 30, 1998.

NEGOTIATING THE AGREEMENT

Gruissem, Buchanan, and Lemaux then began an arduous process of visiting companies—DuPont, Monsanto, Novartis, Pioneer Hi-Bred, Sumitomo Chem-ical, and Zeneca—to discuss whether each would submit a bid for a research alliance. Ultimately, all but Zeneca submitted proposals. It became apparent to Gruissem that there were four interested companies with realistic potential for an alliance—Monsanto, DuPont, Pioneer and Novartis. These companies sought an alliance because the science being conducted in the department was relevant to the companies' developing plant genomics businesses. It was at this time, in the spring of 1998, that Steven Briggs began to formulate the system under which Novartis would engage in plant genomics research. He thought that the Berkeley proposal might be an excellent opportunity to kick-start

NADII's fledgling program. Briggs made overtures to Berkeley through NADII. Prior to that, UC Berkeley had been dealing with NABRI, and Briggs now wanted to shift the relationship over to NADII. He separated himself from both Pioneer and from NABRI and began negotiating with the UC Berkeley department to form an alliance with NADII.

Both Briggs and Gruissem believed they could form a mutually beneficial relationship. They had worked together before, personally trusted and respected each other, were each sensitive to the needs of the other party, and thought that they could achieve their corporate and academic goals through a partnership. Briggs's proposal had indicated to Gruissem that NADII was more interested than other companies in addressing academic sensitivities. Unlike the other companies, NADII proposed to fund the work of any and all of the department faculty. UC Berkeley would have a majority say in which research projects were funded. In addition to the five-year, $25 million funding, Briggs proposed that NADII build a $25 million research facility on campus where plant scientists from the department and NADII could work side by side. Gruissem was impressed by the proposal: no other company was willing to work with the entire faculty, nor allow the faculty almost unfettered ability to conduct the research of their choosing. NADII also offered the access to data bases and tools that Gruissem so highly valued. Having studied other academic-industry collaborations, Gruissem knew this offer was the first of its kind, and he was excited about the prospects for the department.

As for Briggs, he too knew that his offer was unusual, both in the scope of the collaboration and the freedom the faculty would have to conduct research without direction from NADII or Novartis. This kind of freedom was unprecedented as far as Briggs knew. His rationale for believing that the arrangement would result in useful discoveries for Novartis was that the scientists knew "a hell of a lot more than a corporate administrator about how to move the science forward." Scientists would also be far better at generating innovative ideas and discoveries. If that were not the case, he reasoned, then the company could just hire technicians to implement company ideas. Through NADII, Briggs wanted to assist the UC Berkeley faculty with money, information, technologies, and tools. With this support, Briggs expected that the Berkeley researchers would gain a wider perspective on how the research "fits in with the world," including the downstream impact of research on the development of new products. He believed that NADII funding would broaden and accelerate UC Berkeley's research. Briggs also believed that formal direction from Novartis would conflict with the concept of scientists doing cutting-edge discovery work. The arrangement had been a hard sell to Novartis top management—the company had never funded research over which it had so little control. There was a high risk that the discoveries resulting from this work would not be beneficial (or not beneficial enough) to Novartis to make the deal worthwhile. But Novartis was already interested in some of the Berkeley research, and, with the spirit of NADII having been established, Briggs persuaded top management to take a chance.

It seemed that UC Berkeley too was willing to take a chance on an industry alliance. The Department of Plant and Microbial Biology had been looking to find the strongest corporate partner it could in genomics research. Briggs was surprised, however, that Berkeley had chosen NADII's offer over the others'. Novartis's competitors (Monsanto, Pioneer, DuPont) had much bigger genomics research programs, bigger data bases, and more reagents and tools. Novartis only had Briggs. Briggs speculated that UC Berkeley had chosen NADII as a research partner because it took the long view of the relationship. The department did not seem to require year-one technology access. Instead, Briggs guessed that Rausser and Gruissem thought NADII could deliver the most over a period of five years.

Despite the willingness of the three men to develop an agreement, negotiations became complicated once others became involved. There were some difficulties in negotiating the intellectual property rights to the discoveries that would result from the NADII-funded research. At first, the university insisted on full rights to all discoveries even if they resulted from a use of Novartis's proprietary data or tools. Novartis wanted the parties to share in such rights since both faculty effort and company data and materials were involved. Some faculty members were opposed to sharing discovery rights with NADII since that meant less potential royalties for the faculty.[69]

The longest source of delay in coming to an agreement, however, came from the involvement of other campus faculty. Recognizing that such a broad collaboration with an individual company would be controversial, the new university chancellor Robert Berdahl wanted the full University Academic Senate to approve the arrangement. In addition, Dean Rausser opened up the terms of the proposal for public discussion.

OBJECTIONS TO THE PARTNERSHIP

The University Academic Senate took six months to consider the proposal. The senate comprised many nonscience professors unused to even the concept of private industry funding of academic research or the technology transfer system so familiar to the life sciences faculty. Members of the senate immediately raised objections. "There is a troubling feeling that this could put broad influence on the department to redirect its academic activity to please a private company," said Robert Spear, a professor of environmental health and vice chairman of the faculty senate.[70] Others complained that the public interest research mandated by the college's mission would be compromised by the deal. The perception that private interest research detracted from public benefit research was aggravated by the fact that the entire department seemed about to be wedded to the interests of one corporation. Other negative reactions centered on a diminution in faculty integrity, less time spent teaching or attending to administrative duties, and the loss of public trust in the independence of the university. Others felt that the almost exclusive relationship would hinder department faculty from obtaining other research funds from either the public or private sectors. Further, these perceived conflicts of interest would lead to fewer invitations to faculty to serve on prestigious public policy science committees. At one point, the senate sent Dean Rausser a list of three hundred questions to answer about the proposed arrangement.

To complicate matters, a survey of the department faculty was conducted and purported to show that many faculty opposed the deal. A faculty member from the college who was not a member of the department (and who therefore would not be participating in the Novartis deal) spoke of some of the faculty dissatisfactions to the UC Berkeley alumni magazine. He was a forest entomologist who specialized in biological pest control and was wary of Novartis in general. "Novartis is interested in making money. It isn't necessarily interested in solving ecological problems such as sustainability or biodiversity." And he was troubled by some of the company's products. "I just saw the Novartis display at a national meeting in Las Vegas," he said, "and it was all pesticide-oriented. This is what I've been fighting all my life."[71] He was further worried that the Novartis relationship would create resentment within the college since the plant genomics faculty would be getting large amounts of funding and other faculty would not.

Another prominent critic of the Novartis collaboration was Robert Berring, a Berkeley law school professor and alumnus, who wrote a lengthy critique in the February 1999 issue of the *California Monthly*, the school's alumni magazine. In this article, Professor Berring characterized the Novartis deal as part of "a deep and dangerous trend" and asked whether Berkeley was off course when it contracted with Novartis:

To one who has been a student, a faculty member, and an administrator on this campus, this represents a marked change in the very soul of Berkeley. For all the anger, silliness, and lugubrious pretensions of Berkeley campus politics, the one thing that has always impressed me was that it was a faculty-controlled campus. The faculty, driven by its own conceptions of academic freedom and research integrity, exists in constant tension with the administration. But, in the end, it has had the last word. I am not saying it always makes the right call, but the field on which it plays has been the field of academic integrity.

Private fundraising has done little to disturb this universe. The administration can be chided for courting big givers, but everyone understands that buildings need to be built and computers need to be purchased. Besides, the research agenda—the heart of the body—has remained sacred. No one in the administration calls to tell one what to work on. That would violate a sacred taboo. Even the richest alum who can fund a chair in a research area cannot dictate what kind of research should be done by the chair's occupant. The giver does not own the research of the chairholder.

This is where the Novartis arrangement is so different. Here the private sector is making research decisions. There is a voice, even though a small one, helping to chart research. There is a seat at the table for interests who very rightly expect a return on the dollar. Novartis may even invest in the University's infrastructure by putting up a research building in or near campus. This is a turning point.

If the justification for such an arrangement is that only by creating such partnerships can the University of California continue to lead the world in research, we must take that justification seriously. But we must also reflect with care upon the premise that underlies it. We must ask at what point does the University bargain away so much of itself that it ceases to be the University and becomes a partner of the private sector?

These comments and conclusions frustrated Dean Rausser, who believed that the proposal was being misrepresented and that evaluation of the proposal should be based not on speculation of unintended consequences but on whether the agreement adhered to the department faculty principles. He responded to the Berring article with one of his own, emphasizing that Berring's concerns would be alleviated for anyone who took the time to read the collaboration agreement, which was publicly available (see Appendix 6.1 for the research agreement). In his article, Dean Rausser emphasized the benefits of the agreement:

The fact that NADI has "a seat at the table" in reviewing these grant proposals is no abdication of faculty control. In contrast, most privately sponsored

University research is entirely directed by the sponsor, and the funds may be used only for projects selected by the corporate donor. Even taxpayer research funding comes with strings attached. Faculty almost never receive open-ended grants to indulge their curiosity as Professor Berring suggests: they receive limited funding for specified projects. The beauty of the NADI alliance is that it places the choice of research projects under faculty control.

What does NADI receive for its $25-million contribution? Professor Berring describes it as "first rights to particular developments in genomics." What he doesn't say—and may not have realized—is that NADI receives only the right to negotiate to acquire at fair market value a percentage of discoveries that may result from research it helps fund. In other words, if there are no marketable discoveries, or the University doesn't accept NADI's offer to purchase them, NADI will receive no commercial rights at all. Even without this agreement, NADI could negotiate for licensing of any of UC's proprietary rights. The University, on the other hand, will be a winner regardless of outcome. Having obtained not only needed cash and possible intellectual property ownership, it will also, perhaps most important, acquire access to NADI's proprietary genomic databases, which are essential to Berkeley's cutting-edge research in plant and microbial biology.

Despite concerns about the scope of the arrangement, Gruissem remained convinced that the department would be better off if most, if not all, of the faculty were included. The question of which faculty would be included was resolved early in the negotiations with Novartis. Briggs said that all faculty could be included. This prospect pleased Gruissem since it would help to alleviate the Balkanization of his department caused by faculty conducting research for many different companies. Full involvement would also help forge collaborative relationships among the faculty. In addition, his faculty would need to devote less time to fund raising from other sources. Gruissem offered all faculty the choice to join. In the end, all but three members did. The abstainers were a pathologist with no research program and one teacher with a small research program that was not expected to be altered by the NADII deal. A third faculty member had a large research affiliation with another company that had increased his funding so that he would remain devoted to this work instead of NADII's.

To address his own and others' concern about the quality and direction of the research, Gruissem asked for the help of the department faculty to develop peer review guidelines for the selection of the research that NADII would fund. Gruissem wanted recognized quality and merit principles to drive the process. The department adopted guidelines based on standard government agency review criteria: quality and intellectual merit of the proposed research, potential advancement of discovery, and past and present productivity of the researcher. Unlike most agencies or companies that funded research, Gruissem put less emphasis on the feasibility of the research proposals since he wanted his faculty to use NADII funding to "stretch" and innovate in their research.

Some students also had concerns about the Novartis partnership with UC Berkeley. A campus student group, Students for Responsible Research, composed primarily of graduate students in the College of Natural Resources, distrusted corporate funding of academic research and believed the Novartis proposal would promote a narrow focus on profits and involve detrimental biotechnological research. The group held a press conference and passed out leaflets to denounce the Novartis proposal. They also circulated a petition stating their objections, which included that the collaboration had weak oversight, was hurried through while student and faculty concerns were ignored, amounted to tax dollars being used for the research and development of a foreign corporation, and moved the college's research agenda toward developing profitable genetically engineered crops at the expense of its mission. The research that would meet the college mission would be in areas of environmental quality, sustainability of natural resources, food safety, nutrition, and economic development through public good research and the extension of the results to the people of the state. Because of the Novartis agreement, they feared that this kind of socially important research would not take place. In addition to the protests of the Students for Responsible Research, former graduate students from UC Berkeley wrote to the *San Francisco Chronicle* stating that there should have been more faculty, student, and public involvement in the negotiations especially since Novartis had a "questionable" reputation in Europe due to ethical concerns relating to biotechnology and genetic research.[72]

Members of the general public voiced their concerns to the university as well. The Council for Responsible Genetics, a group opposed to patenting life forms, denounced UC Berkeley for participating in a system that created inequalities when corporations owned patents on plants. According to this group, "While centuries of innovation by indigenous farmers have created most of the food crops grown today, the tinkering by agribusiness entitles them to claim a plant as their own invention, and receive all profits from its use. This 'biocolonialism' will continue the pattern of a few transnational corporations profiting at the expense of large numbers of indigenous farmers."[73] A representative of the Green Party of California criticized UC Berkeley for working with Novartis on genetic experiments that could have unintended and devastating environmental consequences. As an example, he pointed to the genetically engineered corn produced by Novartis in Germany, which was alleged to have cross-pollinated with nearby natural corn and thereby corrupted the genetic make-up of this crop.[74] Food First/The Institute for Food & Development Policy in Oakland and the Pesticide Action Network in San Francisco also protested the proposed alliance. In an editorial in the *San Francisco Chronicle*, they stated that the university's corporate alliance would detract from its important public mission projects such as forming partnerships with community organizations to help urban farmers.[75] The picture of one faculty member was posted on the Web site of a protest group with the caption describing him as a "public enemy" for collaborating with Novartis.

UNIVERSITY POSITION

Ultimately closing the prolonged university inquiry process, the chancellor called a meeting of the full Faculty Senate and asked if any of them opposed the deal. Although several of the faculty continued to speak privately against the arrangement afterward, no one expressed objections to the chancellor when he announced at that meeting that the deal would go forward.

CONCLUSION

Briggs was optimistic that the research quality and direction of the partnership with Berkeley would be beneficial for Novartis. Yet the agreement had its risks. Novartis's top management had raised concerns about the usefulness of the arrangement because the company could not specify the kinds of research to be performed. Nor had the decision to consider the agreement been easy for UC Berkeley. Even after it had been ratified, university-based and outside dissenters continued to voice their objections.

As the finalist in UC Berkeley's unusual auction, Briggs considered the responsibilities that would accompany the relationship and the principles that should govern the resulting research. As far as Briggs knew, Novartis was playing a ground-breaking role in developing a partnership to bring minds and technology together for the purpose of advancing discoveries in the life sciences and reaping further benefits by commercializing the results. Clearly there were members of the public, the university community, and political action groups who had views far different from Novartis's and the department's on the benefits of this biotechnology research. As Briggs signed his name to the agreement, he wondered how NADII, now a major patron of an academic research department of a publicly funded university, would safeguard its own interests and those of its partner and deal with external pressures in the face of this exciting research endeavor.

Questions

1. Did Novartis strike the right balance between its needs and those of the university?

2. To what extent, if any, should biotechnology companies in Novartis's position structure academic research collaborations to preserve academic integrity? Why?

3. If this agreement does not produce sufficiently useful discoveries for Novartis, how should the company react? By increasing its control and direction over the research? By unwinding the deal? How should each be accomplished?

Discussion

Novartis's relationship with its academic partner can be viewed as a straightforward business relationship arrived at through the usual contracting process wherein partners with seemingly equal bargaining power negotiate to their best advantage. However, when two parties are inherently different, it is reasonable to question whether bargaining power is indeed equal and whether some advantages can be pushed. For instance, did Novartis have any obligation to cede advantage so as to preserve the academic mission of its partner? A utilitarian analysis would address this question by looking at the benefits and harms of the collaboration for both parties and would also consider whether to broaden the scope of the analysis to include the impact on others such as students and administrators or any outsiders. One prime issue to include in this analysis is whether the arrangement tends to divert department research to meet commercial goals, and, if so, what are the consequences of this change? Who benefits and who is harmed? This kind of analysis can often suggest modifications to the collaboration that would both meet corporate needs and address concerns of both its business partner and others. A rights analysis would lead to questioning whether there were any legitimate rights at stake to be claimed by the university or others that the company had a duty to uphold. Fairness is always a factor in any business contract negotiation, making it reasonable to discuss whether the parties achieved a "just" contract. Are the balances and burdens equally distributed and are both parties likely to receive in return at least the value of the contribution made? In this discussion, Novartis could consider whether the arrangement takes unfair advantage of the need of faculty for financial support (do they give up more than they get?) and what the consequences of that need would be, both short and long term.

The Contract Provisions

In November 1998, the main provisions of the contract that NADII and UC Berkeley were contemplating signing were as follows:

NADII would provide the department with $25 million over five years to conduct plant genomics research. $3.33 million per year would fund research, and $1.67 million would cover university indirect costs. This was the highest indirect cost rate ever for the University of California from a private entity. Also, Gruissem arranged with the university to refund $500,000 of its overhead money back to the department to support student research. From NADII's perspective, the $5 million annual payments would come from its $55 million annual operating budget.

The research funded under this agreement would be selected and monitored by a faculty-NADII peer review research committee composed of three university faculty, the CEO of NADII (Briggs), and a copresident from NABRI. Project selection criteria had been developed by department faculty, and criteria included the quality and intellectual merit of the proposed research, potential advancement of discovery, and the past and present productivity of the faculty investigator.

The research eligible for potential funding under the agreement would be selected by the faculty and submitted to the research committee for evaluation of the proposal. However, the research committee would "not make recommendations to [the department] faculty as to the scope and long term goals of their proposed research projects."

The research funded under the agreement could not be done with the use of any supplemental funds or research material from companies other than NADII/Novartis.

NADII acknowledged that the university

Is an open, academic environment and as a public, non-profit educational institution has no mechanism to guarantee the confidentiality of information and is subject to statutes requiring disclosure of information and records which a private corporation could keep confidential. Notwithstanding this acknowledgment, University and NADII will use their best efforts to ensure that information and materials are controlled in full compliance and accordance with the mutually agreed terms of this Agreement.

NADII would make available to the faculty its proprietary genomics bioinformation data base, research tools, biological materials, and compounds to facilitate the conduct of the research.

Before being allowed access to this proprietary Novartis material, department faculty members would sign access agreements promising not to disclose the proprietary information to any third party without permission from NADII. Faculty use of this information was limited to the faculty research funded under the agreement. Unless NADII gave permission, proprietary information obtained pursuant to an access agreement would receive confidential status for the five-year contract period plus an additional five years.

The department could fully disclose or publish its research results unless the disclosure contained NADII proprietary information, in which case the proprietary information would remain confidential as above unless NADII granted permission for the department to disclose or publish results.

The department would submit to NADII all proposed publications and research disclosures thirty days in advance of submission for publication to determine if the publication would disclose patentable subject matter of interest to NADII. If so, NADII had ninety days to inform the university that it should file for patent protection, during which time no publication or disclosure of the research results could be made.

The department was responsible for keeping adequate records to ensure that evidence of invention was maintained for patent purposes. Each party was required to promptly disclose to the other any invention or discovery made within the scope of the agreement. NADII would then decide which of those inventions it wished the university to patent.

The university owned all of the results of the research and the inventions funded under the agreement except that joint inventions made by university employees and NADII employees without the use of university research facilities were owned jointly, and inventions made solely by NADII employees using university facilities were also owned jointly.

NADII had the right to use for free all research results developed under this agreement for its own research.

If the invention resulted from faculty use of a NADII proprietary genomics bioinformation data base, NADII would obtain an irrevocable, royalty-free, worldwide, nonexclusive license to use the invention.

NADII had ninety days from the university invention disclosure to designate the invention as a "subject invention" for which the university would have to file a patent application.

For all of these subject inventions, NADII had up to 180 days from the filing of the patent application to exercise a first right to negotiate with the university for either an exclusive or nonexclusive royalty bearing worldwide license or option to use, sell, or sublicense the invention.

NADII could exercise this right for only a portion of the subject inventions that resulted from the agreement. This portion would be calculated as the ratio of NADII funding to the total department funding, which comprised NADII funding together with funds that came from other sources (excluding Department of Energy and other private, nonNADII funding). The funds from "other" sources, then, were primarily from the National Science Foundation, NIH, USDA, and the California Agricultural Experiment Station. NADII's selections would be "trued up" at the end of the third, fourth, and fifth contract years, and if NADII had selected more inventions than the contract formula allowed, NADII would have to relinquish rights to the excess selections.

If NADII did not obtain or elect to obtain rights to inventions, the university was free to license to other entities and the university was obliged to give special consideration to licensing to small businesses.

The agreement could be terminated by either party with one year's notice.

In addition, it was contemplated and still under consideration that Novartis would pay for new or renovated department laboratory facilities, and place twenty to thirty Novartis employees on or near campus as collaborators and adjunct faculty. Novartis would contribute an additional $25 million for this aspect of the collaboration.

Notes

1. Dueker KS. Biobusiness on campus: Commercialization of university-developed biomedical technologies. *Food and Drug Law Journal* 1997; 52:453–509.

2. Hall BH, Link AN, Scott JT. *Universities as research partners.* Working Paper 7643. Cambridge, MA: National Bureau of Economic Research; 2000; Eichenwald K, Kolata G. When physicians double as entrepreneurs. *New York Times* 1999 Nov 30; Sect. A:1.

3. Nelson LL. The lifeblood of biotechnology: university-industry technology transfer. In Ono RD, editor, *The business of biotechnology.* Stoneham, MA: Butterworth-Heinemann; 1991. pp. 39–75.

4. Blumenthal D, Causino N, Campbell E, et al. Relationships between academic institutions and industry in the life sciences: An industry survey. *New England Journal of Medicine* 1996; 334:368–73.

5. Bodenheimer T. Uneasy alliance: Clinical investigators and the pharmaceutical industry. *New England Journal of Medicine* 2000; 342:1538–44.

6. *From bench to bedside: preserving the research mission of academic health centers.* New York: Commonwealth Fund; 1999.

7. See Note 5.

8. Kennedy D. Personal interview. 1999; see also Note 1; Note 2, Hall et al.

9. According to the Association of American Universities, almost half of the basic research conducted in the United States is performed by universities and colleges, in contrast with applied research, of which 10 to 15 percent is performed by academia. See www.tulane.edu/aau/USRsrchFactsandFigs.html.

10. Angell M. Is academic medicine for sale? *New England Journal of Medicine* 2000; 342:1516–18.

11. Witt MD, Gostin LO. Conflict of interest dilemmas in biomedical research. *Journal of the American Medical Association* 1994; 271:547–51.

12. Nelson D, Weiss R. Hasty decision in race to a cure? *Washington Post* 1999 Nov 21; Sect. A:1.

13. Bush DL. Gene therapy trials; the role of the NIH and conflicts of interest. *Biotechnology Law Reporter* 2000; 19:576–78; DiStefano JN, Collins H, Vendantam S. Pennsylvania biotechnology researcher negotiates corporate funding. *Philadelphia Inquirer* 2000 Feb 27; Nelson D, Weiss R. Penn researchers sued in gene therapy death. *Washington Post* 2000 Sept 19; Sect. A:3.

14. Firlik AD, Lowry DW. Is academic medicine for sale? *New England Journal of Medicine* 2000; 343:508.

15. Blumenthal D, Campbell E, Causino N, et al. Participation of life-science faculty in research relationships with industry. *New England Journal of Medicine* 1996; 335:1734–39.

16. This statistic was computed by dividing the total number of citations that a journal receives by the number of references the journal gives to other journals in the same field. The average influence of an article in a given journal (the average number of citations a paper in a journal receives, weighted by the influence of the referencing journal) was then computed.

17. Blumenthal D, Campbell E, Anderson M, et al. Withholding research results in academic life science: evidence from a national survey of faculty. *Journal of the American Medical Association* 1997; 277:1224–28.

18. Berg LA, Galbraith A, Rennie D. The publication of sponsored symposiums in medical journals. *New England Journal of Medicine* 1992; 327:1135–40; Rochon P, Gurwitz J, Simms R, et al. A study of manufacturer-supported trials of nonsteroidal anti-inflammatory drugs in the treatment of arthritis. *Archives of Internal Medicine* 1994; 154: 157–63; Cho M, Berg LA. The quality of drug studies published in symposium proceedings. *Annals of Internal Medicine* 1996; 124:485–89; Stelfox HT, Chua G, O'Rourke K, et al. Conflict of interest in the debate over calcium-channel antagonists. *New England Journal of Medicine* 1998; 338:101–6; Friedberg M, Saffran B, Stinson TJ, et al. Evaluation of conflict of interest in economic analyses of new drugs used in oncology. *Journal of the American Medical Association* 1999; 282:1453–57; see also Note 5.

19. See Note 5.

20. Applegate W, Furberg K, Byungton R, et al. The multicenter isradipine diuretic atherosclerosis study (MIDAS). *Journal of the American Medical Association* 1996; 277:297–98.

21. See Note 4.

22. Rose CD. Scripps deal with drug firm approved; Sandoz is partner in scaled-back alliance. *San Diego Union-Tribune* 1994 May 17; Sect. A:1.

23. Ibid.

24. Anderson C. Scripps to get less from Sandoz; Sandoz Pharmaceutical Corp. limits investment in Scripps Research Institute. *Science* 1994; 264:1077.

25. National Institutes of Health. Developing sponsored research agreements: Considerations for recipients of NIH research grants and contracts. *Federal Register* 1994. pp. 55674–78.

26. See Note 5.

27. This case study was prepared by Margaret L. Eaton. The input and assistance of Steven Briggs of NADII, Gordon Rausser and Wilhelm Gruissem of U.C. Berkeley, Donald Kennedy of Stanford University, Robert Rosensweig, and Dan Tangimen of the legal department of Torrey Mesa Research Institute is greatly appreciated. The events described in this case study occurred up until late 1998.

28. In agricultural genetics research, the most advanced science involved the devel-

opment of the complete genetic maps of individual plants and other organisms. These maps listed all the DNA bases in the organism and also contained a list of the identified genes. Such a map was called a genome and gave rise to the term genomics as an area of research. More complete analysis of plant function was possible once the complete genome was available. Plant genomics also involved the related field of functional genomics, which was the understanding of what those genes did to the plant or to insects that fed on the plant.

29. According to the company press release of July 21, 1998, Novartis Group sales in 1997 were 31.2 billion Swiss francs (USD 21.6 billion), of which 18.8 billion (USD 13.0 billion) were in Healthcare/Pharmaceutics, 8.3 billion (USD 5.8 billion) in Agribusiness, and 4.1 billion (USD 2.8 billion) in Nutrition. Market capitalization was approximately 150 billion Swiss francs (USD 104 billion), and net revenues were about 30 billion (USD 21 billion).

Green, D. Prescription for the future: The merger of Sandoz and Ciba is likely to launch a further round of restructuring in the drugs and chemicals sector. *Financial Times* (London) 1996 Mar 8; p. 17.

30. This product was created by inserting a gene into the seed that caused the soya plant to create a protein that made the plant resistant to Monsanto's Roundup® herbicide. As a consequence, farmers could spray Roundup to kill weeds and spare the soybean plant. Because this made weed control easier and more economical, Roundup Ready soybean seeds were popular with farmers. In 1998, about half of the seventy-two-million-acre U.S. soybean harvest came from plants genetically engineered to tolerate Monsanto's Roundup.

Jacob R. Monsanto research finds deep hostility to GM foods. *Financial Times* (London) 1998 Feb 18; p. 10; Pollan M. Playing God in the garden. *New York Times Magazine* 1998 Oct 25; p. 44.

31. Egbert D. Wealth in the weeds, plant genomics start-ups vow to trigger the next biotech revolution. *TechCapital* 1999 Feb 23. Available from www.techcapital.com/.

32. BIO, the Biotechnology Industry Organization, is the organization that represented this industry including the agricultural biotechnology sector.

Prepared testimony of Carl B. Feldbaum, president of the Biotechnology Industry Organization, before the Technology, Environment and Aviation Subcommittee of the House Science, Space and Technology Committee, 1994 Feb 2.

33. Figures are from the Web site of the Biotechnology Industry Organization. Available from www.bio.org.

Figures are from the Web site of the Pharmaceutical Research and Manufacturers Association. Available from www.phrma.org.

34. *Biotech 99: Bridging the gap.* 13th Annual Biotechnology Industry Annual Report. Palo Alto, CA: Ernst & Young LLP; 1999. p. 67.

35. E.I. DuPont 1998 Annual Report, year end 8/31/98; Monsanto 1998 Annual Report, year end 12/31/98; Pioneer Hi-Bred 10-K Report filed 8/31/98; Novartis 1998 Annual Report, year end 12/31/98; figures are year-end market capitalization.

36. See Note 30.

37. Pioneer Hi-Bred 10-K405/A Report filed 12/18/98.

38. Hayenga M. Structural change in the biotech seed and chemical industrial complex. *AgBio Forum* 1998; 1:43–55. Available from www.agbioforum.missouri.edu.

39. Steyer R. Monsanto buys seed business overseas; Cargill operations cost $1.4 billion. *St. Louis Post-Dispatch* 1998 Jun 30; Sect C:6.

40. Monsanto press releases, 5/5/97, 12/1/98; Monsanto 10-K Report of 3/25/99 for fiscal year 1998.

41. Shimoda S. Agricultural biotechnology: Master of the universe? *AgBio Forum* 1998; 1:62–68. Available from www.agbioforum.missouri.edu.

42. E.I. DuPont 1998 Annual Report. Investment Activities. p. 25.

43. Pilling D. The facts of life: Chemical and pharmaceutical companies see their future in biological innovation. *Financial Times* (London) 1998 Dec 9; p. 21.

44. See Note 31.

45. Klotz-Ingram C, Day-Rubenstein K. The changing agricultural research environment: What does it mean for public-private innovation? Washington, DC: U.S. Department of Agriculture, Economic Research Service; 1996. Available at www.ers.usda.gov/briefing/AgResearch/index.htm.

Rausser G. Private/public research: Knowledge assets and future scenarios, AAEA Fellow's Address, Nashville, TN. 1999 Aug 10.

46. Lau E. Cal, Berkeley strike unique deal. *Sacramento Bee* 1998 Nov 23; Sect. A:1.

47. United States Rice Genome Sequencing. Washington, DC: U.S. Department of Agriculture; 2000. Available from www.usricegenome.org/.

48. *Arabidopsis thaliana* is a small, weedy flowering plant that has been intensely studied as a model for plant biology and pathology. It has been a favorite of researchers primarily because it grows rapidly and has a compact genome. Timeline estimates were those of Dean Gordon Rausser, College of Natural Resources, University of California at Berkeley.

49. *United States Code* 3701–3714. See generally, the Council on Government Relations Report, University Technology Transfer. Available from www.cogr.edu/qa.htm.

50. Kuhlman GA. Alliances for the future: Cultivating a cooperative environment for biotech success. *Berkeley Technology Law Journal* 1996; 11:311, 319.

51. *Science & engineering indicators 1998* (NSB 98-1). Washington, DC: National Science Foundation, Division of Science Resources Studies. Available from www.nsf.gov/sbe/srs/seind98/start.htm; *Industry trends in research support and links to public support*. Washington, DC: National Science Board; 1998. Available from www.nsf.gov/pubs/1998/nsb9899/nsb9899.htm.

52. Association of University Technology Managers, AUTM Licensing Surveys, FY 1991–95, 1996, 1997, and 1998. Available from www.autm.net.

See also Note 1.

53. Association of University Technology Managers, AUTM Licensing Surveys, FY 1999. Available from www.autm.net.

54. See Note 1.

55. Although securities analysts had predicted great results from the merger, by mid-

1998, the company was barely making its earnings estimates despite aggressive cost-cutting. The company's largest division (health care) was performing significantly under both the prior year's earnings and the market average. The company CEO Daniel Vasella announced on May 13, 1998, that further cost-cutting was mandatory. See Silverman E. Novartis CEO issues "wake-up call." *Newark Star-Ledger* 1998 June 5; B:47.

56. Standard & Poor's Corporate Descriptions, Novartis AG. Available from Lexis Nexis Academic Universe; accessed 2000 May 1.

57. The Novartis US Foundation was established in 1997 as part of Novartis Corporation's commitment to social investment. Its primary purpose was to support efforts among communities, businesses, and nonprofit organizations on a range of social, health, and education issues related to health care, agribusiness, and nutrition. The foundation supported educational programs that specifically advanced the life sciences. It also sought to assure that America's youth had access to the basic building blocks of development: caring adults, a healthy start, safe and structured environments, effective education for marketable skills, and opportunities to serve their communities. See www.novartis.com.

58. See www.nadii.com/news.html.

59. See www.nadii.com/about.html.

60. See www.berkeley.edu/about_ucb/documents/history.html.

61. See www.cnr.berkeley.edu/index.php3?db=about_cnr&id=1.

62. Rausser G. Public/private alliances. *AgBio Forum* 1999; 2:5–10. Available from www.agbioforum.missouri.edu.

63. Rausser had taken a leave from Berkeley to serve as senior economist on the President's Council of Economic Advisors from 1986 to 1987 and as chief economist of the U.S. Agency for International Development from 1988 to 1990.

64. Tools are such things as gene maps, cell lines, DNA sequences, reagents, etc.

65. University technology transfer is the activity directed to the licensing of patented inventions and technologies developed by the faculty.

66. The purpose of public benefit research was to produce socially optimal technologies; the research would include studies to promote such things as sustainable agriculture, organic farming, environmental protection, access to advanced technology by third world countries, etc.

67. Rausser G, Just R. The governance structure of agricultural science and agricultural economics: A call to arms. *American Journal of Agricultural Economics* 1993; 75: 69–83.

68. See Note 62; Note 45, Rausser.

69. At U.C. Berkeley, if a faculty member was listed as an inventor on a university patent, one-third of the income obtained from licensing the rights to the patent went to that faculty member.

70. Petit CW. Germinating access; Berkeley department's big deal with firm aimed at speeding genetic finds to market. *U.S. News and World Report* 1998 Oct 26; p. 60.

71. Rodarmor W. Dangerous liaison? *California Monthly* 1998 Dec; p. 109. Available from www.alumni.berkeley.edu/monthly/monthly_index/dec_98/talk.html.

72. Epps C. UC should open its books on biotech deal. *San Francisco Chronicle* 1998 Oct 14; Sect A:20.

73. See www.gene-watch.org/programs/patents.html#food.

74. Burress C. UC finalizes pioneering research deal with biotech firm; pie tossers leave taste of protest. *San Francisco Chronicle* 1998 Nov 24; Sect A:17.

75. Rosset P, Moore M. Research alliance debated; deal benefits business, ignores UC's mission. *San Francisco Chronicle* 1998 Oct 23:Sect A:27.

7

Industry-Sponsored Clinical Research and the Use of Placebo Controls

The fundamental goal of any human drug study is to produce scientifically accurate and dependable data that can distinguish the effect of the drug or device from other influences, such as spontaneous change in the course of the disease, placebo effect, biased observation, or chance. These factors are important considerations for companies sponsoring drug research, because the Food and Drug Administration will not approve the marketing of drugs, biologics, or medical devices unless the applications contain data from studies designed to produce reliable data.[1] Thus, the FDA requires that studies provide "substantial evidence" that the drug is effective, established by "adequate and well-controlled investigations." According to the FDA, a fundamental element in an acceptable drug study is a design that permits a valid comparison of the study product with a "control" to provide a quantitative assessment of product effect. Generally, the following types of control are recognized by the FDA for drug studies:

1. Placebo concurrent control. The test drug is compared with a placebo—an inactive (and therefore presumably harmless) preparation designed to resemble the test drug as much as possible.[2]

2. Dose-comparison concurrent control. At least two doses of the drug are compared.

3. No-treatment concurrent control. When objective measurements of effectiveness are available and placebo effect is negligible, the test drug is compared with no treatment.

4. Active treatment concurrent control. The test drug is compared with known effective therapy; for example, when the condition treated is such that administration of placebo or no treatment would be contrary to the interest of the patient.

5. Historical control. The results of treatment with the test drug are compared with data collected in past studies of the natural history of the disease or of past treatment studies. Comparable patients or populations must be identified for these historical comparison studies to be valid. Because historical control populations usually cannot be as well assessed with respect to pertinent variables as can concurrent control populations, historical control designs are normally reserved for special circumstances. Examples include studies of diseases with high and predictable mortality (for example, certain malignancies) and studies in which the effect of the drug is self-evident (for example, general anesthetics, drug metabolism).[3]

Combinations of control elements can also be used in a study. The FDA has the authority to require certain drug study designs or to waive requirements, and will exercise this authority depending on the nature of the drug and disease in question, the need for quality scientific data, and the safety of subjects.[4] The same goes for medical devices and biologics. While regulations do not specify the type of study control required, the FDA will not approve a drug, biologic, or device based on studies lacking a control element, and most often placebo control has been considered the best form of control.

PLACEBO CONTROLS

The introduction of a placebo control in drug, biologic, and device studies came about from the appreciation of the placebo effect in the treatment of diseases.[5] Although physicians had been using inert treatments for patients for centuries when there were no other or no better treatments, the scientific investigation of the placebo effect began in earnest just after World War II when physician Henry Knowles Beecher observed an inexplicable decreased need for morphine among wounded soldiers awaiting evacuation at Anzio Beachhead. Beecher hypothesized that a physiologic effect, most likely driven by a mental process, had occurred in these soldiers that substituted for a drug effect.[6] This hypothesis explained why physicians often observed sick patients to respond to treatment for reasons that could not be attributed to a drug or other medical intervention. Over the years, physicians had noted that patients' health improved seemingly because they had a strong desire to get better, because the physician had prescribed a treatment with enthusiasm and encouraged the patient to be optimistic about the outcome, because patients trusted and wanted to please the doctor, because patients believed that the treatment would work, because getting any treatment seemed to lessen anxiety that contributed to symptoms, or for any number of other reasons. The operation of these effects meant that patients' health could improve without treatment or when an inert treatment (that is, the placebo) was given. However, these effects have been observed to be more powerful when the patients believed that an active therapy had been prescribed. Therefore, when physicians did not disclose to the patient that a placebo was being prescribed, the substance could often produce remarkable therapeutic benefits.

Subsequent research has resulted in the belief that the placebo effect occurs when a patient's beliefs, assumptions, and suggestibility influence behavior or translate into a biochemical effect.[7] Adverse effects can also be seen with the use of placebos. The placebo effect in medicine is well documented, and studies have shown that it is common for as much as 30 percent or more of patients to improve with placebo treatment, depending on the disease. Higher placebo responses are often seen in patients who are in pain, have other symptoms that are difficult to measure objectively (for example, fatigue, nausea, insomnia, stiffness, mental clarity, depression), or have diseases in which symptoms tend to fluctuate. In one analysis of 2,318 patients enrolled in nineteen studies of antidepressant drugs, the authors concluded that approximately one-half of the patient improvement was a placebo effect.[8] In the past, physicians might have used placebos when nothing else worked, to placate anxious patients, or when there were no available treatments for a particular disease. Although placebos are not often used in clinical practice today (most physicians prefer to be straightforward with their patients about what is being prescribed), the practice was justified in the past because placebos were harmless—and they improved patient well-being.[9]

It is easy to see therefore how the placebo effect can bias human drug studies. Without the use of a placebo control group, researchers might not be able to determine whether the effects of a test drug are "real" or a result of the placebo effect. For instance, in a clinical trial, the tendency for subjects to show improvement is probably fundamentally enhanced because of the added medical attention they are receiving or the fact that the placebo intervention creates an atmosphere of healing. Therefore, many human drug trials include at least two groups of subjects: one group receives active therapy and the other (the placebo control group) receives a "dummy" therapy in which the placebo looks exactly like the active product and is given under identical circumstances. Careful trial design requires that the two study groups be treated exactly the same in all respects except for the administration of active or placebo treatment, and the study drug is deemed effective only if it produces statistically valid superior results when compared with placebo treatment results.[10] Drug companies therefore often rely on the use of placebo controls because the resulting study data are considered trustworthy by physicians, and the FDA and companies can learn relatively early if a product lacks sufficient efficacy to justify continued development. For instance, Genentech stopped its costly trials of the cardiovascular drug VEGF (vascular endothelial growth factor), which had been shown in animals to enhance the development of blood vessels that could improve blood flow to damaged hearts, when data showed that study subjects could walk for longer periods of time while taking placebo than they could with either low or high doses of VEGF.[11] This finding was not as unusual as may be expected, because investigators had been observing for years a strong placebo effect in drug trials for many types of cardiovascular disease.[12]

Placebo-controlled drug and device trials are also desirable because they often produce fewer confounding variables, and studies can therefore be conducted more rapidly with smaller populations than clinical trials using active controls. Shorter clinical trials with fewer subjects can save time and money and put effective products on the market more quickly. Moreover, placebo controls are often cheaper to provide than active treatment controls, which typically must be purchased at full price.[13]

Placebo-controlled studies are usually considered the most scientifically rigorous if they are also "double-blinded" and "randomized" to further eliminate bias. Double-blinding a study means that neither the researcher nor the study subject knows if the subject is receiving active treatment or placebo. A subject with Parkinson disease who knows, for example, that he was given the active drug might tend to perceive a benefit (for example, less muscle rigidity), even when there might be no actual improvement. Conversely, the physicians who conduct the drug trial (and may expect or want the drug to work) could also be subject to bias. Knowledge on the part of a physician that a certain Parkinson disease subject received active treatment could prompt that physician to perceive a treatment effect (for example, the subject appeared to be walking steadier) when one did not exist. Therefore, standard scientific precaution calls for subjects and researchers to be "blind" as to which subjects received active treatment or placebo so that no one will be tempted, consciously or not, to bias the study with preconceived expectations.

Studies are randomized when study treatments (either active or placebo) are given to subjects in a random fashion to eliminate the possibility that external factors will influence the outcome. Randomization of treatments improves comparability between test groups and any control groups of pertinent variables such as gender, severity or duration of the disease, use of other therapy, or timing of administration. For instance, if only active drug is administered the first month of a trial and that month happens to have record high temperatures, a drug's effect on weakness caused by Parkinson disease may be subverted by the heat. External biasing factors are also controlled for when subjects who received active treatment are then "crossed over" to a control, and vice versa, in an attempt to eliminate bias caused by the timing of treatment or the variable nature of a disease.

Alternatives to a placebo control are often believed to produce less reliable study data. Use of a no-treatment control group can generate biased data when studying medical conditions strongly influenced by a placebo effect. Drugs in studies such as this tend to appear more beneficial than if compared to a placebo since subjects receiving no treatment do not expect to get better. Active treatment controls require that the study treatment be matched with a comparable treatment to show that the test product is equivalent or better. However, comparable treatment is sometimes not available, or, if it is, it is sufficiently different (for example, less safe, more effective, different side effects, different dosage form, different route of administration) as to raise questions about comparability or to prevent true "double-blindedness." Comparison to an active control also relies on the assumption that the active control is efficacious in its own right and better than placebo. With no prior well-designed placebo control studies on the active control product, this assumption cannot be tested and may not be true. The active control may also produce a significant placebo effect. These problems are recognized in the FDA regulations, which recommend that when an active control is used in a drug study, a placebo control be added: thus there will be more than two arms to a study.[14] Also, some common study problems, such as subjects' noncompliance with treatment, tend to diminish the difference between the two treatments, resulting in a bias in favor of finding that the test and active control products are equivalent.[15] For these reasons, an authoritative textbook on clinical drug trials states, "If a new drug has only been compared to an active control (without a placebo-controlled trial), this is not a convincing proof of efficacy (even if equivalence can be demonstrated)."[16] For initial FDA approval, data comparing the investigational product to active control treatments are not required; companies need only show that their product by itself is sufficiently safe and effective for marketing. If comparison trials were required, it is not only likely that some new products would fail approval, but the company also would run the risk of spending its own money to show that a competitor's product was better. Consequently, companies often prefer to postpone conducting comparative studies until competitive data are needed for business reasons. Finally, historical controls are difficult to interpret because the data are not collected concurrently, leaving open the possibility that conditions in the past were different in a way that influences the data.[17]

ETHICAL ISSUES IN PLACEBO-CONTROLLED STUDIES

Taking all of these factors into account, the "gold standard" well-controlled, scientifically valid clinical trial is usually double-blind, placebo-controlled, randomized, and sometimes cross-over in design.[18] Despite their scientific prominence, however, placebo-controlled trials have generated controversy.[19] From an ethics and science policy standpoint, many have argued that the relevant question to patients is not whether the drug is better than placebo but whether it is better than standard treatment. What good is it, the argument goes, to put a product on the market that is better than placebo but is in fact inferior to existing treatments? Bioethicists and patient advocacy groups also argue that the use of placebos in a medical product study is almost always contrary to the immediate interests of the study patients. Viewed in this light, active treatment controls are preferred since no study subject goes without treatment —the study group receives a potentially effective treatment and the control group receives treatment with established effectiveness. According to a leading biomedical ethicist, "When an effective treatment already exists, the use of placebos is unacceptable. Ethically, it is justifiable to test a new therapy that promises some advantage (in efficacy, side-effects, cost, etc.) over the existing treatment, but not at the cost of withholding the existing treatment from the control group."[20] Reasoning further, only when no other treatment exists is it acceptable to show that a medical product "is better than nothing" by using a placebo control group.

Others acknowledge this problem but counter that the use of placebos is justified so long as potential study subjects are told in advance that they may not receive active product, since subjects make an autonomous choice of whether to participate in the study. According to the 1995 American Medical Association's Council on Ethical and Judicial Affairs, "Ensuring rigorous adherence to the principle of informed consent is perhaps the best possible solution to the ethical difficulties associated with using a placebo control."[21] Nevertheless, ethicists have noted that informed consent cannot be used to justify an inappropriate trial design that exposes subjects to an unreasonable risk of harm.[22] Some patients are not able to make an autonomous choice since they cannot fully appreciate the placebo concept or the full magnitude of potential harm in a study. For instance, studies have found that significantly high proportions of patients enrolled in clinical trials of psychotropic drugs (that is, patients with mental disorders) do not understand placebo control or randomization concepts.[23] Uneducated patients can face the same challenge. Patients, grateful for the medical care received, may enroll in studies simply to please their physician. Other patients, desperate for any treatment, may enroll in a placebo-controlled trial that offers at least some chance that they will not be randomized to the placebo group and will receive the only possibly beneficial treatment in existence. The vulnerability of such patients creates doubts that free, informed decisions to join a study are always present. Because of these problems, FDA regulations require institutional review boards to make independent findings and, regardless of whether patients would consent, approve only studies where the risks are minimized and considered reasonable in light of potential benefits.[24]

Another fundamental argument against the use of placebos challenges the notion that they are harmless. While this may be so for drug placebos per se, the researcher may need to stop subjects' current treatment (a phase of the research called "wash out") to rid the body of any confounding influence of other drugs. Subjects in the wash-out period or who receive only placebos during the study can experience significant deterioration in their health that researchers may not be able to detect before permanent harm is done.

A second possible harm exists if the placebo can cause injury on its own. Such is the case with placebo-controlled surgery trials, where the control group receives placebo or "sham" surgery in which all aspects of the surgery (including anesthesia and surgical incision) are performed except for the vital aspect under consideration. Proponents of placebo-controlled surgical studies have argued that the same kind of statistical rigor is required to establish the efficacy and safety of surgeries as for drugs. Several examples have often been cited as evidence that supposedly "proven" surgical treatments, when subjected to a placebo-controlled study, were shown to be no better than placebo surgery at producing positive effects. These examples included internal mammary artery ligation for angina, bloodletting, routine tonsillectomy, and routine circumcision.[25] Suspicions existed that if other surgical procedures were tested against placebo surgeries, many more would fail, since the few existing trials had shown that just the act of performing some kind of surgery could be curative in itself. Proponents argued further that weeding out ineffective surgeries could spare future patients from costly, unnecessary, or harmful procedures.[26] As a 1994 review on placebo surgery published in the British medical journal the *Lancet* stated, "New technical advances must be assessed carefully. For surgical procedures, as for drugs, the placebo effect must always be taken into account if any assessment is to be objective."[27]

In practice, however, placebo-controlled surgical trials are rare. Surgeons, while recognizing the value of the trials, have balked at the risk—placebo surgeries are not as harmless as placebo drugs. Placebo surgeries require sophisticated surgical skills, and any surgery could be dangerous, with complications ranging from postoperative infection, excessive bleeding, and infection from blood transfusions to injury or death from general anesthesia or intraoperative mishaps. Subjecting patients to potentially serious complications without providing active treatment is untenable to many surgeons raised on the Hippocratic Oath to "prescribe regimen to the good of patients . . . and above all, do no harm," and trained that risks to study subjects should be minimized as much as possible. Many institutional review boards asked to approve surgical research studies have viewed the risks to the placebo group as unreasonable, despite full informed consent.[28]

CHANGING VIEWS ON PLACEBO CONTROLS

Opinions on the placebo control issue became intense during the AIDS crisis. In the United States, AIDS activists and others protested drug company decisions to test experimental anti-AIDS drugs against placebos. The objections were raised by two different groups: AIDS activists, and biomedical ethicists and researchers. AIDS activists objected that since there were no effective treatments available to combat AIDS directly, it was cruel to give placebos to desperately ill AIDS subjects when a potentially efficacious investigational treatment was being given to the other half of the study subjects.[29] This standard objection to the use of research placebos was renewed by biomedical ethicists and researchers, who knew that industry-sponsored Phase III clinical studies occurred only after the company and the FDA were satisfied that the drug had shown sufficient safety and efficacy in earlier trials to justify giving it to a large study population of sick people. Since companies sponsored only those studies that were likely to produce positive results, ethicists argued that the "uncertainty principle" was violated. Under this ethical research principle, a placebo-controlled trial was justifiable only if the researcher and the expert medical community at large were equally uncertain about whether the test product was better than, equal to, or worse than placebo. Biomedical ethicists and some researchers had long complained that industry-sponsored research was often conducted without this necessary state of equipoise.[30] The consequence of ignoring the uncertainty principle was that the subjects who received placebo were denied access to a probably beneficial medical product. Continued experience and research, however, had shown that these problems existed less often than was thought. For instance, years after first objecting to AIDS drug studies, the AIDS patient community acknowledged that corporate insistence on rigorous testing was more beneficial in the long run, since many anecdotally promising new drugs were taken by AIDS patients and only later shown to be useless.[31] Also, biostatistical analyses of industry-sponsored clinical trials were inconclusive about whether these trials generally adhered to the uncertainty principle.[32]

INTERNATIONAL DEBATES

Another debate about the use of placebos in clinical drug trials occurred in the mid-1990s after the publication of sixteen studies on the efficacy of the drug AZT in preventing the transmission of HIV infection from a pregnant woman to her newborn.[33] The studies were sponsored by the U.S. Centers for Disease Control, the NIH, local country governments, and the United Nations AIDS Program and were carried out in eleven impoverished developing countries, mostly in Africa, some in Thailand. Women in these countries were given a shorter and less expensive anti-HIV treatment regimen than was used effectively in Western countries. The studies, which were double-blind and placebo controlled, ultimately determined that the new treatment protocol was better than no treatment but not as effective in preventing infant infection as was the full Western treatment. According to the researchers, the use of placebos was justified because the study women had no access to prenatal care and, if they

did, could not afford (nor could their countries afford) the drug as it was prescribed in the West. Thus, no study women were denied access to any locally
available treatment. The studies offered at least some chance that these women
would receive active treatment.[34]

Heated debates among medical professionals and bioethicists followed publication of the study results.[35] The major objections included the exploitative nature of the research and doubts about whether there was full informed consent
(see the introduction to the VaxGen case study in Chapter 9). But the primary
ethical objections focused on the use of placebos rather than an active treatment
group that received the full and effective Western treatment regimen.

Beginning in 1998, and partly in response to the African AZT study controversy, the American Medical Association and the World Medical Association began work on a revision of the Declaration of Helsinki, a foundational
international guideline for ethical requirements of clinical research.[36] These
modifications included provisions about the use of placebo controls in human
research. The initial declaration was ambiguous about the use of placebo controls, and it was difficult for medical association members to agree on the new
proposed revisions. In October 2000, after substantial and lengthy debates and
several varied proposals, the ultimate revision stated outright that investigational treatments were to be compared to the best available treatments and
that placebos could be used only when there were no other therapies available
for comparison.[37] This change was intended to reflect a widespread interest by
World Medical Association members to place subject safety over concerns
about data certainty. According to country reports submitted at the time of the
contemplated revision, research ethics committees in other countries (United
Kingdom, Germany, Switzerland, New Zealand, France, Spain, and Portugal)
tended to allow only limited use of placebo controls in human studies. These
limitations included restrictions on the use of placebo controls to cases where
the target disease was minor, where standard treatment for the disease was not
available, where effective treatments were not denied to the subject, where the
underlying medical condition would not be prolonged or aggravated, or where
the risk of injury was low. France rejected outright the use of double-blind,
placebo-controlled clinical trials on the conviction that true informed consent
could not be obtained from the subject if neither the subject nor the researcher
knew who would receive the placebo. In Japan, researchers risked civil and
criminal liability if they failed to limit the use of placebo controls to studies of
diseases for which either no standard treatment existed or no harm to the patient was anticipated.

It was not surprising that, given the views within various countries, consensus on the issue was difficult to achieve. By the end of the 1990s, European and international legal bodies (such as the European Agency for Evaluation of Medicinal Products and the International Conference on Harmonization, which was attempting to harmonize pharmaceutical regulation in the United States, Europe, and Japan) had not come to any final conclusions about the appropriate use of placebo controls in human medical product research.[38]

The Declaration of Helsinki revision, however, put the World Medical Association at odds with the ethical guidelines of the American Medical Association and with the FDA regulations and practice, which continued to favor the use of placebo controls in clinical trials. The AMA did recommend that researchers using placebos (1) be extremely thorough in obtaining informed consent from patients in such trials, (2) carefully evaluate study protocols to determine whether placebo controls are necessary or whether alternative study designs would be appropriate, and (3) minimize the time patients are given placebos, and monitor the study and terminate it early when indicated by positive or negative results. Further, the AMA advised that placebo controls would generally not be appropriate where research involved conditions causing death, irreversible damage, or severe or painful symptoms, and that there are situations where placebo controls cannot be ethically justified. The use of placebo controls can more easily be justified, however, where standard therapies are attended by severe side effects.[39]

CONCLUSION

The FDA, in its Code of Federal Regulations governing the determination of adequate and well-controlled drug studies, continues to endorse the use of placebo controls and will accept active-control studies "where the condition treated is such that administration of placebo or no treatment would be contrary to the interest of the patient."[40] What is deemed contrary to the interest of patients is not specified. In speeches and medical publications, FDA officials have also made it clear that they highly value the surety provided by placebo-controlled trials and that active-control trials do not reliably allow the FDA to distinguish between active and inactive treatments.[41]

In such a climate, disagreements about the use of placebos in medical product studies are difficult to resolve. At the time of the following Genzyme case study events, there was no settled consensus about how to balance the need for scientific validity and human subject protection nor how to satisfy the need for either. Guidance terms such as "adequate and well-controlled study," "comparable control treatment," "best interest of the patient," and "unreasonable risk of harm" remained subject to different interpretations. Between the beliefs that it is irresponsible to bypass the scientific rigor provided by placebo controls, that placebo-controlled trials best meet the interests of medical science companies, and that patient interests should not be sacrificed to the goal of study design purity, companies have to engage in a careful balancing act.

Case Study

Genzyme Tissue Repair and the NeuroCell-PD Clinical Trials[42]

September 1997: Tim Surgenor, president of Genzyme Tissue Repair (GTR), a division of Genzyme Corporation, sat back in his chair and watched the autumn leaves starting to fall outside his office in Cambridge, Massachusetts. Favorable Phase I clinical trial results, an important first step in gaining approval from the Food and Drug Administration, had just been announced for Neuro-Cell™-PD. The ground-breaking technology behind this product, developed by Diacrin, Inc., and sponsored by GTR, used fetal "pig cell" neural transplants to treat Parkinson disease. Surgenor was eager to get NeuroCell-PD to market as quickly as possible, and there was tremendous excitement in his division over this new product. Surgenor knew, though, that the path to getting Neuro-Cell-PD approved might be difficult to navigate. Genzyme, an innovative biotechnology company, had often entered uncharted territories in the past and had set precedents in medical research. It was for this reason that Diacrin had decided in 1996 to enter a partnership with Genzyme. Surgenor believed that, in this situation, controversy would likely center on whether GTR would use what some were calling "sham" surgery as a placebo control in its Phase II trials of NeuroCell-PD in Parkinson disease patients, trials intended to demonstrate both the efficacy and safety of the procedure. In sham surgery, a segment of patients in a study would undergo the same aspects of the surgery experience as those receiving the experimental treatment, except that no fetal pig cells—the experimental treatment—would be given.

The decision regarding how to proceed would not be easy for Surgenor to make. A number of different players were involved, each with a point of view that would need to be addressed to gain approval and market acceptance for the treatment. The FDA generally viewed placebo-controlled data as the gold standard for demonstrating that investigational products were safe and efficacious. At the same time, several institutional review boards and physicians would surely oppose sham surgery because of its inherent risks to study patients. And yet, Surgenor believed, these same physicians would want to review placebo-controlled data before they would believe that the product was efficacious. Given the disparity of views, there would have to be a great deal of discussion and negotiation to reach acceptable solutions. Surgenor hoped that ultimately his team would make the "right" decision—right for subjects and patients, right for the physicians who would prescribe and use NeuroCell-PD, and right for GTR and Diacrin, Inc.

PARKINSON DISEASE AND THE NEED FOR NEW TREATMENTS

Parkinson disease (PD) is a neuro-degenerative disorder characterized by a progressive loss of motor (muscle) control. Parkinson patients experience debilitating symptoms that usually start with tremors and a slowness in muscle movement. These symptoms spread to more muscles, and patients typically develop muscle rigidity, a "masked" face (in which the patient cannot move facial muscles), loss of speech control, short and shuffling gait, loss of postural reflexes, unsteadiness, and festination (the need to walk faster and faster to avoid falling over). The disease then worsens, resulting in abnormal and tortured postures, falls, and gait abnormalities that eventually confine the patient to a wheelchair. Swallowing problems can result in choking, making the act of eating a slow and difficult process. Although these motor phenomena constitute the major group of symptoms, there are also nonmotor disturbances that adversely affect the ability to think and alter psychiatric well-being. Some patients develop personality changes that cause them to become more passive, dependent, and fearful. With such psychiatric changes, many people fail to function, and depression is not uncommon. Although disease progression varies, typically it takes more than five years before significant disability occurs, and patients often fear what they know is coming. Parkinson disease is not fatal on its own, but a patient's life span is shortened by the consequences of the disabilities, such as aspiration pneumonia from swallowing problems. Parkinson disease patients are also more prone to other types of infections when they become wheelchair-bound.[43]

Parkinson disease is a costly illness, in both medical and social terms. The economic burden to society has been estimated to be as high as $25 billion per year. This figure is based on a study that estimated the total cost of the disease (medical expenses plus associated social costs: loss of worker productivity and earnings by both the patient and family caregiver) to be $25,000 per patient annually. With the steady increase in the population of elderly individuals, the incidence of the disease and its associated costs and burdens are expected to rise.[44]

It is generally agreed that the symptoms of Parkinson disease are caused by a loss of neurons in the substantia nigra pars compacta area of the brain. This loss leads to decreased production of a chemical called dopamine. Along with imbalances in other brain chemicals, Parkinson disease involves a disorder in the transmission of neurological signals in the brain. The precise cause of Parkinson disease is still not understood; thus there are no curative therapies, that is, no therapy can prevent the underlying brain cell degeneration. Current treatments only relieve symptoms, and, although initially effective, over time medications become less effective.

In 1997, the most popular drug treatment for Parkinson disease was levodopa (brand name Sinemet®), a drug that increases dopamine levels in the brain. Unfortunately, levodopa can lose its efficacy within a few years of initial dosing, during which time the underlying brain cell degeneration continues. Many other drugs were available and prescribed at the time, but none provided consistent or lasting benefit. Levodopa therapy is also associated with many side effects, including psychiatric problems, involuntary muscle movements, and clinical fluctuations (seen in about 50 percent of patients after five years of therapy). The most common form of clinical fluctuation is a wearing-off effect, characterized by end-of-dose deterioration. With prolonged treatment, the duration of benefit from a levodopa dose could be as short as one to two hours. Because of the ineffectiveness and toxicity of existing treatments, intensive efforts were underway by medical researchers to discover alternative approaches to ameliorating this debilitating and frightening disease.[45]

Since the 1980s, doctors had been cautiously testing a new experimental treatment involving the surgical transplantation of fetal dopamine-producing brain cells into the brains of Parkinson patients.[46] Fetal cells were believed to be a promising treatment because their early stage of development allows them to adapt to new environments and regenerate, which adult's cells could not do. In addition, fetal cells are less likely to stimulate rejection by the recipient's immune system. Initially, the fetal cells were derived from aborted human fetuses, and it took six to twelve fetuses to supply enough of the cells to treat one

Parkinson patient. Most of these fetal cell trials enrolled only a few subjects, and although the trial results were variable, some showed promising clinical effects in treated subjects. With refined techniques, research reports kept appearing showing that restoration of motor function could last for months to years after transplantation. There were several problems, however, with this form of treatment. Aborted human fetuses were difficult to collect and were often in short supply, the aborted material could harbor infectious agents, and, if they were a result of spontaneous abortion, could be defective in some way. In addition, there were many ethical concerns about the use of this tissue, particularly from those in the antiabortion movement and from those with a general concern about the mistreatment of fetal remains.[47]

Because of these difficulties, some researchers were exploring the use of animals as a source of fetal cells for the treatment of Parkinson disease. While free from some of the restraints associated with human fetal cells, the use of animal cells raised other issues. It had been determined that pig fetal cells were better suited for this type of use, since pigs were relatively easy to raise and had large litter sizes and short gestation periods.[48] However, animal cells were more likely to be rejected by humans (human cells recognize pig cells as foreign and attack them). It was also known that pigs could carry undetectable viruses or viruslike organisms embedded in their DNA that might infect and cause disease in human recipients, sometimes years later.[49] Both of these problems had to be solved before fetal animal cells could be used for human therapy. One company, Diacrin, Inc., had made significant progress in developing a promising pig fetal cell therapy product for Parkinson disease.

DIACRIN, INC., GENZYME TISSUE REPAIR, AND THE DEVELOPMENT OF NEUROCELL-PD

Diacrin, a small biotechnology company in Charlestown, Massachusetts, was founded in 1989 with the goal of developing proprietary platform technology for the production, harvesting, and transplantation of pig cells into humans. These cell transplantations might effectively treat diseases that are characterized by human cell dysfunction or cell death and for which current therapies are inadequate and human donor cells not easily available. With no products on the market in 1996, Diacrin was focusing its efforts on developing cell types for transplantation in the treatment of Parkinson disease, Huntington's disease, focal epilepsy, and cognitive disorders. The company was developing hepatocytes (liver cells) for the treatment of familial hypercholesterolemia, cardiac myocytes (heart muscle cells) for the treatment of cardiac disease, and pancreatic islet cells for the treatment of diabetes. Of these, the cell transplant product for Parkinson disease was the furthest along in 1996.

At that time, Diacrin had already succeeded in removing one significant roadblock in the treatment of Parkinson disease: cell rejection. The company had licensed technology from the Massachusetts General Hospital for suppression of immune rejection.[50] Animal studies had shown that grafts of fetal pig neural cells could integrate into the brain tissue of the recipient and restore damaged neural circuitry. Phase I safety trials in humans had begun in March 1995. In August 1996, the FDA, which has regulatory oversight for animal-to-human transplant products (called xenotransplant products), developed draft guidelines to protect against human infections from transplanted animal tissue.[51] To ensure that they minimized the risk of viral infection, the Diacrin scientists followed these guidelines in selecting and raising the donor pigs, but there was insufficient experience to ensure that the draft guidelines were effective in preventing the risk of zoonotic infection in human recipients or those whom they might subsequently infect. Because some pathogens (like HIV or the prion that causes Mad Cow Disease) that had infected humans from animal sources had long latency periods before symptoms appeared, infected tissue recipients might harbor the virus and infect others for years before the infection was discovered.[52] To compound the problem, no reliable tests were available to detect all of the potential pig pathogens that might infect humans.[53] It was likely that the FDA approval process would be very complicated with such a novel product that had unknown and maybe unknowable risks. Diacrin was inexperienced in dealing with the regulatory and clinical research processes required to gain approval to take a product to market. To successfully commercialize its Parkinson disease product, it looked for a corporate partner, skilled in navigating the regulatory process, and found one in its regional neighbor, Genzyme.

GENZYME

Genzyme Corporation, a biotechnology and health-care products company that describes itself as focused on developing innovative products and services for major unmet medical needs, was founded in 1981 and has been public since 1986. In 1997, Genzyme Corporation had three divisions, each with its own common stock intended to reflect the divisions' separate value and costs and to allow the performance of each unit to be tracked individually. Genzyme

General, the oldest and biggest division, develops and markets a large variety of products and services: therapeutic products (including those made from recombinant DNA processes), gene therapies, diagnostic testing kits and genetic diagnostic services, biomaterials and surgical products, and specialty pharmaceutical components. In 1997, the second division, Genzyme Tissue Repair, was developing biological products for the treatment of cartilage damage, severe burns, chronic skin ulcers, and neurological disorders. Genzyme Molecular Oncology was created to develop molecular approaches to cancer diagnosis and therapy through genomics, gene therapy, and genetic diagnostics, and this division also had a small-molecule combinatorial chemistry drug discovery program.[54] The assets of Genzyme Corporation were distributed among these divisions, but these divisions did not mix or mingle assets. For tax purposes, any division that made money could use the losses of another division as an offset. This corporate structure was unique within the biotechnology industry at the time and gave Genzyme great flexibility in managing its various businesses. According to Elliott Hillback, Genzyme's senior vice president for corporate affairs, the main advantages of this structure are that it:

- Allows the smaller units to spend more on R&D in early years without negatively affecting general division profitability
- Provides freedom for each business to maintain a unique focus
- Creates efficiency of shared resources in areas such as capital formation, research and development, clinical and regulatory affairs, and manufacturing
- Offers opportunities for shareholders to invest selectively in the businesses of interest
- Allows each business to raise capital separately
- Provides greater opportunity to provide the management of each division with incentives to increase shareholder value[55]

Genzyme was recognized as one of the world's top five biotechnology companies, with 1997 revenues of $530 million and a market capitalization close to $3 billion (see Table 7.1). The company had gained this distinction over the preceding decade under the leadership of Henri Termeer, who brought an unorthodox approach and a pride in innovation that soon filtered down through the company. The company was known for its ability to develop novel products, successfully compete in tough markets, and take risks—especially with orphan products that other companies avoided.[56]

Perhaps most representative of Termeer's and Genzyme's bold and innovative approach is what they did with Ceredase® and Cerezyme®, two drugs used to treat a very rare genetic enzyme deficiency disorder called Gaucher's disease. This disease was seriously debilitating, sometimes fatal, and until Genzyme introduced new drug products, there were no safe and effective treatments for the disease.[57] Genzyme General, which manufactured the drug, estimated that there were only five thousand Gaucher's disease patients in the world. Despite the low numbers, Genzyme developed the treatment and entered the market. The company obtained orphan drug status for the product and charged patients about $170,000 a year for the treatment. In 1996, sales of Ceredase totaled $264.6 million and were growing. Genzyme's ability to make Ceredase a money-maker was indicative of the company's lack of fear in developing products and entering markets that other companies would not touch. Sales of its Gaucher's disease drugs represented 62 percent of consolidated product sales in 1996. Genzyme Corporation depended heavily on the sale of these two drugs to sustain its other operations.

Genzyme was widely considered to be a well-managed company. For four consecutive years the *Wall Street Transcript* had hailed Henri Termeer as an industry executive committed to shareholder value. Termeer was named Entrepreneur of the Year by Merrill Lynch and Ernst & Young in 1992 for his achievements in establishing an innovative, successful, and growing business. In 1995, *Success Magazine* named him Renegade of the Year, honoring business leaders whose "guts and vision" had paid off for their companies.[58]

Genzyme had also earned a reputation for responsible corporate citizenship, an extension of Henri Termeer's personal interest in public concerns. Termeer had been recognized with the Torch of Liberty Award for his leadership in human rights and for promoting understanding among people of diverse religious, ethnic, and racial backgrounds. At Genzyme, he had been instrumental in establishing college education scholarships for youth, summer internship programs, and a matching grant initiative with the Tactical Training Initiative Program, which retrained displaced workers for manufacturing positions in the biotechnology industry.[59]

GENZYME TISSUE REPAIR

Led by Tim Surgenor, GTR was focused on developing, manufacturing, and marketing technologically advanced products for the treatment and prevention of serious tissue damage. Its essential core technologies included autologous cell processing, therapeutic protein development, and biomaterials. The GTR division of Genzyme Corporation was formed in December of 1994 with the acquisition of BioSurface Technology.

In March of 1995, GTR went to market with its principal product, Carticel® (autologous cultured chondrocytes), which was used to treat damaged knee cartilage. To make this novel product, GTR employed a proprietary process to harvest and grow a patient's own (autologous) cartilage cells, which were then surgically implanted into the patient's damaged knee. In addition to cartilage cell processing, GTR trained orthopedic surgeons to harvest cartilage and implant its product, collected and analyzed surgical outcomes data, and assisted physicians and patients in obtaining reimbursements from third-party payers for the product and the surgical procedure.[60] GTR was counting on Carticel sales and services for its future success but the marketing of the product was initially complicated.[61] At the time Carticel was first marketed, the FDA regulations dealing specifically with autologous tissue products and services were not yet final, although the company knew that it would have to comply with new and unknown regulations by late 1997. In August 1997, the FDA granted GTR a biologics license under the new regulations; this license allowed the company to continue marketing Carticel. GTR acquired some breathing room with this FDA decision, since it would take other companies possibly eight years to meet the new regulatory requirements to obtain a biologics license. The successful commercialization of Carticel and its related services would also depend heavily on GTR's ability to obtain approval for reimbursement from public and private medical insurers. These approvals were slow in coming, and by 1997 the company was still struggling to improve reimbursements (see Table 7.1, p. 227, for company financial information).

Diacrin chose GTR as a partner to further develop and market the Neuro-Cell products because of GTR's expertise with cell and tissue therapies, its proven ability to get products to market, and its corporate backing. In September 1996, GTR and Diacrin established Diacrin/Genzyme LLC, a joint venture to develop NeuroCell cell therapies for the treatment of Parkinson and Huntington's diseases. Under the terms of this joint venture, GTR would provide 80 percent of the next $50 million in funding for the two products; after that, all costs would be shared equally. The joint venture planned to manufacture the products, and GTR would provide sales and marketing services on a cost-reimbursement basis. Profits from the joint venture would be shared equally. Genzyme Corporation agreed to allocate up to $20 million in cash from its general division in exchange for GTR stock allocated to Genzyme General.[62] To launch the joint venture, Genzyme General provided $1.9 million in cash, and in December 1996, GTR borrowed $18.0 million under Genzyme's $225.0 million revolving credit facility to fund the operations of Diacrin/Genzyme LLC. On February 27, 1997, GTR raised $13 million through the private placement with an institutional investor of a 5 percent convertible note due February 27, 2000. For both companies, the NeuroCell products represented a significant investment. NeuroCell-PD would involve the most expensive clinical trials of any product Genzyme had yet conducted, and Diacrin's very survival rested heavily on its success. NeuroCell-PD had the potential to revolutionize the treatment of Parkinson disease, so a great deal was at stake, and both sides entered into the agreement with a tremendous sense of excitement and hope.

Genzyme's research had revealed that Parkinson disease was a sizeable market; the disease is among the most common seen in clinical medical practice in patients over fifty. At the time, it was estimated that approximately five hundred thousand people in the United States had Parkinson disease, and fifty thousand new cases were diagnosed each year. GTR decided that it would seek approval to market NeuroCell-PD for the over one hundred thousand patients who had reached the later stages of disease for which the current therapies provided little benefit.[63] This way, the company could take advantage of the orphan drug protections and have a clear shot at the market. Although medical payer reimbursement would be a hurdle, GTR planned to emphasize the cost-saving potential of NeuroCell-PD: arresting the degeneration from the disease would save costs of care, including medical expenses and nursing home care, which for Parkinson patients in the United States was estimated to be between $6,000 to $9,400 per patient per year.[64]

Tim Surgenor knew that the Parkinson disease market had attracted a number of new biotechnology competitors who were attempting to develop novel therapies to fill the therapeutic gap. Although years behind Genzyme, the privately held NeuralStem Biopharmaceuticals in Maryland was developing a fetal human neural stem-cell therapy for Parkinson that, if successful, would directly compete with Genzyme. Though production of these cells required access to aborted human fetuses, NeuralStem's cell culture technology had dramatically reduced the number of fetuses needed—from eight to twelve fetuses for each patient down to one fetus for tens of thousands of Parkinson patients.[65] Other experimental therapies under development for Parkinson disease included surgical destruction of certain portions of the brain (pallidotomy), implantation of stimulating electrodes ("deep brain stimulation"), gene therapy, the use of growth factors, and neuro-protectant therapy. All of these therapies were in early-stage development and were unproven. Even with some competition, Surgenor and his team believed that NeuroCell-PD could be successful with a segment of the Parkinson market. GTR was therefore in a unique position to produce the first cell therapy for patients, which would confer a huge business advantage.

PHASE I SAFETY TRIALS OF NEUROCELL-PD

The first transplant surgery of the Phase I clinical trials for NeuroCell-PD was performed in April 1995.[66] Eleven more followed over the next eighteen months. These trials were conducted at the Boston University Medical Center and the Lahey-Hitchcock Clinic (also in the Boston area).

For each of these transplants, company technicians would kill one artificially inseminated pig that had been pregnant exactly twenty-seven days with multiple fetuses. These fetal pigs were then surgically removed. This method of retrieving the fetal pigs was used to prevent any infections from developing in the fetal pig or its brain tissue. The brains of six to seven pig fetuses were used to gather twelve million dopamine-producing cells, enough for one subject. In these Phase I safety studies, the biggest concerns were rejection of the cells by the immune system or the risk of viral infections passed on from the pig cells. To help avoid rejection of the transplant, half of the subjects received the drug cyclosporine to suppress the immune system. The other half received pig cells that were treated prior to transplant using the antirejection masking technology from the Massachusetts General Hospital, so that the patient's immune system would not recognize the pig cells as foreign and attack them. The most advanced tests available were used to test for the presence of animal viruses in the extracted cells. Once the cells had been tested and treated, they were shipped to the research hospital, and less than seventy-two hours later, they were transplanted into the brain of one of the study subjects.[67]

The twelve subjects recruited for these safety studies were patients with moderate-to-severe Parkinson disease. One subject who volunteered in 1996 was Jim Finn, a forty-eight-year-old man who had had Parkinson disease for seventeen years. He kept an on-line diary of his experience with the Neuro-Cell-PD safety study.[68] In one early entry, he said, "After 15 years of dealing with Parkinson, it was obvious that I was entering the 'end stage' of this hideous disease. [My decision to participate in the trial] was an act of desperation. . . . I was to the point of committing suicide. I had to crawl on my hands and knees from room to room. I couldn't button a button on my shirt. I couldn't cut the food on my plate." Finn told a reporter that his fatigue was so profound that he slept nearly eighteen hours each day. His limbs shook uncontrollably, he had lost the use of his hands, and his speech was often unintelligible.[69] Of his experience with the existing medications, Finn said in his diary, "The only one that is of any use (and that has become very limited) is Sinemet. And even that is highly unpredictable with severe 'on/off' performance. Eldepryl, while it did provide some relief, had to be stopped because of horrible side-effects (sudden projectile vomiting)."[70]

Finn's motivation to join the NeuroCell-PD safety study came from the desperation caused by his ruinous disease. Yet his after-the-fact accounts of the procedures required for the trial were remarkably upbeat. Finn had more complaints about the pretrial work-up, in which he had to endure long-distance travel to get to the research clinic for a battery of tests, there were weeks of delay, and he suffered during the special brain scan needed to assess the degree to which Parkinson had damaged his brain tissue. This brain scan, he said, was "similar to an MRI but you will have your head tied down while you're in the machine for two and a half HOURS. To make matters worse, they will inject a substance into a vein in one arm while they draw blood out of an artery on the other. This will take place after you've been without medication for eight to twelve hours and without food for at least that long. I had a bad reaction to some pre-scan pills; severe diarrhea and blacking-out. At the end of that day I was a complete wreck." Finn knew that this scan would be repeated periodically after the cell implants, and he was not happy about this.

In his diary, Finn described the cell implant procedure, which involved the administration of a relaxing drug followed by local anesthesia to the head. Once these drugs took effect, a stereotactic metal frame was bolted onto his head to mark and maintain positions where the cells would be injected. The frame was attached at four points with aluminum screws that kept the frame in place by pressure on his skull. The areas where the screws contacted the skin, which tended to get cut and swollen, were numbed by the local anesthetic. Burr holes were then drilled through his skull at three sites on one side of the brain, located just below the part of the cortex where Parkinson disease was doing its damage. The twelve million treated fetal pig cells were injected into the brain through these burr holes.[71] The holes were then sewn up, and he was held at the hospital for postoperative care for twenty-four hours after surgery.

Excerpts from Finn's diary account contain his perceptions of what took place:

I was the eleventh person in the world to have this particular implant procedure. . . . I was given a sedative to help me relax and a shot of local anesthetic
to the skull. Yes, you are AWAKE during the operation! And you are fully
aware of what's going on. Every now and then I was asked to move my toes
or hands. Anyway, they opened up my skull and went in with the needle.
No, you don't feel anything at all! It's just amazing. About two hours later
they were finished and sewed me up. Naturally, I was a bit groggy when
I was returned to the post-operative holding area. But I felt fine and
HUNGRY. Eventually I was sent up to my room. The floor staff couldn't
believe that the doctor ordered my supper. I ate every scrap of it and slept
well that night. They gave me a couple of shots of codeine for my headache.
The next morning (are you ready for this?) I was discharged! It sounds
impossible, doesn't it? And I did well on the trip home. But it was short-
lived. I developed a headache unlike any before it. I very rarely get them;
this one was agony and lasted for nearly a week. Also, for several days I
couldn't keep food down. I was really very ill. Dr. S [the physician who
performed the procedure] called and said it would all pass. And it did. But
for a couple of weeks after the operation I was even more tired and weak
than usual.[72]

Study subjects were monitored on a continual basis after the surgery for
significant adverse events and neuropsychological damage. Although this was
a safety study, GTR did not want to lose the opportunity to collect efficacy
data as well, even though the dose of the cells given was only one-quarter of
what was to be used therapeutically. To determine if the small doses had any
effect on muscle movement, the subjects' ability to perform several different
types of movements was measured on a standardized scale and compared to
performance prior to surgery. The safety and efficacy data would be collected
on these subjects for up to five years. Additionally, all patients enrolled in the
study would be followed for safety (including tests for zoonoses) for the rest of
their lives.[73]

PHASE I TRIAL RESULTS

By December 1996, the last of the Phase I surgeries was complete, and the results began to generate considerable excitement in the Parkinson community.
The very first patient to undergo the surgery showed significant symptom improvement, approximately 50 percent of which persisted a year after surgery.[74]
In September of 1997, after fifteen months of tracking the Phase I subjects,

Genzyme and Diacrin finally announced that the NeuroCell-PD transplants had been well tolerated and that there was even evidence of clinical improvement in some patients.[75] Although adverse events were possible and had been seen in other trials where human fetal cells had been implanted, there were no reported significant adverse events, and preliminary data indicated that the patients showed an average improvement of 15 percent at six months after surgery on a standardized scale that measured a patient's ability to perform a variety of movements and timed movements.[76] These data were from ten patients, two of whom showed significant improvement (32 percent and 50 percent). These patients were tested when they were on their levodopa medication (their current therapy) and when its effects had worn off. The results were statistically significant compared to an evaluation that was taken prior to surgery. Two patients were excluded from the group data, as they had been too sick prior to surgery for data to be collected.[77] One of the patients died suddenly of an unrelated pulmonary embolism seven months after surgery. Following his death, his brain tissue was studied to see if any effects of the surgery could be detected. Histological studies indicated that some porcine cells survived, including a small number of dopamine cells. These results were published in the March 1997 issue of the prominent medical journal *Nature Medicine*.[78]

Jim Finn gave an account of his progress at six months:

> Here is some truly amazing news. Even WITHOUT medication for 15 hours, I was quite mobile and able to walk (rather well) from the parking lot to the doctor's offices; over 2 blocks away. I didn't even take my cane! Also, the staff was very pleased with the results of their examinations. Again, the word "amazed" must be used. They made note of such things as better walking, facial expression, voice, and the like. . . . I am certainly in better condition since the operation; that's been properly documented. Just as important; I FEEL better, too. However, I do NOT feel as though I've been cured. There are still problems to deal with. In my case, fatigue is at the top of the list. But, I see a glimmer of hope for the first time in the 17 years of dealing with Parkinson.[79]

After one year, Finn's dramatic results peaked and then held steady.[80] Finn also regained some of the deteriorated fine motor skills that had forced him to curtail his electronics repair business, and he resumed his sports car hobby. Genzyme wrote about Finn's experience in their 1997 annual report:

> Jim Finn was first diagnosed with Parkinson disease when he was 32 years old. Over the next 16 years, the symptoms progressively worsened. Jim

suffered from tremors, stiffness, and fatigue. Walking, bathing, cooking, talking, and handwriting all represented significant challenges. In recent years, the standard therapies for Parkinson disease provided only minimal relief. In 1996, Jim accepted his doctor's invitation to participate in a clinical trial for a new type of therapy, under development through a joint venture between Genzyme Tissue Repair and Diacrin Inc. This therapy, NeuroCell-PD, is based on the transplantation of fetal porcine neural cells to replace cells destroyed by Parkinson disease. A related product, NeuroCell-HD, is directed at Huntington's disease, also a devastating neurological disorder. Within two months after surgery, Jim began to experience noticeable progress. He had more energy and better coordination. Motor skill tests indicated a 50-percent improvement. Today, more than a year after surgery, Jim continues to improve.

The annual report also included photos of a dapper-looking Finn happily working on the engine of his TR 7 sports car.[80]

The promising Phase I trial results led the FDA to grant NeuroCell-PD orphan drug status in January 1997.[81] In the meantime, the joint venture had been preparing for the pivotal Phase II trials that would assess both the safety and efficacy of the product. Efficacy trials usually require that the experimental product be compared to a placebo to ensure that the data are reliable. While the concept of a placebo-controlled clinical trial was not new for experimental drugs, the fact that this clinical trial would involve brain surgery made the decision to proceed quite difficult.

NEUROCELL-PD AND A PLACEBO-CONTROLLED PHASE II TRIAL DESIGN

If GTR decided to proceed with placebo-controlled Phase II trials for Neuro-Cell-PD, the study procedures would differ markedly from Phase I. The number of cells delivered would be much higher—three pregnant pigs and twenty-six fetuses to produce forty-eight million dopamine-producing cells. The surgery would be more extensive—a total of twelve implantation sites through two burr hole sites on both sides of the skull. As a consequence, the procedure would take up to six hours and subjects would be put under general anesthesia instead of local anesthesia and sedation. The use of general anesthesia alone added an element of risk to the study.[82]

Both experimental and control groups would forgo their medications for various times during the trial and the pretesting. Both groups would undergo the same surgical procedure. They would be fitted with a stereotactic frame, bolted to the skull to guide the injections (similar to the procedure used in Phase I). The experimental group would then receive injections of porcine fetal neural cells through twelve needles passed into the brain through two drilled burr holes. The control group would remain under general anesthesia for roughly the same duration of time, would have two burr holes drilled partially through the skull but no needles would be passed into brain tissue and no material introduced into the brain. There had been considerable discussion about this placebo procedure among Genzyme employees. Some at the company favored a partial-thickness burr hole believing that drilling all the way through the skull was too risky. Others believed that the added risk was acceptably low and that, to adequately test for the placebo effect and remove doubts on the part of the FDA and physicians, partial thickness burr holes would be too weak a control procedure. This last view prevailed until late in the protocol development process, when it was decided that the risk of infection with full-thickness burr holes was too high.

After surgery, both groups would undergo treatment and evaluation by investigators not connected with the surgery. Experimental subjects would receive standard antirejection drugs and antibiotics. While control subjects would receive a fake antirejection drug pill, it turned out to be impossible to make antibiotic pills that looked, smelled, and tasted like real antibiotic pills. Therefore, to avoid unblinding of clinical investigators and subjects (which would introduce a risk of bias), control subjects would also receive real antibiotics for the first several months. As a result of participation, it was possible that subjects in this trial might be excluded from future research studies of other promising Parkinson therapies. The subjects who received active treatment would be followed for the rest of their lives and tested for the presence of zoonotic infections.

The subjects would be informed of all of the anticipated risks involved in the study, including the risks from taking the postprocedure antibiotic, the risks of lifelong antirejection medication, and the unknown risks associated with zoonotic infections.[83] The benefits to the study subjects assigned to a placebo control group (or "imitation surgery" group) included receiving the thorough pretest medical work-up at no cost and being spared the risks associated with cell transplant if it proved to be unsafe or ineffective. At the end of the study, subjects would be told whether they had received active or placebo treatment and, if the fetal cell treatment proved to be safe and effective, those in the placebo group would be offered free fetal-tissue transplant.

CONSIDERATIONS ON THE USE OF A
PLACEBO CONTROL GROUP

Some reports in the scientific literature of fetal cell therapy studies in Parkinson disease patients suggested that placebo control was not necessary to assess the efficacy of this experimental treatment. In these "open label" studies that used no placebos, the researchers concluded that it was unlikely that benefits observed following cell transplants were solely due to a placebo effect, since benefits were not detected immediately and determinations of clinical improvements were based on tracking brain function on brain scans. Also, in some cases, clinical improvement was so robust that it seemed unlikely that the degree of improvement could be caused either by a placebo or by the "natural history" or fluctuation of the disease. Also, some researchers saw improvement primarily on the opposite side of the patient following a unilateral transplant. Researchers believed that a strong placebo effect would have produced none of these findings.[84] Still other surgeons believed placebo-controlled surgical trials were not reliable because of differences in the skills of individual surgeons and because of the confounding effect of increasing experience in performing the procedure.[85]

A placebo design would also cost considerably more (upwards of $40 million) and take longer to recruit patients for the trial. It was reasonable to assume that some Parkinson disease patients would not want to participate in a study where there was a 50 percent chance of facing the risks of placebo surgery without the trade-off of the potential benefit from administration of the product. In addition, the academic investigators who would be running these trials might refuse to perform the placebo surgery, thus limiting the number of sites where the research could take place. Some physicians and patient advocates were generally opposed to the use of placebos, and favored trials using active controls where the experimental treatment is compared with an approved treatment.[86] Other investigators were concerned about the risk of placebo surgery and also about the coercive nature of any trial involving Parkinson patients. Many investigators were acutely aware that patients who volunteer for clinical trials often do so out of desperation. According to Mary Mowry, executive director of the San Diego Parkinson Corporation, a Parkinson patient advocacy group, "Most Parkinson disease patients are desperate enough to agree to a 50/50 chance of receiving a fetal cell implant when they are considering this surgery. To them the chance for long-time relief of symptoms is worth the risk taking." Another concern might be that patients who enrolled in the trial hoping to receive the active product would become frustrated and disappointed if they received the placebo, and it was possible that, as a consequence, their disease would worsen. The company also had to consider the possibility of patients filing lawsuits if harm was caused by the placebo surgery or follow-up treatments.

Despite the risks, three interrelated reasons could be used to justify the need for a placebo-controlled trial—the nature of the disease and the needs of Parkinson patients, the FDA requirements, and gaining acceptance in the market.

Patients' Needs

In the downward spiral that is characteristic of the disease, Parkinson patients have good and bad days or weeks, and a patient's mood or sense of well-being can often determine which kind of day it will be. Patients can improve their ability to walk, for instance, if they have a positive encounter with their physician at a check-up. Thus, the fact that this disease is prone to psychosomatic influences makes placebo control important. Some researchers found that one group of Parkinson subjects assigned to the placebo control group of a drug study had a 20 to 30 percent increase in their muscle movement scores that lasted the entire length of the six-month study.[87] It was reasonable to expect, then, that a surgical intervention alone could have powerful and long-lasting effects on a patient's motor function. If that were so, how could Genzyme determine whether any improvements experienced by its study subjects were caused by the surgery or the cell therapy?

Jim Finn had a definite opinion about whether there should be a placebo control in the future NeuroCell-PD trials. Eighteen months after having received the low doses of NeuroCell-PD he wrote:

> We all despise the use of 'double-blind' studies. But most of us recognize the necessity of them. Until something better is developed it's likely that they'll be with us for a long time. . . . As far as ethics are concerned; it seems to me that it is UNETHICAL to NOT continue this important research. It is morally wrong to deny the possibility of a cure (or, at least an improved life) for those of us who suffer from this hideous disease. I strongly suspect that these somewhat Holier-Than-Thou ethicists would sing a different tune if they were struck with Parkinson Disease.[88]

FDA Requirements

Placebo-controlled trials are considered the "gold standard" method to assess the safety and efficacy of experimental treatments.[89] Although in practice, the FDA shares this view, the Food and Drug regulations do not require the use of placebo controls in clinical trials.[90] The FDA's position is that it requires the best scientific evidence to support product claims. Whether Genzyme would need placebo-controlled data to obtain NeuroCell-PD marketing approval was therefore uncertain from a regulatory standpoint. In addition, Surgenor suspected that the FDA would be influenced by the fact that NIH-sponsored trials (the results of which were not yet completed or published) were using sham surgery as a placebo control in an assessment of human fetal-tissue transplantation in patients with Parkinson disease.[91]

To get a better feel for the FDA views on the need for placebo control, Surgenor and his team (now with CEO Termeer's involvement) invited FDA officials to attend meetings with investigator groups regarding NeuroCell-PD. However, the FDA always declined these invitations, stating its need for objectivity (a standard FDA operating procedure). Despite the lack of direct FDA input at the time, according to Surgenor, the company managers felt that, if the FDA eventually suggested that GTR include a sham surgical control in its study design, that suggestion "would not be at all controversial."

Gaining Acceptance in the Marketplace

From discussions taking place at medical meetings, Surgenor knew that, despite the fact that they would probably be opposed to using placebo surgery on their patients, neurologists and neurosurgeons would require rigorous scientific evidence that NeuroCell-PD was safe and effective before they would prescribe the product or conduct the transplant surgery. GTR's internal debate about whether to include placebo controls in the NeuroCell-PD clinical trials was informed by its experience with its earlier product, Carticel. According to Surgenor, Carticel was marketed in 1995 prior to any FDA requirements governing the marketing of this type of product and service. Although fifteen hundred patients worldwide had been treated with Carticel, data about its efficacy came from uncontrolled Swedish clinical studies. However, at least one study had shown that those subjects who had received placebo knee surgery in a study of surgical procedures for arthritic knees had improved.[92] It was likely, then, that some physicians would be skeptical about Carticel's efficacy without placebo control data.

Later, when the FDA developed a protocol for reviewing human autologous tissue and cell therapy products, GTR submitted a biologics license application and worked closely with the FDA to set the quality standards for this field. In August 1997, Carticel became the first such therapy to be approved. However, as a condition of approval to continue marketing the product, GTR was required by the FDA regulators to conduct two confirmatory postmarketing studies to gain a better understanding of Carticel and to assess longer-term clinical results.[93] Some of these surgical studies were required to have a placebo control arm, presumably because the regulators had decided that placebo controls would produce the best scientific evidence of safety and efficacy. This posed a great dilemma for the company, since it would now be very difficult to recruit subjects as well as convince investigators to give their patients a placebo surgery and deny them what was believed to be effective and approved therapy. Surgenor asked, "What patient would want to subject himself to this experiment when the real product is approved and can be used?" At the time, Surgenor was in the process of negotiating with the FDA to get its need for controlled data satisfied some other way.

Still later, GTR experienced slow market acceptance of Carticel because of resistance from orthopedic surgeons. Despite the fact that close to two thousand surgeons had been trained on Carticel use by the end of 1997 (the second full year after marketing), fewer that 240 patients were treated that year. Even though there was no precedent for sham surgical trials with other products in the cartilage repair field, Carticel was still facing criticism and resistance to use, Surgenor thought, because there was no placebo control data. Without the data from such a carefully controlled trial, physicians were uncertain whether the product was reliably beneficial.

TIM SURGENOR'S DILEMMA

The frustrating Carticel experience reminded Surgenor of the need for overwhelmingly convincing tests to prove NeuroCell-PD's effectiveness. A surgical placebo-controlled trial seemed an attractive way to test NeuroCell-PD as definitively as possible and, in effect, curb skeptics' arguments before they were voiced. However, GTR had to consider whether incorporating a placebo group would accelerate or slow NeuroCell-PD's release to market. What GTR could not tolerate would be the time and expense of having to redo uncontrolled clinical trials if the FDA decided that placebo control data were needed in order to obtain market approval for the product. If Surgenor and his team did go forward with a placebo-controlled design, it would have to be now.

Questions

1. Should the company proceed with the clinical trials that include placebo brain surgery? Why or why not?

2. If the company proceeds, how should the consent form be worded and how should subjects be recruited for the studies?

3. What responsibility does the company have to those subjects who are harmed from study participation?

4. How should the company react to those medical practitioners who protest the company's research program?

Discussion

According to one editorial written on the subject of sham surgeries:

An essential ethical standard for research is to minimize the risk of harm to subjects. Therefore, to avoid the risks from sham surgery, one may select an alternative research design (e.g. historical control cohort), but to do so requires trading off high methodological quality for high ethical standards. Such a trade off may not be in the best interests of society because the estimate of the treatment effect derived from the trial would be less accurate and lead to inferences that may be incorrect. Too many surgical procedures are supported on the basis of anecdotal evidence. Thus, it is now time to introduce into surgical trials the level of rigor to which medical trials are accustomed. However, the benefits and risks must be balanced to achieve a favorable ratio.[94]

This statement offers keys to responding to the ethical dimensions of this issue. A utilitarian view can often justify conducting clinical research, since the few who may be harmed serve to benefit many other subjects and sick patients who will either be spared a toxic product or benefit from a desperately needed new treatment. In addition, the research, whether it produces positive or negative results, will doubtless benefit medical science and society. Whether the research benefits the company depends on how wisely the company balances the various competing interests. The rights of the few subjects who may be harmed (the right to autonomy, to be spared the risk of unreasonable harm, to be free of duress and exploitation, and so on) deserve serious consideration as does the justice question since the burdens of research are born by relatively few ill patients. A threshold question to ask is whether enough is known about the investigational treatment and the underlying disease process to justify exposing human subjects to the potential risks of the contemplated research. Companies and research subjects can be harmed by a "full steam ahead" mindset that can develop based on the results of a few subjects who participated in Phase I open label trials. The inherent uncertainties that exist in attempting to predict results of cutting-edge biotechnology research make it imperative that study protocols are designed cautiously, attempting as much as possible to maximize the rights of subjects and minimize the burdens.

TABLE 7.1

Genzyme Financial Data

(in thousands of dollars for years ended December 31)

	Genzyme Corporation					
	1992	*1993*	*1994*	*1995*	*1996*	*1997*
Revenues	219,079	270,371	311,051	383,783	518,754	608,841
Operating costs/expenses	247,152	301,826	276,909	347,987	594,078	567,596
Operating income (loss)	(28,073)	(31,455)	34,142	35,796	(75,324)	41,245
Other income (expenses)	16,560	18,901	(3,358)	7,503	5,702	(15,516)
Net income (loss)	(30,317)	(6,095)	16,303	21,650	(72,817)	13,629

	Genzyme General				
	1993[a]	*1994*[a]	*1995*[a]	*1996*[a,b]	*1997*
Revenues	265,687	310,727	378,563	511,442	597,203
Operating costs/expenses	273,320	260,805	319,391	544,894	501,225
Operating income (loss)	(7,733)	49,922	59,172	(33,452)	95,978
Other income (expenses)	18,901	(3,387)	6,157	6,145	(5,351)
Net income (loss)	8,456	30,194	34,823	(47,513)	57,026
Tax benefit allocated from Genzyme Tissue Repair	9,564	1,860	8,857	17,011	17,666
Tax benefit allocated from Genzyme Molecular Oncology					2,755
Net income (loss)	18,020	32,054	43,680	(30,502)	77,447

(continued)

TABLE 7.1 *(continued)*

| | *Tissue Repair Division* | | | | |
	1993[a]	1994[c]	1995	1996	1997
Revenues	4,684	324	5,220	7,312	10,856
Operating costs/expenses	28,506	16,104	28,596	49,184	48,204
Operating income (loss)	(23,822)	(15,780)	(23,376)	(41,872)	(37,348)
Other income (expenses)		29	1,346	(443)	(8,636)
Net income (loss)	(24,115)	(15,751)	(22,030)	(42,315)	(45,984)

| | *Molecular Oncology Division* | | | |
	1994[a]	1995[a]	1996[a]	1997[d]
Revenues				782
Operating costs/expenses	37	464	1,003	19,923
Operating income (loss)	(37)	(464)	(1,003)	(19,141)
Other income (expenses)				(1,529)
Net income (loss)	(37)	(464)	(1,003)	(19,578)

[a] Pro forma
[b] Losses in 1996 were primarily attributable to $136.3 million in acquisition-related charges.
[c] Tracking stock division formed in 1994.
[d] Tracking stock division formed in 1997.
SOURCE: Genzyme Financial Reports

Notes

1. For drugs developed in the United States, the regulations that specify the requirement for reliable study data are found at 21 *Code of Federal Regulations* 314.126. Similar regulations for medical devices are found at 21 *Code of Federal Regulations* 860.7.

2. From ecclesiastical Latin, the term *placebo* means "I shall please."

3. See Note 1.

5. Benson H, Epstein M. The placebo effect: A neglected aspect on the care of patients. *Journal of the American Medical Association* 1975; 232:1225–27.

6. Kopp VJ. Henry Knowles Beecher and the development of informed consent in anesthesia research. *Anesthesiology* 1999; 90:1756–65.

7. Since the placebo effect is attributable to these "human" causes, a placebo effect cannot be tested in the laboratory because animals are not known to respond to placebos.

8. Kirsch I, Sapirstein G. Listening to Prozac but hearing placebo: A meta-analysis of antidepressant medication. *Prevention and Treatment* 1998; 1. Available from http://journals.apa.org/prevention/volume1/pre0010002a.html.

9. Kapp MB. Placebo therapy and the law: Prescribe with care. *American Journal of Law and Medicine* 1983; 8:371–405; Harrington A, editor. *The placebo effect: An interdisciplinary exploration*. Cambridge, MA: Harvard University Press; 1999.

10. See Note 9, Harrington.

11. Talbot M. The placebo prescription. *New York Times* 2000 Jan 9; Sect. 6:34.

12. Bienenfeld L. The placebo effect in cardiovascular disease. *American Heart Journal* 1996; 132:1207–21.

13. Jost TS. The globalization of health law: The case of permissibility of placebo-based research. *American Journal of Law and Medicine* 2000; 26:175–86.

14. When describing an "adequate and well-controlled" study using an active control arm, the FDA regulations (21 *Code of Federal Regulations* 314.126(b)(2)(iv)) state: "Active treatment concurrent control. The test drug is compared with known effective therapy; for example, where the condition treated is such that administration of placebo or no treatment would be contrary to the interest of the patient. An active treatment study may include additional treatment groups, however, such as a placebo control or a dose-comparison control. Active treatment trials usually include randomization and blinding of patients or investigators, or both. If the intent of the trial is to show similarity of the test and control drugs, the report of the study should assess the ability of the study to have detected a difference between treatments. Similarity of test drug and active control can mean either that both drugs were effective or that neither was effec-

tive. The analysis of the study should explain why the drugs should be considered effective in the study, for example, by reference to results in previous placebo-controlled studies of the active control drug."

15. Temple R, Ellenberg S. Placebo-controlled trials and active control trials in the evaluation of new treatments: Part 1: Ethical and scientific issues. *Annals of Internal Medicine* 2000; 133:455–63.

Ellenberg S, Temple R. Placebo-controlled trials and active-control trials in the evaluation of new treatments: Part 2: Practical issues and specific cases. *Annals of Internal Medicine* 2000; 133:464–70.

16. Rothman KJ, Michels KB. The continuing unethical use of placebo controls. *New England Journal of Medicine* 1994; 331:394–98.

17. See Note 9, Harrington.

18. See Note 16.

19. Clark PI, Leaverton DE. Scientific and ethical issues in the use of placebo controls in clinical trials. *Annual Review of Public Health* 1994; 15:19–38; see also Note 13.

20. Capron AM. Human experimentation. In Veatch RM, editor, *Medical ethics.* Boston: Jones and Bartlett ; 1989. pp. 154–55.

21. Council on Ethical and Judicial Affairs. *Ethical use of placebo controls in clinical trials.* American Medical Association; 1995.

22. Macklin R. The ethical problems with sham surgery in clinical research. *New England Journal of Medicine* 1999; 341:992–96.

23. See Note 13.

24. 21 *Code of Federal Regulations* 56.101 et seq.

25. In the mammary artery ligation sham surgery, the patient's chest was opened and a ligature (cord) was placed around the internal mammary artery (a blood vessel located on the inside of the chest cavity beside the sternum), but the artery was not ligated (tied) as it was in the true operation. The sham surgery studies revealed that actual surgery was no better than sham surgery at improving angina.

Freeman TB, Vawter DE, Leaverton DE, et al. Use of placebo surgery in controlled trials of a cellular-based therapy for Parkinson's disease. *New England Journal of Medicine* 1999; 341:988–92.

26. Beecher HK. Surgery as placebo. *Journal of the American Medical Association* 1961; 176:1102–7; Daya S. Issues in surgical therapy evaluation: The sham operation. *Evidence-based Obstetrics & Gynecology* 2000; 2:31–32. Available from MD Consult at http://home.mdconsult.com.

27. Johnson AG. Surgery as placebo. *Lancet* 1994; 344:1140–42.

28. See Note 22.

29. Greenberg MD. AIDS experimental drug approval, and the FDA new drug screening process. *New York University Journal of Legislation and Public Policy* 1999–2000; 3:295–350.

30. Freedman B. Equipoise and the ethics of clinical research. *New England Journal of Medicine* 1987; 317:141–45.

31. See Note 29.

32. Djulbegovic B, Lacevic M, Cantor A, et al. The uncertainty principle and industry-sponsored research. *Lancet* 2000; 356:635–38; Halpern S, Karlawish J. Industry-sponsored research. *Lancet* 2000; 356:2193.

33. Bayer R. The debate over maternal-fetal HIV transmission prevention trials in Africa, Asia, and the Caribbean: Racist exploitation or exploitation of racism? *American Journal of Public Health* 1998; 88:567–70.

34. Perinatal HIV Intervention Research in Developing Countries Workshop Participants. Consensus statement: Science, ethics, and the future of research into maternal infant transmission of HIV-I. *Lancet* 1999; 353:832–35.

35. Angell M. The ethics of clinical research in the third world. *New England Journal of Medicine* 1997; 337:847–49; Lurie P, Wolfe SM. Unethical trials of interventions to reduce perinatal transmission of the human immunodeficiency virus in developing countries. *New England Journal of Medicine* 1997; 337:853–56; Resnik DB. The ethics of HIV research in developing nations. *Bioethics* 1998; 12:286–300.

36. World Medical Association. Declaration of Helsinki. *Journal of the American Medical Association* 1997; 277:909–14.

37. Enserink M. Helsinki's new clinical rules: Fewer placebos, more disclosure. *Science* 2000; 290:418–19.

38. See Note 13.

39. Council on Ethical and Judicial Affairs. *The use of placebo controls in clinical trials.* American Medical Association; 1996. Opinion No. E-2.075. Available from www.ama-assn.org/ama/pub/catagory/2513.html.

40. See Note 1.

41. See Note 15, Temple, Ellenberg.

42. The initial case study was prepared by Tara Thiagarajan and Mark Hong under the guidance of and with later revisions by Margaret Eaton. The input and assistance of Tim Surgenor and Elliott Hillback of Genzyme and Jim Finn is greatly appreciated. The events described in this case study occurred up until fall 1997.

43. Jankovic J. Parkinsonism. In Cecil RL, Goldman L, Bennett JC, editors, *Cecil textbook of medicine.* 21st ed. Philadelphia: W.B. Saunders; 2000. pp. 2079–83.

44. Scheife RT, Schumock GT, Burstein A, et al. Impact of Parkinson's disease and its pharmacologic treatment on quality of life and economic outcomes. *American Journal of Health-System Pharmacy* 2000; 57:953–62.

45. Manyam, BV. Practical guidelines for management of Parkinson disease. *Journal of the American Board of Family Practice* 1997; 10:412–24; see also Note 43.

46. Freed CR, Breeze RE, Rosenberg NL, et al. Survival of implanted fetal dopamine cells and neurologic improvement 12 to 46 months after transplantation for Parkinson's disease. *New England Journal of Medicine* 1992; 237:1549–55; Lindvall O, Widner H, Rehncrona S, et al. Transplantation of fetal dopamine neurons in Parkinson's disease: One-year clinical and neurophysiological observations in two patients with putaminal implants. *Archives of Neurology* 1992; 31:155–73.

47. Bell NM. Regulating transfer and use of fetal tissue in transplantation procedures: The ethical dimensions. *American Journal of Law and Medicine* 1994; 20:277–94.

48. Friedrich MJ. Fetal pig neural cells for Parkinson disease. *Journal of the American Medical Association* 1999; 282:2198–99.

49. Such animal-to-human infections, called zoonoses, were responsible for such diseases as influenza (from pigs or birds), AIDS (from chimpanzees), and BSE or Mad Cow Disease (from cows). In some cases, the human symptoms of infection appeared rapidly, but in other cases, such as for AIDS and BSE, years would pass before signs of infection occurred.

50. Diacrin and Massachusetts General Hospital receive U.S. patent for immune system "masking" technology; technology may allow cell transplantation without lifelong immunosuppression therapy. Genzyme press release. 1998 July 21. Available at www.genzyme.com.

51. Genzyme Tissue Repair, Diacrin form joint venture to advance NeuroCell products for Parkinson's, Huntington's diseases. Genzyme press release. 1996 Sept 26. Available at www.genzyme.com.

42 *United States Code* §§ 201–99.

Draft guideline on infectious disease issues in xenotransplantation. 61 *Federal Register* 49,920; 1996 Sept 23.

52. Fredrickson JK. He's all heart . . . and a little pig too: A look at the FDA draft xenotransplant guideline. *Food and Drug Law Journal* 1997; 52:429–51.

53. Stephenson J. Xenotransplantation workshop ponders science, safety of animal tissue grafts. *Journal of the American Medical Association* 1995; 274:285–88.

54. Genzyme Corporation corporate information. Available at www.genzyme.com/company/welcome/htm.

55. Genzyme Web site, investor information. Available at www.genzyme.com/ir/welcome.htm.

56. Orphan drugs were drugs and other treatments that lacked a viable market since they were used to treat medical disorders that afflicted very few people. The U.S. Orphan Drug Act provided incentives to manufacturers to develop and market drugs for rare diseases and conditions affecting fewer than two hundred thousand persons in the United States. The first developer to receive FDA marketing approval for an orphan drug was entitled to a seven-year exclusive marketing period in the United States for that product. In 1997, there were several legislative attempts to shorten the term of exclusivity and to allow more than one company to obtain orphan drug marketing rights.

57. Ceredase was obtained from a large pool of human placental tissue collected from selected donors. It was administered intravenously over 1–2 hours several times per week. The supply and quality of placental tissue limited Genzyme's ability to supply all that was needed. Genzyme had consequently developed a recombinant DNA form of the drug called Cerezyme, and was completing a domestic manufacturing facility that would allow the company to produce an unlimited supply and to expand its market for this product.

Genzyme Web site; Ceredase® prescribing information. Available at www.genzyme.com/prodserv/specialty_therapeutics/ceredase/welcome.htm.

Gaucher's Disease was a rare, inherited disorder characterized by decreased levels of an important enzyme. The disease was characterized by an enlarged liver or spleen, anemia, bleeding problems, bone and joint pain, fatigue, and orthopedic complications such as repeated fractures and bone erosion. Balicki D, Beutler E. Gaucher Disease. *Medicine* 1995; 75:305–23.

58. Genzyme Web site; Henri A. Termeer, president and chief executive officer. Available at www.genzyme.com/company/henri.htm.

59. Ibid.

60. Genzyme Tissue Repair 1997 Annual Report. Available at www.genzyme.com/ir/gtrar/carticel/carticel.htm. Tim Surgenor also provided background information on company research and products.

61. The procedure cost ranged from $17,000 to $38,000, with an average cost of approximately $26,000 per procedure. Genzyme Tissue Repair charged $10,360 per procedure for the cells. See www.genzyme.com/carticel/welcome.htm.

62. Genzyme Tissue Repair, Diacrin form joint venture to advance NeuroCell products for Parkinson's, Huntington's diseases. Genzyme press release. 1996 Sept 26. Available at www.genzyme.com.

63. Genzyme Tissue Repair Annual Report, 1997. Available at www.genzyme.com/ir/gtrar/neurocel/neurocel.htm.

64. See Note 44.

65. Spalding BJ. Nature's brain specialist: Neural stem cell research on the rise. Biospace.com 2000 Mar 8. Available at www.biospace.com/articles/030900_print.cfm.

66. Phase I human trials are intended to study the safety of an experimental medical product, but many times these trials also give the company early information about whether the product will be effective.

67. Enserink M. Can the placebo be the cure? *Science* 1999; 284: 238–40.

68. Callahan MC. Parkinson's patient gets story told on TV. *Newport Daily News* 1998 June 20. Available at www.geocities.com/jimcfinn/1998/043379.html.

Jim Finn's pig cell diary. Available at www.geocities.com/SoHo/Village/6263/pienet/finn/index.html. Used with Jim Finn's permission.

69. Grondahl P. Rescued from the edge: Parkinson's sufferer makes dramatic improvement with fetal pig brain cell transplant. *Albany Times Union* 1999 Sept 27. Available at http://neuro-www.mgh.harvard.edu/forum_2/ParkinsonsDiseaseF/10.13.9910.53AMNewspaperi.html.

70. See Note 68, Jim Finn's pig cell diary.

71. As Phase I trials are intended purely to test safety, the doses of cells injected were low. The trial was also completely unblinded, which meant that doctors knew what they were giving and patients knew exactly what they were getting.

72. See Note 68, Jim Finn's pig cell diary.

73. Genzyme Tissue Repair 1997 Annual Report. Available at www.genzyme.com/ir/gtrar/carticel/carticel.htm. Tim Surgenor also provided background information on company research and products.

74. Genzyme Tissue Repair, Diacrin announce NeuroCell-PD Phase I results. Genzyme press release. 1997 Sept 29. Available at www.genzyme.com.

75. Ibid.

76. Adverse events could include bleeding at the site of cell injection, mental status changes like confusion or hallucinations, and worsening muscle movements. Freeman TB, Olanow CW, Hauser RA, et al. Bilateral fetal nigral transplantation into the postcommissural putamen in Parkinson's disease. *Annals of Neurology* 1995; 38:379–88.

77. Genzyme Tissue Repair, Diacrin announce NeuroCell-PD Phase I results. Genzyme press release. 1997 Sept 29. Available at www.genzyme.com.

78. Deacon T, Schumacher J, Dinsmore J, et al. Histological evidence of fetal pig neural cell survival after transplantation into a patient with Parkinson's disease. *Nature Medicine* 1997; 3:350–53.

79. See Note 68, Jim Finn's pig cell diary.

80. See Note 69.

81. Genzyme Tissue Repair, Diacrin announce orphan drug designations. Genzyme press release. 1997 Jan 8. Available at www.genzyme.com.

82. The significant risks of general anesthesia, although rare, included cardiopulmonary arrest, respiratory difficulties, heart attack, malignant hyperthermia (very rare but deadly), airway problems, and anesthesia mistakes. Side effects after the procedure included nausea, vomiting, chills, and other similar discomforts. Fleisher LA. Risk of anesthesia. In Miller RD, editor, *Anesthesia*. 5th ed. London: Churchill Livingstone; 2000. p. 795.

83. At the time of the study, the antirejection medication that would be used was cyclosporin, a drug that suppresses the immune system and prevents the body from rejecting foreign cells. This drug was known to cause such side effects as hypertension, reduced kidney and liver function, nausea, tremors, increased body hair growth, numbness and tingling in the hands and feet, bleeding gums, and an increased risk of infections and cancer.

84. See Note 76.

85. Bonchek LI. Are randomized trials appropriate for evaluating new operations? *New England Journal of Medicine* 1979; 301:44–45.

86. See Note 16.

87. See Note 19.

88. See Note 68, Jim Finn's pig cell diary.

89. See Note 19.

90. 21 *Code of Federal Regulations*, Food and Drugs, Parts 300 to 499. Revised 1993 Apr 1.

91. See Note 25, Freeman et al.

92. Moseley JB Jr, Wray NP, Kuykendall D, et al. Arthroscopic treatment of osteoarthritis of the knee: A prospective, randomized, placebo-controlled trial: Results of a pilot study. *American Journal of Sports Medicine* 1996; 24:28–34.

93. Genzyme Tissue Repair 1997 Annual Report. Available at www.genzyme.com/ir/gtrar/carticel/carticel.htm. Tim Surgenor also provided background information on company research and products.

94. See Note 26, Daya.

8

Mitigation of Harm to Subjects Injured in Clinical Research

Clinical research by its very nature involves some level of risk. Given that even the most rigorous preclinical testing in tissues and animals cannot accurately predict the risk of adverse events in humans, it is necessary for researchers to expose subjects to some level of risk to assess the safety and effectiveness of novel experimental agents. Because risks are unknown, bioscience companies must conduct product research in humans in progressive phases, the first of which is to test the product in a small number of healthy people at various dose levels to discover whether the product is safe enough to use in increasing numbers of diseased human subjects. Careful research design, subject selection, and study monitoring are necessary to reduce risk or detect injury early, so as to harm the fewest number of subjects. Including a full disclosure of reasonably foreseeable research risks in the informed consent process, along with the fact that some risks are unknown, allows subjects to decline to participate in research they consider too risky. Together, these mechanisms act as risk-reducing measures and also uphold the right of subjects to know the nature of the risk they face prior to entering a clinical trial.

If research subjects are harmed, however, the question arises whether and how to compensate them. There are no mandatory or comprehensive compensation programs to cover injuries resulting from publicly or privately sponsored clinical research, and no laws have ever required compensation. Medical insurance typically covers no experimental or research treatments. Consequently, practice on this matter has varied. During the 1970s in the United States, however, a consensus began to evolve among medical ethicists that compensatory justice principles required that subjects who were injured as a result of participating in clinical research were entitled to full compensation for both medical and nonmedical related costs. Policy reasoning that supported this conclusion stemmed from the view that society as a whole had a direct stake in the conduct of scientific research, including the benefits that came from experimental failure, which could lead to insights that in turn led to modifications and improvements in medical products. If society shared the benefits, so should it share the financial burden of the research activity by paying for the costs of research-related injuries. Legal and ethical commentators argued that even if these injuries occurred through no fault of the researcher or sponsor, accountable public policy required that responsibility be fixed wherever it will most effectively reduce the hazards to life and health inherent in the research endeavor. If research sponsors were committed in advance to pay for injuries, the tendency to engage in excessively dangerous research would be minimized and research sponsors would take more care in designing safe trials, monitoring for injury, and stopping trials as soon as the data revealed excessive risk. Also, researchers were most often in a better financial position to bear the costs of research injury. Product manufacturers were especially able to spread the loss caused by injury-producing products among all of those who benefit by including the cost of injury compensation in the price of the product. Finally, people would more likely consent to participate in research if they knew they would not be responsible for the costs of any injuries. Many proponents of this view also argued that since the primary goal of compensatory justice was to restore the injured person as much as possible to his or her original condition, injury compensation should include medical and nonmedical costs of injury, the latter including such things as lost wages or services provided while the injured subject was disabled.[1]

HISTORY OF ATTEMPTS TO DEVELOP
COMPENSATION POLICIES

The question of whether to provide mandatory compensation for research injuries was addressed periodically by various agencies of the U.S. government, which conducted, sponsored, or regulated a vast amount of human research.[2] Several attempts have been made to set policy in this area.

U.S. Army

In the late 1940s, the Army debated, but ultimately rejected, suggestions to establish a program for compensating prisoner volunteers who were injured during experiments involving malaria and hepatitis.

National Institutes of Health

In the 1970s, the National Institutes of Health, the U.S. agency that sponsors or conducts the largest amount of clinical research, submitted three proposals to its parent agency, the Department of Health, Education and Welfare (DHEW; now the Department of Health and Human Services, or DHHS) that would have authorized the federal government to indemnify all injured research subjects for both medical and nonmedical expenses if the subjects were injured in studies sponsored in whole or in part by federal money. The secretary of DHEW rejected all of these proposals but agreed to study the question further.

Department of Health, Education and Welfare

In the mid-1970s, DHEW established a Task Force on Compensation of Injured Research Subjects to study the question of whether the government should provide mandatory no-fault compensation for all subjects injured as a result of participating in DHEW-sponsored research.[3] No-fault compensation was considered because the department experts agreed that when injury did occur, it often was not the result of any fault on the part of the subject or the researcher, but simply a natural consequence of the undertaking. Attempting to base compensation only on cases in which the researcher had done something wrong would ignore those subjects who were just as deserving of compensation. In addition, a no-fault compensation program would provide more uniform compensation and would be more efficient and less destructive of relationships than litigation, since it eliminated the need to show misconduct by the researcher or the sponsor.

The task force eventually recommended that DHEW provide compensation to subjects whose injury (whether physical, psychological, or social) was directly caused by DHEW research and when the injury exceeded that reasonably associated with the subject's illness or treatments at the time the subject first participated in the research. These recommendations were endorsed by DHEW Secretary Joseph Califano, and new regulations were prepared to implement them. However, the week that Califano was to sign the proposed regulations and forward them to Congress, he was fired by President Carter, and his successor decided that instead of signing the regulations, he would ask DHEW's Ethics Advisory Board to further investigate the recommendations. The ethics board was dissolved before it could complete the task, but did forward a recommendation that the new President's Commission for the Study of Ethical Problems in Medicine and Biomedical and Behavioral Research continue to consider the issue.[4]

President's Commission for the Study of Ethical Problems in Medicine and Biomedical and Behavioral Research

The President's Commission was created in 1981, during the Reagan administration, and took on the compensation question as part of its work. In 1982, after extensive investigation, the commission generated one of the most comprehensive reports on compensation for clinical research injury.[5] In the opening section to this report, the commission wrote that

> the suggestion of compensation for research injuries has been a mainstay of ethical and public-policy discussions of research with human subjects for many years. The failure to resolve the issue exposes the entire research enterprise to the public recriminations that could follow from one or a series of serious, uncompensated injuries to subjects. The importance of biomedical and behavioral research for this country is manifested in the many billions of dollars that such research receives each year in an attempt to conquer disease and to relieve human suffering. The formal ethical standards and individual consciences of investigators, as well as Federal rules and guidelines developed in the past two decades, have done much to protect research subjects and to reduce the risk of injury to them. Some risk remains nevertheless—risk that though statistically small may manifest itself in serious ways for individuals. A social policy experiment is needed to see whether compensation programs might provide a feasible means to further reduce the risk of unremedied injury.

Despite their convictions, the commission members found it difficult to reach agreement on whether and how to compensate for research injury. The difficulty was associated with the lack of data about the magnitude of the problem and also with disagreements about how to characterize the role of the research subject. After interviewing over twenty federal agencies and representatives from academia and the pharmaceutical and insurance industries, the commission concluded that "surprisingly little" was known about the incidence of the problem. No federal agency collected data on the number of subjects injured in government-related research, not even the Public Health Service, which supported approximately 80 percent of the federally funded biomedical research conducted in the country.[6] Since there were no published data on the incidence of research-related injury, the commission was required to seek them out. The few institutions that had collected data for internal purposes provided information that gave the commission what it called "only suggestive evidence" of the magnitude of the research injury problem, and from this it made the following "modest, but important" conclusions:

1. The incidence of serious injury and the absolute numbers of people seriously injured are small

2. Most injuries are trivial in nature and require no medical intervention

3. Of those injuries that require intervention, most are only temporarily disabling

4. Most serious injuries and fatalities associated with research are more likely to result from underlying disease than from the research per se

5. Patient-subjects in therapeutic research are more likely than normal subjects in nontherapeutic research to suffer injury

6. The existence of compensation programs does not stimulate excessive or unmerited claims of injury[7]

The commission debated whether prospective studies should be conducted to verify these conclusions, but decided that such studies would be too costly and time consuming to perform.

The commission also concluded that the decision to compensate injured research subjects was dependent on how their role was perceived. Were research subjects heroes deserving of public gratitude since they volunteered to perform a valuable public service? The space shuttle astronauts were one example of this view. Should research subjects be viewed as victims—easily misled and used as a means to derive research data? This view of a research subject was supported by those who saw the Tuskegee syphilis study not as an aberrant phenomenon but as an example of the need to constrain the normal scientist's tendency to let scientific and medical goals drive research practice.[8] Or were subjects like employees or contractors, where research participation and injury compensation were more a matter of negotiation between two freely contracting parties? This last view was endorsed by those who believed that contracting allowed people to make choices that maximized individual welfare, and that therefore, the rules of contract should govern human relationships whenever possible. Depending on the circumstances, research subjects could fill any of these roles, making it difficult for the commission to decide how to characterize the role of subjects and thus whether subjects' informed consent should be viewed as relieving researchers of responsibility for any injuries caused by the research.

The commission also investigated whether any existing programs were adequately compensating research subjects. Medical insurance was the most obvious source for compensation, and the commission's studies led it to conclude that while some medical treatment costs were being covered, individual health insurance was not universal or comprehensive and would not cover nonmedical costs, such as wage loss. Health insurance, therefore, was only a partial solution. Insurance executives informed the commission that it would not be feasible to issue policies to individual subjects to cover the risk of research injury, but that it was feasible to issue policies to research institutions, since if the institution were willing to collect data, the costs and claims experiences could be tracked and serve as a basis to set premiums.

In 1982, the commission sent to President Reagan its report, *Compensating for Research Injuries: A Report on the Ethical and Legal Implications of Programs to Redress Injuries Caused by Biomedical and Behavioral Research.*[9] In this report, the commission endorsed the proposals of the prior DHEW task force and stated that redress should be made for many research injuries. However, the commission recommended that no program be instituted at that time but that subjects be told as a part of the informed consent process if any compensation were available should they become injured. In the meantime, the commission recommended further studies to determine if a formal compensation program was needed and, if so, the fairest and most efficient means of providing compensation. The letter to the president concluded with the statement, "The Commission is pleased to have had an opportunity to assist in the resolution of this important topic." DHHS subsequently concluded that the recommended studies were not feasible and decided not to initiate them.[10]

Recombinant DNA Advisory Committee

In January 1993, the Recombinant DNA Advisory Committee asked NIH director Bernadine Healy to investigate or ask President Clinton's health care reform task force to consider covering the medical costs of research-related, nonnegligent injuries. The request letter stated that it was "unfair to expect individuals, their families, or their insurers to absorb unpredictable and potentially substantial medical costs arising out of these individuals' participation as research subjects."[11] No efforts were made to implement this request.

Advisory Committee on Human Radiation Experiments

In 1994, President Clinton created the Advisory Committee on Human Radiation Experiments, a cabinet-level committee to investigate and report on the use of human subjects in federally funded research using ionizing radiation.[12] As part of its task, the advisory committee addressed the compensation question, again framed as a matter of justice—"Why it should be research subjects, rather than others, who are to be expected to absorb the financial, as well as the unavoidable human costs of the societal research enterprise which benefits everyone?"[13] In making the argument that satisfactory resolution of this unresolved and long-standing social issue was required, especially with regard to medical care costs for injured subjects, the advisory committee went further than other groups that had issued recommendations on this issue:

> The Advisory Committee urges not only consideration of a compensation policy for physical injuries attributable to research but also that consideration be given to appropriate remedies for subjects who have suffered dignitary harms, even in the absence of physical injury. Subjects so wronged have little recourse in the current system; litigation in the absence of physical injury is unlikely to provide relief to people who have been used as subjects without their adequate consent. If it is determined that financial compensation is not generally an appropriate remedy in the absence of physical injury, consideration should be given to other remedies that would be fitting.[14]

While no direct action was taken on the general recommendation for a federal government compensation policy, the government did provide financial compensation to those subjects (or the next of kin of subjects) injured in human radiation experiments in cases where subjects were misled, not fully informed of the intent of the research or the risks involved, and where the secrecy had the effect of denying individuals the opportunity to pursue potential grievances.

National Institute of Medicine

A similar recommendation that NIH review and resolve the matter of compensation for research-related injury was made in 1994 by the Institute of Medicine (IOM) when it published a report about the health consequences of underrepresentation or exclusion of women from clinical research.[15] After studying the issue, IOM found that although many injured subjects received emergency or short-term medical care for research injuries, no federal program exists in which injured subjects are offered long-term care as a matter of course. The report recommended that NIH address this problem since it was often the most severely injured subjects who needed long-term care.

National Bioethics Advisory Commission

The most recent national attempt to address the question of research subject compensation came from President Clinton's National Bioethics Advisory Commission (NBAC), which assumed as one of its tasks making ethical and policy recommendations for the conduct of human clinical trials. With regard to compensation, NBAC's report concluded as follows:

> Participants who are harmed as a direct result of research should be cared for and compensated. This is simple justice. The fact that they offered to participate in no way alters the view that mere decency calls for us to take care of these volunteers. Unfortunately, this is a greater challenge than it might appear. For those who endure harm while participating in research, it is often very difficult to separate injuries traceable to the research from those that stem from the underlying disease or social condition being studied. For others, appropriate care and compensation would be far beyond the means of the researchers, their sponsors, and their institutions. Two decades ago, the President's Commission for the Study of Ethical Problems in Medicine and Biomedical and Behavioral Research called for pilot studies of compensation programs—a recommendation that was not pursued. It is time to reconsider the need for some type of compensation program and to explore the possible mechanisms that could be used were one to be adopted. Regardless of individual motives, research participants are providing a service for society, and justice requires that they be treated with great respect and receive appropriate care for any related injuries. It should always be remembered that it is a privilege for any researcher to involve human participants in his or her research.[16]

The NBAC report was completed and published during the more conservative Bush administration, not long before the NBAC charter was to expire. Commentators believed that it was unlikely that this recommendation would be implemented in any form.

INDUSTRY RESEARCH PRACTICE

As with the governmental regulatory bodies, no drug or medical device companies have adopted policies for mandatory or no-fault compensation for clinical research injuries. Generally, industry fears that such a policy would expose companies to the uncertainty of an open-ended financial risk, for which no insurance is available.[17] Instead, pharmaceutical and biotechnology companies, depending on their size and resources, insure their clinical trials risk under professional liability and general liability policies or purchase separate clinical trials insurance policies for each study. Premiums are fixed according to the insurer's assessment of the risk of engaging in clinical trial work, which includes the risk that injured subjects will file claims for injury compensation. Although premium costs vary, they typically are not a large part of the cost of any particular clinical trial.[18] These policies are fault-based, meaning that the insurance provides compensation to the subject only when the insured entity is considered to be negligent in causing the research injury. Backstopped with this coverage, the custom in the industry has evolved to include the following practices: subjects are informed that medical treatment will be made available for any injuries experienced as a result of research participation. Sponsors often voluntarily pay for emergency and short-term treatment if they conclude that the injury was directly caused by the research. Otherwise, the subject pays for his or her own medical expenses, hopefully with reimbursement from medical insurance coverage. Subjects typically are informed in the consent process that no (or no other) compensation for injuries is available.

Some subjects, especially those with severe injuries or large expenses, have not been satisfied with this arrangement and have filed legal claims against the researcher or sponsor.[19] Companies have often attempted to settle these claims, and the settlement process can encompass anything from offering no money (if the company believes that the alleged injury did not exist or was not caused by the research intervention) to full compensation for medical and nonmedical costs (if the company believed that it was at fault and especially if misconduct had occurred). If attempts to settle fail, litigation proceeds. Insured or not, and even if the company ultimately prevails, no company welcomes a lawsuit from one of its research subjects. These lawsuits tend to harm corporate reputations, can lead to doubts about the safety of the product, and can sometimes oblige the company to defend itself by blaming the injury on physician researcher misconduct, which in turn can discourage other physicians from conducting research for the company. Litigation is also costly and the outcome often uncertain. One lawsuit can prompt plaintiffs' lawyers to seek other potentially injured subjects for follow-on or even mass tort litigation.[20]

Relying on the legal system is also not a uniformly satisfactory process for the injured subject, and there are many reasons why the subject would have difficulty prevailing. Not all research subjects have the resources to initiate a lawsuit. If a lawsuit were filed, it could be difficult for the subject to prove two critical elements of negligence, that the researcher should have foreseen the injury and that the injury was proximately caused by the product. Because there is little clinical experience with any investigational product, it is not easy for experts to foresee injuries or determine causation. These two elements are especially hard to prove with fetal or birth injuries, the causes of which are notoriously difficult to diagnose under any circumstance.[21] In some cases, such as under the federal medical device laws, subjects claiming injuries as a result of a defect in the experimental device were denied legal remedies under strict liability and could only prevail if they proved that the researcher was negligent in conducting the study.[22] Factors unrelated to the research injury, such as disparity between the parties in information, financial resources, and quality of legal representation, could influence the outcome of the litigation. Also, jury verdicts could seem arbitrary and more related to the bias of jury members or their inability to understand and weigh complicated medical evidence. Depending on the claims made in the lawsuit and the jurisdiction where the suit was filed, manufacturers defending themselves against claims of harm have been able to take advantage of certain defenses. If the plaintiff sued because of inadequate consent (in battery or under a strict liability claim for failure to warn), the broad language of the consent form could defeat the claim. Proving that the language of the consent form was inadequate to warn of risks is especially difficult since a local IRB or the FDA most often approved the language.

Also, depending on the jurisdiction, if the plaintiff sued claiming negligent conduct of the sponsor or researcher, two defenses, one called contributory or comparative negligence and the other typically called "assumption of the risk," might be used to defend against the claim. Proving contributory negligence means that the subject's recovery would be reduced by the degree to which he or she was found to have contributed to the injury through his or her unreasonable conduct, such as when a subject ignores the researcher's instructions. Assumption of risk is a legal concept whereby injured plaintiffs are not entitled to legal compensation or compensation will be reduced if, knowing in advance of a risk, the plaintiffs willingly consented to expose themselves to the risk.[23] Again, the warnings and broad risk language used in consent forms would make it difficult for the subject to get around these defenses.[24]

TENTATIVE RESPONSES AND RENEWED CALLS FOR MANDATORY COMPENSATION PROGRAMS

Aside from suggestions for renewed study, the U.S. government deliberations and recommendations in this area have had two primary effects. The first was that compensation was made to subjects for past research misconduct in the

Tuskegee and Cold War radiation experiments when it was determined that subjects had been misled, exploited, and injured. Also, DHHS implemented regulations requiring that, for all research involving more than minimal risk, subjects should be told in advance whether medical treatments or compensation for injury are available and about any anticipated expenses to the subject for participating in the trial. This became a standard informed consent requirement for clinical drug and medical device studies and was also adopted as a regulatory requirement by the FDA.[25] By the end of the 1990s, the practice of NIH, which sponsors more human research than any other government agency, was to pay for acute care costs for hospitalization required by research injuries. However, compensation was paid only for the duration of the specific research protocol because the Office of Management and Budget contains no funds to indemnify subjects for injuries that extend beyond any NIH research contracts.

From time to time, medical research ethics commentators who felt that the insurance and legal systems were inadequate means to compensate for research injuries have renewed objections and called for a comprehensive response. Publicized reports of catastrophic research injuries also often served as a catalyst for critics of the current compensation status quo. Criticisms were based on the claim that the typical informed consent process for human research is often flawed and does not result in a fully informed agreement to accept the known and unknown risks of research. In these circumstances, forcing the subjects to accept both the physical and financial risks of research injury is considered unfair. Further, the financial risks of injury are often unpredictable, and the consent form sentence that states that no compensation for injuries will be provided could easily be overlooked. Others claimed that it was unfair not to provide and pay for all medical care for injured subjects since they are rendering a service to the research sponsor.[26] In the late 1990s, several research injury cases led to renewed demands that the government strengthen the budgets and roles of research review boards, institute better monitoring programs for clinical trials, and develop research injury compensation programs.[27] The fact that an estimated three million Americans volunteer annually to participate in fifty to sixty thousand ongoing clinical trials meant that significant numbers of research injures would occur, some of which were likely to be catastrophic, thus further guaranteeing that these issues would remain a matter of public debate.[28]

Case Study

Adiana, Inc., and the Development of a Female Sterilization Device[29]

In December 1999, Paul Goeld, president of the Redwood City, California-based medical device startup Adiana, Inc., faced several decisions about the company's sole product, a new female sterilization catheter. The catheter had proved to be extremely successful in both animal and preliminary human clinical trials in Mexico. Adiana planned to request approval from the Food and Drug Administration for an investigational device exemption (IDE) to begin full-scale human testing of the device. Before proceeding, however, Goeld had several decisions to make about how the company would treat the women who enrolled in the clinical trials. Specifically, he needed to decide what would constitute adequate consent for the sterilization study and what responsibility the company would assume for women for whom the device failed to prevent pregnancy.

ADIANA, INC.

Adiana was founded in July 1997 by Peter Breining, vice president of operations, and Doug Harrington, vice president of research and development. Prior to founding Adiana, Breining and Harrington had worked at Medtronic, a medical device company. Adiana was launched after Breining and Harrington, with an initial concept for the catheter product and its potential market in hand, made presentations to graduates of the Stanford Graduate School of Business and requested assistance with their business plan. The business plan attracted the attention of venture capitalists, and Adiana received $3 million in private funding. Stanford University also made a small direct investment in the company. With these funds, Breining and Harrington began their research and development effort to create what they believed to be a revolutionary innovation in the field of female sterilization. Soon after the company was started, the founders discovered that Dr. Thierry Vancaille, an obstetrician-gynecologist and researcher from Sydney, Australia, had already done work in this field and in fact had a patent covering closely related technology. Realizing the value of using Vancaille's experience and benefiting from his patent, Breining and Harrington recruited Vancaille to their venture. Consequently, Vancaille also became an Adiana founder.

ADIANA'S FEMALE STERILIZATION CATHETER

Adiana's novel catheter device was the brainchild of Breining and Harrington. The two founders saw an opportunity to capture the market for female sterilization with the new tool and procedure. The Adiana procedure offered many advantages over the traditional method of female sterilization, which was surgical tubal ligation. Adiana's procedure was much shorter—lasting a total of about five minutes—and could be performed in a doctor's office. There was no requirement for any presurgical preparation or anesthesia except a paracervical block (local anesthesia on the cervix). Since no general anesthesia was necessary and the procedure was easier to perform than tubal ligation (although physicians would have to be trained in the new procedure), the Adiana principals were confident that their catheter would allow a much safer sterilization than the traditional surgical approach.

The device that enabled the procedure was a disposable catheter, about twelve inches long and extremely thin, with a handle and a port that connected it to a power generator. The catheter was placed into the vagina and then through the cervix into the uterus by a hysteroscope (an optical diagnostic device used to view the uterus). In order for this device to be inserted, the uterus first needed to be inflated with fluid. Once the catheter was inside the uterus, the surgeon guided it into one of the two fallopian tubes. At the very entrance to the fallopian tube, a small electrical charge would be delivered, raising the temperature of the inside lining of the tube to about 45 degrees C (113 degrees F) for about one minute. This charge would be sufficient to cause something like sunburn in the fallopian tube, resulting in an acute inflammatory reaction. The catheter would then be withdrawn, leaving a biologically inert plug inside the tube. When the tissue recovered from the inflammatory reaction, it would regenerate and grow into the plug, effectively blocking the path for eggs to move from the ovary to the uterus. Two catheters were required, one for each fallopian tube.

The procedure was projected to cost about $1,500: an estimated $750 for the two catheters, with the doctor's fees constituting the other half. The company had ascertained that insurance companies and other payers would cover the cost of the entire procedure. Given the changes in the health-care sector—rising price pressures as well as the shift to nonhospital care—Adiana's president Goeld had high hopes that the product would be successful if he could get it to market. However, although the device had been shown to have 100 percent efficacy in short-term trials in rabbits, it had not yet been studied for effectiveness in preventing human pregnancies. The traditional surgical tubal ligation procedure, in contrast, had been established as being about 98 percent effective in preventing pregnancies. This figure represented a benchmark against which Adiana needed to compete, since the costs of a failed sterilization could be great.

In 1999, Goeld led Adiana's team of motivated professionals. Goeld had an M.B.A. from the Kellogg and Pepperdine graduate schools and brought with him nearly twenty-five years of experience in the medical device industry. He had helped start, fund, and manage several medical device startups, and Adiana was his ninth company. Under his leadership was a team comprising three executives, one scientist, four engineers, three technicians, and an office manager. Goeld's challenge was to guide the company through the legal, ethical, and regulatory hurdles it had to face in order to convince U.S. regulators that Adiana's catheter and procedure was superior to traditional methods of female sterilization.

FEMALE CONTRACEPTION VIA SURGICAL
STERILIZATION: 1960 TO 1999

Female contraception had undergone a revolution since pharmaceutical and medical device technology had expanded in the early 1960s to give women more options than the difficult-to-negotiate condom or the notoriously unreliable rhythm method. In the United States, where more than half of all pregnancies (3.5 million pregnancies annually) were unintended, the benefits of effective and safe contraception were myriad.[30] For women who could not tolerate pregnancy because of medical problems, contraception prevented injury and death. For the rest of women users, contraception enhanced the quality of life by allowing couples to choose whether and when to have children, and how many. In the late 1990s, choices abounded for women who wished to temporarily prevent pregnancy. However, there was only one commonly used method to permanently sterilize women, and that was surgical tubal ligation.

Female sterilization via tubal ligation involved mechanically blocking or interrupting the fallopian tubes to prevent an egg from descending to where it would encounter, and be fertilized by, sperm.[31] The procedure could be conducted using laparotomy or laparoscopy procedures, and physician skill and training usually governed which procedure was used. Laparotomy (the more traditional procedure) involved making incisions in the abdomen to directly view and access the fallopian tubes for the surgery. In laparoscopy, a small, lighted, telescoping microscope was passed through small abdominal incisions (1.0 to 1.5"), allowing the surgeon to indirectly view the fallopian tubes by watching a projected image on an external monitor connected to the microscope. Very small surgical tools were passed through another small incision, and the surgeon manipulated these tools while looking at the site on the external monitor.[32] Once the fallopian tubes were accessed, ligation ("tube tying") or sealing the fallopian tubes was accomplished in a number of ways—tying a loop of tube and removing a middle section of the loop, cutting the tube and burying the ends in surrounding tissue, variations of these techniques, or using clips, rings, or electrocautery to obstruct or seal the tube.

Prior to the procedure, women were most often evaluated for medical appropriateness and the steadfastness of their decision to become permanently sterilized. Although it varied, the process of informed consent under most standards of care required a discussion of the benefits and risks of the procedure and alternate methods of contraception, including male sterilization of the women's partners.[33] For U.S. patients who had medical care coverage from a federal source (for example, Medicaid), a mandatory written informed consent process followed by a thirty-day waiting period was required before the procedure could take place.[34] Many states also had particular informed consent requirements, all intended to ensure that patients fully comprehended the consequences of this usually irreversible procedure. In the United States, tubal ligation procedures typically were performed in an outpatient setting using general anesthesia. The procedure took at least half a day, including the time for anesthesia, the surgery itself, and recovery from anesthesia. After the procedure, patients were instructed to rest for twenty-four hours at home, take pain medication if needed, refrain from bathing for forty-eight hours, and avoid sexual intercourse and strenuous lifting for one week to allow the incision to heal. Most patients were advised to take a few days to a week off from work. At least one postoperative incision check was generally required.[35]

In the late 1990s, the frequency with which women elected surgical sterilization was high. It was estimated that almost half of all couples in the world were using some form of contraception, and that almost half of these had undergone sterilization, making sterilization the most frequently used form of contraception worldwide.[36] In the United States, rates of tubal ligation procedures began increasing in the 1970s when laparoscopic procedures were developed. In 1995, the National Center for Health Statistics reported that 41 percent of ever-married U.S. women/couples between the ages of fifteen and forty-four were sterilized.[37] Other studies at the same time showed that between 20 to 25 percent of U.S. women at risk for pregnancy (that is, those not sterile from surgical, medical, or age-related causes) had been sterilized.[38] The incidence of U.S. female sterilization was higher for Hispanic women (21 percent) and black women (25 percent) than for white women (16 percent) and others (11 percent).[39] All told, studies estimated that, by the late 1990s, approximately seven hundred thousand to one million tubal ligation surgeries were performed yearly in the United States.[40] About half of all tubal ligations were performed in hospitals, and most of these were done with regional anesthesia immediately following childbirth. The rest of the procedures, of which 95 percent were done under general anesthesia, were performed in outpatient settings.[41]

The most frequently cited reasons women chose tubal ligation as their form of contraception in the mid-1990s were that Baby Boomer women were completing their families and wanted a permanent form of contraception; more women were becoming alarmed at the long-term risks associated with other forms of contraception (for example, hormones or intrauterine devices— IUDs); stigma associated with sterility was reduced; and women wanted to avoid contraception failure.[42] Sterilization was an increasingly preferred means of contraception for women who never wanted children, had completed their families, or for other reasons had firmly decided that they wanted no more children. Sterilization was also beneficial since it was highly effective in preventing pregnancy, eliminated contraception compliance problems (as with daily pill taking), did not require interruption of sexual intercourse (as with condoms), and eliminated repeated physician visits (as with injectable or implantable drugs or IUDs).[43]

ADVERSE EFFECTS OF SURGICAL TUBAL LIGATION

Surgical sterilization via tubal ligation was considered a safe procedure, with an average complication rate for both major and minor problems of about 1 to 2 percent. The lowest complication rates were associated with laparoscopy (0.9 to 1.7 percent), and much higher rates were associated with laparotomy performed on obese women or on women with significant medical problems.[44] The most common complication occurred in about 1 percent of cases, when surgeons could not complete a laparoscopic procedure and had to revert to the more traditional open surgery, which, because of longer anesthesia time and larger incisions, caused longer and more difficult postoperative recovery. Other complications included damage to surrounding tissue and organs, inadequate ligation of the fallopian tube, and anesthetic complications.[45] The risks of general anesthesia, although rare, were not insignificant—they included cardiopulmonary arrest, respiratory difficulties, heart attack, malignant hyperthermia (very rare but deadly), and anesthesia mistakes. Side effects after the procedure included nausea, vomiting, and other postanesthetic complications, as well as pelvic pain, bleeding, and infection. Between a third to one-half of patients complained about intense pain and/or nausea and vomiting after the procedure.[46] The only consistently reported long-term side effect of tubal ligation was a higher risk for hysterectomy.[47]

Deaths resulting from surgical tubal ligation procedures were very rare, occurring in about 4 per 100,000 cases in the United States and 6 per 100,000 cases internationally.[48] Death was most often related to anesthetic, operative, or infection complications, and the incidence of death was higher in women with pre-existing medical conditions. In the United States, 10 of 27 sterilization-related deaths occurred in women with underlying medical conditions. In contrast, death as a result of pregnancy or childbirth ranged from 7 to 28.2 per 100,000 women age fifteen to forty-four years.[49]

Nonphysical adverse reactions to female sterilization were most often caused by postoperative regret. Most studies showed that the women who regretted being sterilized were those who remarried, were undergoing marital strife, were younger than thirty years old, were sterilized at their partner's request, had no children, or chose sterilization because of financial, health, or emotional difficulties.[50] These same studies showed that Hispanic women and women with lower educational levels were more likely to report regret than white women or those with a higher level of education. In some studies, the incidence of regret was as high as 25 percent.[51] Those women with the highest level of regret (between 1 to 2 percent of all women sterilized in the United States) sought to reverse the sterilization. However, sterilization reversal was not easy—between 30 to 70 percent of women were candidates for the procedure, and, of those who did have the procedure, only about 50 percent subsequently became pregnant. The reversal procedures (recanalization surgery or *in vitro* fertilization) were also costly and associated with a much higher complication rate than the initial sterilization.[52]

EFFECTIVENESS OF SURGICAL TUBAL LIGATION

Pregnancy after surgical sterilization was believed to be a very rare event, resulting from conception occurring immediately before surgery or from an initial failure to fully occlude the fallopian tube.[53] Until the mid-1990s, the incidence of pregnancy after surgical sterilization was thought to be between 0 and 0.4 percent (or 0 to 4 per 1,000 patients), and all surgical failures were thought to occur within the first year under the belief that ligated fallopian tubes (once fully severed or occluded and scarred over) would remain closed. However, newer studies began to show that the incidence of failure had been underreported because follow-up had been limited to one year, or the prior studies had surveyed only those physicians who had performed the procedures and had excluded other physicians who would have diagnosed and treated these same women for subsequent pregnancies. In 1996, the Centers for Disease Control published a study that eliminated these flaws.[54] This Collaborative Review of Sterilization (CREST) study was a large, multicenter, prospective study of tubal sterilizations on 10,685 women conducted between 1978 and 1986 at sixteen U.S. hospitals. Women in the study were interviewed before sterilization, one month after surgery, and annually thereafter. Data from this study showed that failure rates varied by surgical method, timing of surgery, and age and race of the woman (younger and nonwhite women were at higher risk). The overall ten-year cumulative failure rate for all forms of tubal sterilization was calculated to be 18.5 per 1,000 surgeries, with a range of 7.5 to 36.5 per 1,000 surgeries depending on the procedure. Pregnancies occurring years after the procedure were believed to be the result of the fallopian tube reconnecting or the development of an uteroperitoneal fistula (an abnormal passage connecting the abdominal cavity with the uterus).[55]

Prior to the CREST study, it was known that pregnancies following tubal ligation were often ectopic.[56] However, the CREST study data allowed researchers to calculate the ten-year cumulative probability of this risk as being

7.3 per 1,000 procedures for all methods of tubal sterilization. Again, the incidence of ectopic pregnancy varied with the method of tubal ligation and the age and ethnicity of the women. These same researchers found that the annual rate of ectopic pregnancy for all tubal sterilization methods combined in the fourth through tenth years after the procedure was no lower than that in the first three years. From this finding, the researchers concluded that a history of tubal sterilization did not rule out the possibility of ectopic pregnancy even many years after the procedure.[57]

An analysis of the many individual studies and of the CREST study led one physician reviewer to recommend that women who sought sterilization should be informed that the pregnancy rates following tubal ligation can be similar to some reversible contraceptive methods, such as the IUD and injectable long-term hormones, especially for younger and nonwhite women.[58]

ALTERNATIVES TO FEMALE STERILIZATION

Men could be sterilized with vasectomy, a procedure performed under local anesthesia, which involved cutting the vas deferens (the tube that carries sperm) through a small abdominal incision. Studies had shown that male sterilization via vasectomy was more effective, safer, and cheaper than female tubal ligation.[59] The only identified benefit of tubal ligation over vasectomy was its immediate sterility. The male who had undergone vasectomy could continue to be fertile until sperm had been eliminated, which took about fifteen ejaculations.[60] Despite the benefits of male sterilization, since the advent of laparoscopic tubal ligation, women were two to three times more likely to be sterilized than men in the United States.[61] The reasons for this ratio were most often cultural (more white men than nonwhite men have vasectomies) or were due to the fact that women are more highly motivated than men to avoid having "extra" children.[62]

Reversible contraceptives were the alternative to sterilization surgery for women who wanted to avoid pregnancy but who did not want to undergo a surgical procedure or permanently lose their fertility. The U.S. market for these contraceptives was very well developed with many products available, including contraceptive tablets taken daily, Norplant® by Wyeth-Ayerst (implantable rods inserted directly under the skin that slowly released contraceptive hormones and were replaced every three to five years), and Depo-Provera® by Pharmacia-Upjohn (slow-release progestin hormone injections given every three months).[63] Intra-uterine devices (small devices inserted into the uterus) could also be used, but product liability litigation had reduced the number available to only two: one with copper, which lasted five years, and Progesta-sert®, a device that released a small amount of locally effective hormone, which required annual replacement. The hormone-based products were considered to be 96 to 99 percent effective when used properly, the IUDs were 98 to 99 percent effective, and both types had a wide margin of safety but did cause side effects in some women.[64]

U.S. MEDICAL CARE COVERAGE

Although third-party medical insurance payers were the primary beneficiaries of any cost savings resulting from pregnancy prevention, not all U.S. contraception insurance coverage practices were governed by considerations of cost effectiveness. Most private and public medical insurance payers would cover the costs of sterilization procedures, but there was a wide variation in coverage practices for other forms of contraception.

Many private health care insurers would not cover any of the costs of reversible contraception, and most public payer coverage was so low that reversible contraception access was limited for covered individuals of lower economic status.[65] Most private and public payers would cover the costs of ectopic pregnancy, spontaneous abortions, births, and newborn hospitalizations. Most private insurers would cover the costs of induced abortions, but very few public insurers did so. In an economic modeling study of tubal ligation, vasectomy, and the reversible contraceptive methods, all were more effective in preventing pregnancy and less costly than no method. Because of the high cost of tubal ligation, it was not one of the most cost-effective contraceptive methods in the initial years following the procedure. But the fact that continuing costs were nil after year one increased its long-term cost effectiveness.[66] These health-care coverage practices for contraception led the medical economist who performed the modeling study to comment:

> For a woman choosing between tubal ligation and other long-term alternatives such as the copper-T IUD or implants, insurance coverage is likely to be a factor in her decision and is likely to favor sterilization surgery. This pattern in insurance coverage may explain in large part why 24.8% of women at risk of pregnancy in the United States have been surgically sterilized, while only 1.8% use IUDs. Despite its apparent popularity, tubal ligation is much more costly than a copper-T IUD or implants. Using a copper-T IUD for 10 years costs $528 (or $1106 for 30 years), using implants for 10 years costs $1516, but tubal ligation costs more than $2500.[67]

Pregnancy care was one of the most frequent U.S. medical insurance expenses, with costs as high as $8,600 for prenatal care, delivery, and newborn hospitalization. Payments associated with problematic newborns could be astronomical and represented the single largest reimbursement liability for medical insurance companies. Reversible and surgical contraception saved health-care resources by preventing unintended pregnancies and any resultant complications of pregnancy or birth. Compared to contraception, pregnancy was very costly.[68]

ADIANA'S HUMAN TRIALS

After completing trials of the new catheter procedure in animals, Adiana moved into safety trials on human subjects. The point of these trials was to test the safety and perfect the mechanical features of the device, not to test for efficacy. The safety studies had been carried out on perihysterectomy patients to determine if the plug had been placed in its correct position in the fallopian tube. The patients in these studies were undergoing hysterectomy (removal of the uterus) for some other medical reason and were tested with Adiana's device during the surgery. Since the uterus was removed immediately after the Adiana procedure, only mechanical features of the device and procedure could be studied, not whether sterility had been achieved. These safety studies were conducted by obstetricians and gynecologists skilled in hysteroscopic procedures. All surgeons involved in the safety studies received special training in the use of the Adiana device, which generally took a few hours. Two qualified surgeons were present at every research procedure.

These safety and procedure development trials took place in a gynecology medical facility in Monterrey, Mexico. The site, a well-known center for early stage, pilot gynecological clinical studies, was chosen for many reasons. Adiana's company advisors had worked well with this center and with its associated physician group in previous clinical studies. Prior research data collected at this facility had been accepted by FDA in previous submissions by other companies. In addition, the personnel at the facility had a reputation for being adept at educating patients on the consequences of trials before obtaining consent to proceed with any research. (The consent form used in this study is contained in Appendix 8.1.) To facilitate enrollment of women in the studies, Adiana paid for the full costs of the device studies as well as the hysterectomy surgeries for women who volunteered. The surgeons and staff were also paid for their time. Because Adiana had determined that the additional catheter procedure did not pose a safety risk or any additional burden above and beyond the hysterectomy, the study patients received no compensation other than the cost of their surgery and follow-up care. Paul Goeld explained why Adiana chose to conduct trials in Mexico rather than in the United States:

> We went to Mexico because we have a "non-significant risk" device and regulations permit us to perform limited studies in this setting. In Mexico, there are strong ethical requirements, highly skilled operators and good facilities, good clinical follow-up, relatively easy patient recruitment, and the results are accepted by FDA.[69]

The Mexican studies showed that the Adiana procedure did not pose any additional risks or potential complications over and above those associated with hysteroscopy. As with any hysteroscopic procedure, there was the risk of perforation of the uterus if the hysteroscope was mishandled. Additional risks associated with the use of the Adiana catheter could include burning of the bowel and the uterine wall if the current was applied in an unintended portion of the local anatomy. Although small, there were also the risks associated with diagnostic hysteroscopy, such as fluid overload due to excessive absorption of the fluid used to inflate the uterus. None of these complications had been observed in the Mexican safety studies. Therefore, Adiana could conclude that the safety studies showed that their catheter product had performed very well and there were no complications resulting from the use of the new device. However, there were some potential long-term problems that this study could not evaluate because all of the tissue affected by the Adiana procedure (including the uterus and fallopian tubes) was immediately removed from the patients. These potential problems could range from persistent pelvic pain, dysmenorrhea (painful periods), or amenorrhea (no periods) to infection or pelvic inflammatory disease. Other than the failure of the device resulting in a normal pregnancy, there was also the risk of ectopic pregnancy if the tubes were not adequately blocked.

With the safety data in hand, Adiana began to plan for expanded U.S. clinical trials to evaluate efficacy as well as safety of the device and the procedure. Because these studies were crucial to the success of the product, they had to be carefully designed. The trials would take about six months of recruiting, with a one-year follow-up, at an estimated cost of $2 million. Although Adiana classified the risk profile of the device as "non-significant risk" for the purpose of the initial safety studies, the pivotal efficacy trial would need FDA preapproval. The company anticipated the complications of the procedure to include infection, bleeding, pelvic pain, painful or interrupted periods, and other complications normally associated with diagnostic hysteroscopy. There was also the risk that the device would be ineffective in preventing pregnancy and that some of the resulting pregnancies would be ectopic.

Based on animal studies, the company believed that the fallopian tubes would be completely blocked within weeks of the procedure. However, to be on the safe side, Adiana planned to advise the women in its clinical trials to wait one month after the procedure before discontinuing contraception protection. The efficacy of the procedure and the device would be tested after that first month. Because of the need for this additional contraception, Adiana had to select the study subjects carefully to prevent contraception noncompliance from confounding the efficacy data. The company planned to exclude from the study any women with a prior history of inability to comply with contraception. The subjects also had to be well-educated about the implications of the trial, and would be required to follow up with the study physician at intervals of one, three, six, and twelve months after the procedure. Goeld was confident that because of the regular visits, the physicians would be able to detect a pregnancy before any complications developed.

As the company made progress developing the clinical trials, several venture capitalists began to exhibit interest: Adiana received more than $10 million in a second round of venture funding from well-known Silicon Valley firms Abingworth Management, Alloy Ventures, Charter Ventures, Delphi Ventures, and Forward Ventures.

ADIANA'S STRATEGIC PARTNERSHIP

At the time Adiana was designing its efficacy trials, the company was planning to enter into a strategic partnership with a major health maintenance organization to conduct late phase (termed Phase III by FDA) human clinical trials in the United States. The ideal HMO would be a medical facility that performed thousands of sterilizations every year and could effectively conduct clinical research. This expertise was needed since Phase III trials were the expanded trials intended to demonstrate ultimate product efficacy, as well as to collect further safety data. Investigational use of the devices at such a large facility was attractive to Adiana because it would also establish market inroads for the product. Adiana intended that both parties would benefit from such a partnership. Adiana would use the HMO's clinical research resources, expertise in conducting trials on human subjects, and data base of available subjects.

The managed care firm could reduce the overall cost of female sterilization surgeries by 50 percent by using Adiana's catheter. Adiana also planned on offering a reduced price on the marketed catheters to the HMO as one of the company's most favored customers.

TUBAL LIGATION MARKET AND MARKET ENTRY

With the multiple advantages that its catheter promised, Adiana's management believed the company had the potential to garner a significant portion of the market for female sterilization, the most prevalent surgery performed worldwide—an estimated seven million surgeries annually. Adiana was confident that if the device received U.S. regulatory approval, the company would be able to market it in other developed countries. Western Europe, Canada, Australia, and Japan combined had an estimated market potential of more than three million patients.

At the time, about half of all female sterilization surgeries were performed in the developing nations of India, China, Taiwan, and Thailand. Due to the price of the catheters, however, Goeld did not think that the device would be commercially viable in third world countries. Other drawbacks included the fact that hysteroscopy equipment was expensive, and physicians would have to be trained in the new procedure, which Adiana could not readily manage in a third world setting. Poor education and awareness levels about contraception among women in third world countries were also believed to create an increased risk that postprocedure contraception would fail. However, owing to the educational programs sponsored by the World Health Organization and other agencies, women in these regions had begun to accept contraceptive practices and a third world market for Adiana was expected to grow eventually. In spite of the opportunities in the global marketplace, Adiana decided to focus on overcoming the hurdles of getting to market in the United States.

FAILED DEVICES

To enter the U.S. market, which it estimated to be about $1.5 billion in size, Adiana had to recognize and address the problems associated with earlier attempts at developing a similar device. Over the years, other physicians and companies had attempted to develop nonsurgical tubal ligation devices that would access the fallopian tubes via the vagina, but these attempts had all failed. Reasons included failures to fully occlude the fallopian tubes and a high rate of infection caused by the devices dragging bacteria from the vagina into the deeper reproductive tissues.[70]

EMERGING COMPETITION

Adiana also had some emerging competition to take into consideration. One competitor, Valleylab, Inc., of Boulder, Colorado, was in the process of animal testing a new computer-controlled bipolar cautery probe. The probe was passed through the cervix and delivered a target temperature to close the fallopian tube. In a trial with sixty rabbits, Valleylab's device was found to be effective and safe.[71] In addition, a platinum microcoil delivered to the fallopian tubes via the cervix was also undergoing testing.[72] One public company, Conceptus, had developed a metal coil device intended to be inserted nonsurgically into the opening of the fallopian tubes through the vagina. This firm had already started Phase II human clinical trials on about 150 women, with no reported pregnancies to date. Approximately 94 percent of the procedures had been performed without general anesthesia, and the average procedure took only twenty-one minutes. Based on this information, Goeld figured that Conceptus was probably six months ahead of Adiana in the product development cycle.[73]

FDA REGULATORY PROCESS

The FDA regulatory process constituted another hurdle. In order to receive FDA approval to market the device in the United States, Adiana had to prove that the device was safe and effective for sterilization. This could be achieved in two different ways. In the first, Adiana could set a hurdle rate for itself and prove that the device met the rate by presenting results from a clinical study. For example, Adiana could file an IDE request with FDA claiming that the device had 97 percent efficacy in preventing pregnancy.[74] The company would then have to provide FDA with proof from clinical trials. Meeting this preselected target would allow FDA to grant marketing approval for the device with the proven claim. A second strategy involved conducting clinical trials using historical controls. The CREST study had frequently served as a benchmark against which other sterilization devices/drugs were tested. Following this strategy, Adiana would do single group trials and then compare its results with those of the study. However, Adiana was unclear which of the CREST study benchmarks it needed to meet or exceed. The CREST study examined the efficacy and safety of various techniques and devices used to sterilize patients, such as clips, rings, and cautery. Each of these was associated with different contraceptive rates, but none was sufficiently similar to Adiana's device to allow the company to select comparative data. For this reason, Adiana might choose not to use any concurrent controls to compare its device to another method.

Because of the difficulty of selecting a study that would meet FDA approval, Goeld decided to make the decision on what study design was appropriate after discussing his options with the regulatory agency. Goeld knew that his competitor Conceptus was meeting with FDA soon after his meeting, and he hoped to learn more about FDA's view from how it treated Conceptus.

ETHICAL AND LEGAL ISSUES RELATED
TO THE EFFICACY TRIALS

Having arrived at the stage where the company needed to design the first efficacy trials, Goeld found himself facing some ethical and related legal issues. He decided that he needed to resolve three major issues before he went ahead with his meeting at FDA. Foremost in his mind was the company's responsibility for subjects who became pregnant after undergoing the experimental sterilization procedure. From the success rates seen with the catheter in animal trials, Goeld expected that the probability of pregnancy in the human test group would not exceed 1 percent, that is, not more than five out of a total test group of about five hundred women subjects would become pregnant during the trials. However, despite the low probability figures, Goeld was concerned about the corporate responsibility for dealing with these possible pregnancies.

The costs of medical care for women who became pregnant after undergoing sterilization with the Adiana device was a relevant issue. In their economic modeling study, researchers Leveque and Koenig had calculated that the managed care payment costs for pregnancies resulting from contraception failure (including from tubal ligation) were as follows: $4,994 for ectopic pregnancy, $416 for induced abortion, $1,038 for spontaneous abortion, $5,512 for maternal prenatal and delivery care of a term pregnancy, and $3,107 for newborn hospitalization.[75] These costs could be much higher for difficult pregnancies and births. The costs of subsequent childcare would vary depending on the women's circumstances, and could also be very high. Finally, the anticontraception and antiabortion views of some religious and other groups needed to be taken into consideration. Goeld knew that strong reactions from such organizations were a risk of conducting these clinical trials and managing any subsequent pregnancy.

Sitting at his desk and contemplating these concerns, Goeld drew a small decision tree and outlined a three-pronged approach to the problem. He decided that if a pregnancy occurred in a study subject, the company would: (1) pay for termination of the pregnancy if the woman so elected and/or (2) pay for the cost of a traditional surgical tubal ligation procedure if the woman so elected. The company planned to have the subjects execute an agreement in which Adiana promised, in the event of sterilization failure, to pay for an abortion and traditional surgical tubal ligation procedure for a specified time period (up to five years, for instance) at the subject's request. Goeld's third prong concerned Adiana's financial and moral responsibility for pre- and postnatal care should a woman elect to bring the pregnancy to full term. On this question, he decided that Adiana would not pay for any prenatal, perinatal, or postnatal care or any expenses associated with the delivery of the child. Finally, Goeld considered the company's obligation in the event the baby was born with a congenital defect. Since the Adiana procedure only modified a reproductive conduit, the physicians consulting with the company were confident that it was extremely unlikely that the catheter procedure would directly cause congenital deformities. But Goeld knew that a certain number of pregnancies resulted in the birth of abnormal children, and despite the lack of direct causation, there were always attorneys who could fashion a causation argument and would use a congenital defect as an opportunity for financial gain in a lawsuit.[76] Under this scenario, Goeld was undecided about what Adiana should do. Goeld wanted to "do the right thing," and he considered this to be the company's biggest and most challenging ethical and legal dilemma.

If a woman held Adiana legally responsible for causing the birth of a defective child, a lawsuit would be difficult for the company. Goeld knew that the cost of lawsuits against the major pharmaceutical companies had increased considerably in the last few years, and some juries were awarding larger and larger settlements to people who had developed serious or even minor side effects with current contraceptive methods. For instance, American Home Products Corporation (AHP), the parent of Norplant maker Wyeth-Ayerst Laboratories, had recently decided to settle a class action lawsuit after five years of litigation. It was reported to have paid $50 million to more than thirty-six thousand women to settle claims that the implantable contraceptive device caused primarily minor side effects such as headaches, irregular menstrual bleeding, nausea, and depression, all of which had been included in the warning section of the product labeling. AHP made the decision to settle based on economic considerations even though it had won three jury trials and twenty pretrial verdicts, and had obtained dismissals of fourteen thousand lawsuits. The litigation simply had been too costly.[77] Goeld was also mindful of the fact that most companies that had manufactured IUDs had either abandoned the market or gone bankrupt following an onslaught of product liability lawsuits. The IUD litigation had lasted over ten years and resulted in billions of dollars in payments to plaintiffs.[78] Such increasingly large legal damage awards and settlements were of great concern to Adiana, since given its small size and reliance on venture funding, a similar legal hit, even on behalf of a small number of women, could easily wipe out the entire enterprise.

Paul Goeld turned his attention back to his decision tree as he considered how the courts and religious groups would view the various outcomes to the clinical trials that he had sketched out. He wondered about the outcomes he could not foresee and how his competitors would decide to address similar challenges.

Questions

1. What are the responsibilities of a U.S. company conducting premarketing clinical studies on Mexican women? Did the company address these issues appropriately?

2. How should the recruitment and consent process for the upcoming device efficacy studies be handled?

3. What responsibilities does Adiana have for the women in the upcoming efficacy studies who become pregnant?

Discussion

This case study has two aspects to it. The issues dealing with conducting clinical research in foreign countries (ensuring quality and conformance with general principles of research ethics and managing questions of cultural relevance) can also be explored in the VaxGen case study in Chapter 9. The primary question that this study addresses is whether and to what extent Adiana has a duty to compensate women harmed in its contemplated U.S. study of its investigational device. The inherent uncertainties related to research results and the costs of compensation or litigation defense make the utilitarian analysis difficult for Adiana. However, the exercise will be worthwhile since it requires a consideration of the positive and negative consequences of Adiana's various courses of action with the goal of identifying the course of action that produces the maximum social good. Regarding a rights analysis, it is undisputed that women are entitled to full, unbiased benefit, risk, and compensation information prior to consenting to participate in these trials. But is supplying information the limit of the company's responsibility? The answer to this question may depend on whether human research subjects are viewed as free agents equally capable of making autonomous choices, as vulnerable and easily exploited individuals, or as courageous volunteers who make knowing sacrifices for the benefit of medical science. The justice question involves asking which parties should bear the burdens of unintended pregnancy. Notions of fairness lead to questions such as, who can best bear the burdens, and who caused the problem? In addition, Nozick's views, with its focus on fair process, can be contrasted to a Rawls's approach that focuses on equality of liberty, fair opportunity, and lessening the differences between parties when equality cannot be achieved.

Appendix 8.1

Consent Form for Adiana Clinical Trial Conducted in Mexico

(translated from the Spanish)

Voluntary Consent Form for Participation in a Research Study

Protocol: Implant Sterilization System/Radio Frequency
Principal Investigator: Dr. _____
Location: _____ Hospital, _____, _____
Sponsor: Adiana, Inc.

1. INTRODUCTION

This form is known as a consent form. You should read it carefully and clarify any and all doubts you may have before consenting to participate in this study. You may take all the time you consider is necessary before making a decision. Before giving your consent to participate in this study, Dr. _____, or one of his representatives, will discuss with you all information contained in this consent form. If there is unfamiliar medical or scientific terminology, please be sure to ask the person obtaining your consent for an explanation.

2. PURPOSE OF THE STUDY

The purpose of this study is to evaluate the new device designed by the Adiana Company for the treatment of female sterilization. This protocol will evaluate this new device with respect to its safety and feasibility on humans. This new method developed by the Adiana Company could become a new noninvasive method of female sterilization to be utilized in a medical/clinical setting. You are being asked to participate in this study because you are scheduled for a hysterectomy. At least sixteen patients will participate in this study.

3. PROCEDURE

Selection Visit

A physical exam will be performed on you, and you will be asked to provide us with exact and complete information regarding your medical history. Blood tests (hematic biometry and biophysical profile) will also be performed to rule out infections, and an electrocardiogram and chest x-ray will also be done. If any of the results from the tests performed are positive, you will not be able to be participate in this study.

Placement of the Adiana Device

The device will be placed immediately before your hysterectomy. It is estimated that this procedure will add approximately one hour to your hysterectomy procedure.

A. Before the procedure, antibiotics will be given to you to prevent infection. This is a routine procedure done before a surgery is performed.

B. You will be given an anesthesia, as is normally done before a hysterectomy.

C. Before the hysterectomy, a hysteroscope (thin telescope) will be introduced into your uterus by way of your vagina and cervix so that the inside of your uterus and entrance to your fallopian tubes can be viewed.

D. The Adiana device consists of a plug adhered to a catheter. The catheter will be introduced via the hysteroscope, and the plug will be placed at the entrance of the fallopian tube. A current will then be administered to the plug. This plug is removed from the catheter, and the catheter will be retracted. The procedure is then repeated on the other fallopian tube.

E. The actual hysterectomy is performed in the usual manner (the plugs are removed along with the uterus).

F. After the hysterectomy, the doctor will examine your uterus to evaluate the performance of the Adiana device.

4. RISKS

The following are possible complications that are associated with the use of the Adiana method; however, not all the risks are recognized.

A. *Anesthesia; adverse reactions and overdose*: The anesthesia and other medications can cause reactions such as low blood pressure or difficulty breathing. Appropriate equipment and medications will be available during the surgery to counteract these possible reactions. The doctors participating in this study are experienced in the proper use of anesthesia and other medicines.

B. *Uterine perforation*: Uterine perforation is a risk associated with placement of any type of device into the uterus. The Adiana device has been designed and tested to minimize the risk of perforation. The doctors participating in this study are experienced with and understand hysteroscopy.

C. *Damage to adjacent organs (i.e., intestines)*: The use of current in the uterus and fallopian tubes poses a risk of burns to the intestine. Various medical devices that utilize heat in the uterine tissue are available on the market. The complications produced by excessive heat are rare, but if it occurs, it can produce thermal damage to adjacent organs. The Adiana device has been designed to work at temperatures lower than those of other devices on the market, further lowering the associated risks. The Adiana system automatically controls the amount of current that is transmitted so that the temperature of the tissue can be controlled.

D. *Fluid overload*: It is possible that an excess of fluids can be absorbed through the blood during the hysteroscopy procedure. To control this risk of fluid overload, the investigator will monitor the fluid balance (entering versus leaving) during the procedure. It is very improbable that this could occur because the blood vessels aren't severed during this process.

E. *Infection*: Any surgery has its risk of infection. The device will be sterilized and will be maintained sterilized until its use. The doctors will utilize sterile techniques to minimize the risk of infection.

F. *Bleeding*: Bleeding can occur at any time during the procedure; however, there will be no surgical incisions. Thus, the risk is minimal. In the case of any complication, the study will terminate and the proper treatment will be administered, without cost to the patient.

I understand that it is my right to solicit whatever clarification and obtain information regarding the procedure during any time of this entire process. In addition, I understand that I am at liberty to withdraw from the study whenever I choose, and that this action will not affect any treatments I may receive at the _____ Hospital in the future.

I understand that the information obtained from this study will be kept confidential and that under no circumstances will my privacy be violated.

In addition, Adiana Inc. will provide me with medical or surgical treatment, without cost to me, in the case that directly or indirectly, I suffer damage from the procedures of this research project, and that in case of permanent damage, I will have a right to be indemnified according to the damages I may suffer.

Patient	Date
Witness	Date
Researcher	Date

Notes

1. Levine RJ. Compensation for research-induced injury. In *Ethics and regulation of clinical research.* New Haven: Yale University Press; 1988. pp. 155–61; U.S. President's Commission for the Study of Ethical Problems in Medicine and Biomedical and Behavioral Research. *Compensating for research injuries: The ethical and legal implications of programs to redress injured subjects.* Vol. 1. Washington, DC: Department of Health and Human Services; 1982. Available at www.gwu.edu/nsarchiv/radiation/dir/mstreet/commeet/meet16/brief16/tab_b/tab_b.html; Jortberg LK. Who should bear the burden of experimental medical device testing: The preemptive scope of the medical device amendments under Slater v. Optical Radiation Corp. *DePaul Law Review* 1994; 43:963–1003; O'Reilly JT. Elders, surgeons, regulators, jurors: Are medical experimentation's mistakes too easily buried? *Loyola University of Chicago Law Journal* 2000; 31:317–68.

2. Mariner WK. Compensation for research injuries. In Mastroianni A, Faden R, Federman D, editors, *Women and health research: Ethical and legal issues of including women in clinical studies.* Washington, DC: National Academy Press; 1994. pp. 113–26; Appendix D: Compensation systems for research injuries. In Mastroianni A, Faden R, Federman D, editors, *Women and health research: Ethical and legal issues of including women in clinical studies.* Washington, DC: National Academy Press; 1994. pp. 243–52.

3. *Secretary's task force on the compensation of injured research subjects: Report* (OS) 77–003. Washington, DC: Department of Health, Education and Welfare; 1977.

4. See Note 2, Mariner.

5. See Note 1, U.S. President's Commission for the Study of Ethical Problems in Medicine and Biomedical and Behavioral Research.

6. Neither did agencies have data on the number of subjects enrolled in federal studies. However, the commission estimated that in the late 1970s, about eight hundred thousand subjects per year were involved in Public Health Service supported clinical trials (i.e., controlled studies of new therapies). This estimate did not include the large numbers of subjects participating in studies of basic physiology, normal growth and development, and a variety of other inquiries utilizing normal volunteers. It was also estimated that 375,000 subjects per year were participating in FDA-regulated research designed to test new drugs. This figure did not include subjects involved in the testing of medical devices.

7. Information excerpted from U.S. President's Commission for the Study of Ethical Problems in Medicine and Biomedical and Behavioral Research. *Compensating*

for research injuries: the ethical and legal implications of programs to redress injured subjects. Vol. 1. Washington, DC: Department of Health and Human Services; 1982. Available at www.gwu.edu/nsarchiv/radiation/dir/mstreet/commeet/meet16/brief16/tab_b/tab_b.html. The data collected by the commission on research injuries were from different institutions and difficult to compare, since each institution used different metrics and different definitions of "adverse event" and "injury." Nonetheless, the programs were considered large enough to generate data suggestive of the extent and nature of research-related injury. The University of Washington had collected data both prior to and after instituting a liability insurance program in 1976 that covered research injuries. Their data showed that during the period of 1972 to 1981, an estimated 356,000 subjects had been enrolled in more than 5,300 protocols for biomedical research. Data on "nontrivial" adverse effects were reported and showed that over a period of eight years, 144 injured subjects (or 0.04 percent of the estimated total) experienced temporary disability, none were permanently disabled, and two patient-subjects died. Most of those who experienced injury were patient-subjects with existing disease. The university believed that these were not accurate figures since there was not universal compliance with the reporting system, and a significant number of research physicians only reported unanticipated adverse effects. Over a period of 9.5 years, only eighteen subjects had submitted formal claims for injury compensation to the university's insurance program. University officials attributed the low number to the facts that research subjects were not told about the existence of the compensation program, most reports were filed by physicians, and informal mechanisms may have eliminated the need for further compensation.

Another institution, the Quincy Research Center in Kansas City, Missouri, was a drug-testing facility whose subjects had been covered by a workers' compensation program since 1975. Data had been collected from 151 Phase 1 (nontherapeutic) projects involving 2,596 normal volunteers, and 78 Phase 2–4 (therapeutic) projects involving 2,478 patient volunteers. These data showed that the total number of adverse events and the number of serious adverse events were greater in Phase 2–4 studies (which used patients) compared with Phase I studies of normal volunteers. Patient-subjects were more likely than normal subjects to withdraw from protocols because of significant adverse events, and although the incidence rates were very low, patients were more likely to be hospitalized (1.43 percent vs. 0.2 percent) and to die (0.24 percent vs. 0). It appeared that most of the clinically significant side effects occurred because of pre-existing disease in patient-subjects rather than as a direct consequence of the experimental drugs or participation in the research. The Quincy official concluded that none of the six deaths and only seven of the thirty-six hospitalizations could conceivably have been research related, whereas three of the five hospitalizations for normal volunteers could have been as a consequence of the research.

Michigan State Prison had an active research program in Phase I drug testing in normal prisoner volunteers. For over twelve years, from 1964 to 1976, records were reviewed for 805 protocols involving 29,162 participants over 614,534 subject days. Prison officials reported fifty-eight adverse drug reactions and six additional "complications" temporally related to the drug study, forming a total of sixty-four subjects (.2 percent) who experienced "significant medical events." None of the adverse reactions and only one of the complications were permanently disabling; one subject on placebo died of cerebrovascular hemorrhage while asleep. Thus, a clinically significant medical event occurred once every 9,602 days of subject exposure or about once every 26.3 years of individual subject participation.

The only federal attempt to collect and analyze data on research injuries was a special study conducted for the HEW secretary's Task Force on the Compensation of Injured Research Subjects. In a telephone survey, investigators were asked to report the number of subjects involved in therapeutic and nontherapeutic studies, the nature and incidence of injuries "that could be attributed to the conduct of the experimental regimen," and whether those injuries were experienced by subjects of therapeutic or nontherapeutic research. Injuries were classified as trivial, temporarily disabling, permanently disabling, and fatal. This survey included data on a total of 132,615 subjects. Overall, 3.0 percent of the subjects experienced trivial adverse effects, 0.7 percent experienced temporarily disabling injuries, less than 0.1 percent were permanently disabled, and 0.03 percent died. (All of the fatalities occurred in patient-subjects in therapeutic research.) Of the more than thirty-nine thousand subjects participating in therapeutic research studies, 10.8 percent experienced adverse affects or injuries, most of which were trivial in nature. Only 2.4 percent of subjects were temporarily disabled, less than 0.1 percent were permanently disabled, and approximately 0.1 percent died. Most of the forty-three fatalities were not clearly related to the research. In fact, thirty-seven (86 percent) of the reported deaths were in cancer chemotherapy trials. In the other categories as well, many of the "injured" were cancer patients who experienced familiar side effects of standard treatment. The incidence of injury for subjects participating in nontherapeutic research was even lower. Of 93,399 subjects, only 8.8 percent experienced injuries, most of which were trivial. Thirty-seven people (0.1 percent) were temporarily disabled, one person was permanently disabled, and there were no fatalities.

8. The Tuskegee Study of Untreated Syphilis in the Male Negro was started by the Public Health Service in 1932 to study the natural progression of untreated syphilis. Hundreds of African-American men, mostly poor sharecroppers from Macon County, Alabama, were recruited for the study with promises of free medical care. The "medical care" was primarily to obtain research data and no treatment for syphilis was provided. Public disclosure in a *New York Times* article caused the study to end in 1972, which was twenty years after penicillin was known to be an effective treatment for syphilis. According to the Report of the Tuskegee Syphilis Study Legacy Committee, "In the almost 25 years since its disclosure, the Study has moved from a singular historical event to a powerful metaphor. It has come to symbolize racism in medicine, ethical misconduct in human research, paternalism by physicians, and government abuse of vulnerable people." Report of the Tuskegee Syphilis Study Legacy Committee Final Report. 1996 May 20. Available from www.med.virginia.edu/hs-library/historical/apology/report.html.

9. See Note 7, U.S. President's Commission for the Study of Ethical Problems in Medicine and Biomedical and Behavioral Research.

10. See Note 2, Appendix D.

11. Ibid.

12. Documents declassified since 1994 showed that dozens of government-sanctioned Cold War radiation experiments were conducted between 1944 and 1974 on military personnel, A-bomb plant workers, patients, children, pregnant women, and prisoners who were not fully informed and who were misled about the nature of the experiments, what was being administered, or the risks of the interventions. Some subjects were not even told they were participating in an experiment, and many subjects were from vulnerable populations such as the poor, elderly, mentally retarded, infants, and hospitalized patients with terminal diseases. These studies were attempts to determine the effects of radiation on human beings and were considered highly important given the perceived threat of nuclear war. At the time the studies were done, researchers understood that exposure to radioactive materials could cause cancer. Many such experiments resulted in valuable medical advances such as radiation treatments for cancer and the use of isotopes to accurately diagnose illnesses. This advisory committee made the first public disclosures of this research.

13. Advisory Committee on Human Radiation Experiments. Washington, DC; 1994. Available from www.gwu.edu/nsarchiv/radiation/.

14. Ibid.

15. See Note 2, Mariner; Note 2, Appendix D.

16. *Ethical and policy issues in research involving human participants: Report and recommendations of the National Bioethics Advisory Commission.* Volume 1, 2001 Aug, p. 123. Available from http://bioethics.georgetown.edu/nbac/pubs.html.

17. Secondary policy reasons for not requiring mandatory compensation included that the added financial burden could discourage manufacturers from developing new products and would effectively imply that the FDA was irresponsible in allowing the clinical study to proceed.

See also Note 1, Jortberg; Note 1, Levine.

18. Personal communication from Virginia Paton, Pharm.D., director, clinical operations, Cerus Corporation, to ML Eaton, author. 2001 June 18.

19. The FDA required that companies inform research subjects that by signing the consent form, subjects did not waive their legal rights nor did they release the sponsor or researcher from liability for negligence. 21 *Code of Federal Regulations* 50.20.

Factual claims were most typically that the research injuries resulted from inappropriate selection of persons as test subjects, deficiencies in the product or process tested, failure to obtain adequate informed consent, errors or omissions by research personnel, or unreasonable and dangerous conduct by the researchers. Either or all of these failures could be alleged in a lawsuit for research-related injuries. The legal bases for these lawsuits were either in the laws of battery (failure to obtain informed consent), strict liability (the injury was the result of a defective product or inadequate manufacturer's warning), or negligence (the conduct of the sponsor or researcher was unreasonable under the circumstances). To prevail in negligence, a plaintiff must prove that the defendant owed the plaintiff a legal duty of care, that the defendant breached that duty, that the plaintiff suffered an injury, and that the injury was caused by the breach of the defendant's duty. See Dobbs DB. *The law of torts*. St. Paul, MN: West Group; 2001.

20. See Note 1, O'Reilly.

21. See Note 2, Mariner.

22. See Note 1, Jortberg.

23. The defense of assumption of risk usually required a showing that the subject knew that the risk was present, must have understood its nature, and that the subject's choice to incur the risk was free and voluntary. See Note 19, Dobbs. Whether companies could avail themselves of this defense in a research injury lawsuit was an evolving question of law. It might also be difficult to persuade a jury that the research subject fully understood the nature of the research risk as well as the company did. In addition, since the company could not inform subjects of the full nature of all possible risks (otherwise, why do the research?), it might seem unfair to a jury to assert the defense against a research subject.

24. Merton V. The exclusion of pregnant, pregnable, and once-pregnable people (aka women) from biomedical research. *American Journal of Law and Medicine* 1993; 19:369–451; Marstroianni AC. HIV, women, and access to clinical trials: Tort liability and lessons from DES. *Duke Journal of Gender Law and Policy* 1998; 5:167–91; see also Note 1, O'Reilly; Note 1, Jortberg.

25. 21 *Code of Federal Regulations* 50.25(a)(1).

Guideline for good clinical practice, informed consent of trial subjects. International Conference on Harmonisation of Technical Requirements for Registration of Pharmaceuticals for Human Use; 1996. pp. 15–18. Available from www.ifpma.org/pdfifpma/e6.pdf.

26. See Note 2, Mariner.

27. Research injuries that led to litigation and publicity included the death of eighteen-year-old Jesse Gelsinger in a company-sponsored gene therapy trial at the University of Pennsylvania; a class action lawsuit (brought on behalf of eighty-two subjects by the same attorney as in Gelsinger) against Seattle's prestigious Fred Hutchinson Cancer Research Center and a biotechnology company where at least twenty subjects were alleged to have died from experimental cancer treatments; a lawsuit against the University of Oklahoma (brought by the same attorney) where nineteen subjects were alleged to have been injured in a melanoma study; the death of a young woman in a Johns Hopkins University asthma study; the death of a healthy college student at a University of Rochester bronchoscopy study; and the death of five of fifteen subjects in an NIH-sponsored study of hepatitis B. Nelson D, Weiss R. Penn researchers sued in gene therapy death, teen's parents also name ethicist as defendant. *Washington Post* 2000 Sept 19; Sect. A:03; Weiss R, Nelson D. FDA halts experiments on genes at university; probe of teen's death uncovers deficiencies. *Washington Post* 2000 Jan 22; Sect. A:01; Brower V. Gene therapy's wake-up call; adenoviral vectors not ready for prime time. Biospace.com 2000 Jan 3. Available from www.biospace.com; Wilson D, Heath D. Class-action suit filed against "The Hutch." Protocol 126 broke laws, say families of

cancer patients. *Seattle Times* 2001 Mar 27; Sect. A:1; Altman LK. Volunteer in asthma study dies after inhaling drug. *New York Times* 2001 June 15; Sect. A:16.

Greenberg D. Our flimsy surveillance of science. *Washington Post* 2000 Jan 31; Sect. A:19.

Menache A. Healthy human volunteers and informed consent. *Medicine and Law* 2000; 19:523–25.

28. See Note 27, Menache.

29. The initial case study was prepared by Anjali Reddi and Aradhana Sarin under the guidance of and with later revisions by Margaret Eaton. The input and assistance of Paul Geold, president, Adiana, and of Doug Kelly, partner, Alloy Ventures, is greatly appreciated. We also thank the following people who provided information and advice: Thomas Murphy of Everest Medical Corporation; Gene Segre formerly of Syntex Corporation; Tim Wells of the FDA (OB/GYN Medical Devices); and Brad Marinder of the FDA, Pacific Region. The events described in this case study occurred up until late 1999.

30. Lee PR, Stewart FH. Failing to prevent unintended pregnancy is costly [editorial]. *American Journal of Public Health* 1995; 85:479–80.

31. Fallopian tubes are the tubes that connect the two ovaries to the uterus and serve as a conduit to move the egg to the uterus.

32. Newkirk GR. Permanent female sterilization (tubal ligation). In Pfenninger JL, Fowler GC, editors, *Procedures for primary care physicians*. 1st ed. St. Louis, MO: Mosby-Year Book; 1994. pp. 678–98.

33. Ibid.

34. 42 *Code of Federal Regulations*, section 50.210.

35. See Note 32.

36. Hendrix NW, Chauhan SP, Morrison JC. Sterilization and its consequences. *Obstetrical & Gynecological Survey* 1999; 54:766–77.

Relevant to this case study, Mexico ranked in the top ten of the world's developing countries with an incidence of 21.4 percent of married women of reproductive age having been sterilized. By comparison, South Korea had the highest incidence, with 47.6 percent of women having been sterilized. See Hendrix, supra.

37. Chandra A. Surgical sterilization in the United States; prevalence and characteristics, 1965–1995. National Center for Health Statistics. *Vital Health Statistics* 1998; Series 23, No. 20. Available from www.cdc.gov/nchs/data/sr23_20.pdf.

Of the 15.3 million women represented by this statistic, 26 percent had a tubal ligation, 7 percent had a hysterectomy, and 12 percent were currently living with a husband or partner who had had a vasectomy.

38. See Note 32.

39. Chandra A. Surgical sterilization in the United States; prevalence and characteristics, 1965–1995. National Center for Health Statistics. *Vital Health Statistics* 1998; Series 23, No. 20. Available from www.cdc.gov/nchs/data/sr23_20.pdf.

40. Westhoff C, Davis A. Tubal sterilization: Focus on the U.S. experience. *Fertility & Sterility* 2000; 73:913–22.

41. Ibid.

43. See Note 40.

42. See Note 39.

44. See Note 36.

45. These adverse events included cutting blood vessels or perforating the uterus, bladder, or intestines, events that could cause bleeding or infection and often required cutting open the patient's abdomen to perform surgical repair.

46. See Note 32.

47. See Note 36.

48. See Note 40.

49. Ory HW. Mortality associated with fertility and fertility control: 1983. *Family Planning Perspectives* 1983; 15:15–63. Available from MDConsult, Drug Information, Contraceptives, referencing Mosby's *GenRx*®, 10th ed. St. Louis, MO: Mosby; 2000, prescribing information for ethinyl estradiol/norethindrone, accessed at http://home.mdconsult.com/das/drug/view.

50. See Note 32; Note 39.

51. See Note 39.

52. Total cost of tubal re-canalization procedure alone was about $13,000, and the cost of producing a child via *in vitro* fertilization could range from $66,000 to $800,000. See Neumann PJ, Gharib SD, Weinstein MC. The cost of a successful delivery with in vitro fertilization. *New England Journal of Medicine* 1994; 331:239–43; see also Note 32; Note 36.

53. See Note 40.

54. Peterson HB, Xia Z, Hughes JM, et al. The risk of pregnancy after tubal sterilization: Findings from the US Collaborative Review of Sterilization. *American Journal of Obstetrics and Gynecology* 1996; 174:1161–70.

55. Pisarska MD, Carson SA, Buster JE. Ectopic pregnancy. *Lancet* 1998; 351:1115–20.

56. Ibid.

Ectopic pregnancy is a union of egg and sperm that lodges outside of the uterus. This type of aberrant pregnancy is a risk any time the fallopian tubes are impaired. Some of these pregnancies spontaneously abort on their own and are never detected. But because of the potential harm to the mother (e.g., hemorrhage, infection) and the fact that these pregnancies always fail, diagnosed ectopic pregnancies most often require urgent medical attention to surgically or medically terminate the pregnancy. As of 1992, ectopic pregnancy was associated with a 9 percent incidence of maternal death. Ectopic pregnancies continued to be the leading cause of maternal death in the first trimester. See Pisarska MD, Carson SA. Incidence and risk factors for ectopic pregnancy. *Clinical Obstetrics & Gynecology* 1999; 42:2–8.

57. Peterson HB, Xiz Z, Hughes JM, et al. The risk of ectopic pregnancy after tubal sterilization. U.S. Collaborative Review of Sterilization Working Group. *New England Journal of Medicine* 1997; 336:762–67.

58. See Note 40.

59. Compared with a vasectomy, female tubal ligation is twenty times more likely to result in major complications, twelve times more likely to result in death (a rare event for either procedure), and ten to thirty-seven times more likely to fail. Female

sterilization costs three times more than vasectomy, is costly to reverse, and is associated with lower reversal success rates. See Note 36.

60. See Note 36.

61. See Note 32; Note 39.

62. See Note 36; Note 39.

63. Oral contraceptive pills are used daily by over seventy million women worldwide, and by approximately eighteen million women in the United States. See Osathanondh R. Conception control. In: Ryan KJ, Berkowitz RS, Barbieri RL, et al., editors, *Kistner's gynecology & women's health.* 7th ed. St. Louis, MO: Mosby; 1999. pp. 287–97.

64. Rare but serious side effects for hormone-based contraceptives are: conception caused by noncompliance (highest with the tablets that must be taken daily), blood clots (which can cause leg swelling, pulmonary embolism, heart attack, stroke, or vision loss), gallbladder disease, aggravation of diabetes, possible birth defects in offspring, and possible increase in the incidence of estrogen-dependent cancers of the breast and reproductive organs. Less serious but more common side effects with hormone-based contraceptives are: unpredictable menstrual bleeding, acne, weight gain, breast tenderness, mood changes, nausea, headache, and elevated blood pressure. IUDs have no systemic side effects but can cause serious local effects: infection and pelvic and inflammatory disease (which, if serious, can cause infertility), uterine perforation, and ectopic pregnancy. Unexpected pregnancy with an IUD in place can cause miscarriage or premature delivery. Death resulting from the use of these contraceptive methods is a very rare event, ranging from 0.3 per 100,000 in nonsmoking women ages fifteen to nineteen years on oral contraceptives to 117 per 100,000 in women who smoke, ages forty-one to forty-four years on oral contraceptives. In comparison, deaths that occur from pregnancy and childbirth range from 7 to 28.2 per 100,000 women, ages fifteen to nineteen years to forty to forty-four years old, respectively. From Osathanondh R. Conception control. In Ryan KJ, Berkowitz RS, Barbieri RL, et al, editors, *Kistner's gynecology & women's health.* 7th ed. St. Louis, MO: Mosby; 1999. pp. 287–97.

65. Trussell J, Leveque JA, Koenig JD, et al. The economic value of contraception: A comparison of 15 methods. *Obstetrical & Gynecological Survey* 1996; 51:61S-72S.

66. Ibid.

67. Ibid. Other studies gave cost estimates for tubal ligation ranging from $1,500 to $3,500. See Note 32.

68. See Note 30.

69. A *nonsignificant risk* device is an FDA term under the investigational device exemption (IDE) regulations at 21 CFR part 812, for a nonapproved, low-risk medical device that does not require FDA approval prior to beginning human clinical trials. However, a local investigational review board (IRB) is required to preapprove the study and all subjects must give informed consent prior to entering the clinical trial. The Mexican safety study could be considered a nonsignificant-risk device study since the device manipulation did not add risk to the hysterectomy procedure. See Information Sheets for Institutional Review Boards and Clinical Investigators. Food and Drug Administration; 1995 Oct 1; 73–86.

70. See Note 40.

These methods and devices include the use of laser or radiofrequency current or methylcyanoacrylate glue (commonly called Crazy Glue) to seal the tubes or quinacrine pellets, rings, or clips inserted into the fallopian tubes.

71. Hurst BS, Ryan T, Thomsen S, et al. Computer-controlled bipolar endotubal sterilization is successful in a rabbit model. *Fertility & Sterility* 1999; 71:765–70.

72. Post JH, Cardella JF, Wilson RP, et al. Experimental nonsurgical transcervical sterilization with a custom-designed platinum microcoil. *Journal of Vascular & Interventional Radiology* 1997; 8(Pt 1):113–18.

73. Conceptus shares zoom on word of female contraceptive device's success. *Dow Jones Business News* 1999 Dec 23 [on-line].

74. An investigational device exemption (IDE) allows manufacturers to ship and use unapproved medical devices intended solely for investigational use involving human subjects. The IDE regulations (21 *CFR* part 812) apply to most clinical studies in the United States that are undertaken to gather safety and effectiveness data about a medical device. There are two categories of devices covered by the IDE regulation: (1) significant risk devices and (2) nonsignificant-risk devices (21 *CFR* 812.3(m) and 812.2(b)). Significant risk devices require both FDA and institutional review board (IRB) approval prior to initiation of a clinical study. Nonsignificant risk devices require only IRB approval prior to initiation of a clinical study. Adiana's large-scale human efficacy trials fit the definition of a significant-risk device study, and the company was therefore obliged to seek both FDA and local IRB approval before commencing the studies. Approval was contingent on finding that the study design ensured that risks to subjects were minimized and did not outweigh the anticipated benefits to the subjects and the importance of the knowledge to be gained.

75. See Note 65. Calculations were based on estimating the ectopic pregnancy rate for each of fifteen contraception methods (including tubal ligation) and then assuming the following distribution for the other pregnancy outcomes: 47.5 percent induced abortion, 12.4 percent spontaneous abortion, and 40.1 percent term delivery. Costs were estimated as of 1991.

76. Women cannot waive legal entitlements to sue on behalf of their children, and in most U.S. jurisdictions a child can bring a lawsuit against the entity that caused his or her birth defects if the child is born alive.

77. AHP offers to settle all Norplant suits for more than $50 million. *Medical Devices Litigation Report* 1999; 6:3.

78. Steyer R. Searle nearing end of lawsuits over Copper 7 contraceptive. *St. Louis Post Dispatch* 1995 Oct. 15; sect E:1.

9

Conducting Clinical Research in Developing Countries[1]

Increasingly in the 1990s, American and European pharmaceutical and bio-technology companies began conducting human research studies outside of their own countries. Several factors accounted for this trend. Some countries (like Japan) required research data on their own citizens as a precondition for product approval. Also, an overall increase in the number of clinical trials meant that companies were finding it difficult to recruit sufficient numbers of domestic subjects. The burgeoning existence of contract research organizations (CROs) willing to assist with research using foreign subjects improved the ability to recruit these subjects.[2] In a newsletter devoted to supporting the CRO industry, one article entitled "Latin American Fever" made the enthusiastic comment, "A valuable untapped opportunity is waiting . . . a changing clinical trials market in Latin America may offer a unique opportunity to reach much larger numbers of study subjects."[3] Foreign countries also were becoming attractive research sites as their research infrastructure and technologies became more sophisticated, and better-trained foreign scientists were available and anxious to become more involved as commercial research partners. For these foreign scientists, collaborating with Western medical science companies was often the only way to obtain the funds, medical products, and experience to conduct the research that would allow them to combat local health problems. Finally, less onerous regulatory restrictions, lower costs, and the possibility of gaining inroads into large markets were also motivating factors to conduct research abroad.[4]

However, when Western pharmaceutical and biotechnology companies conduct research on foreign human subjects, especially those in the third world, questions arise about which research practice standards should govern such investigations. Political, legal, and economic systems, customs and culture, poverty and educational levels, and social and medical turmoil can all influence how these standards are applied. From an ethical perspective, questions arise about whether to impose Western values and standards (which can lead to charges of imperialism) or to follow the "when in Rome, do as the Romans do" philosophy, which has been called cultural relativism. If abiding by cultural relativism, an outsider's behavior in a country or within a culture is determined by that country's laws and customs.

Given the differences between first and third world countries, it can be difficult to decide how to proceed. For instance, is it acceptable to engage in a certain legally condoned practice in one country if the practice is considered unethical in the home country? Are there circumstances where ethical standards can justifiably differ? Certainly from a utilitarian perspective, facts and circumstances can change what is considered the best course of action to achieve net social benefit. The costs and benefits of covering the medical care for injured study subjects, for example, would certainly differ between first and third world countries. But for questions about rights or justice, the answers are more complex. Are standard business goals alone (for example, lower cost, improved efficiency, lighter regulatory restrictions) suitable reasons to conduct human research abroad? Should the research be relevant to the health needs of the developing country? What inducements to engage in research are too coercive in a third world setting? Should researchers provide better medical care (if it is available) to human subjects than is generally available in the community from which the subjects are drawn? Are there responsibilities owed to the research subjects or others in the host country outside of the research study? Other standards, such as the requirement for full, informed consent, seem to be universally agreed on but can fall apart in practice. What, for instance, is required to obtain voluntary and fully informed consent from an illiterate tribal African, an intravenous drug user in Bangkok, or a woman in whose culture a husband or tribal chief makes medical decisions on her behalf? Finally, whose responsibility is it to monitor and enforce ethical research conduct? For some insight into these questions, see Appendix 9.1. For U.S. and foreign human research, institutional review boards (IRBs) are required to review and approve only studies designed to ensure that research risks to subjects are minimized and commensurate with potential benefits. However, commentators have questioned whether these boards, composed mainly of research physicians, uniformly place the interests of subjects ahead of those of researchers and whether they can adequately represent the interests of research subjects in another country. At the local level, conflicts of interest can exist when research members of IRBs are also seeking funds and sponsors to conduct local research, therefore having a vested interest in seeing that research protocols proceed.[5]

HIV TRANSMISSION RESEARCH IN HAITI

Differences in opinion abound on how to address these perplexing questions. As an example of how they can manifest, consider the Haitian AIDS studies performed by researchers from the U.S.-based Cornell Medical College. The studies were a collaboration between U.S. and Haitian researchers, using about $7 million in U.S. health agency funds. At the time in the early 1990s, Haiti was one of the poorest countries in the world, health-care services were unavailable to most, and AIDS had become a countrywide epidemic. These factors combined to make Haiti a fruitful place to gather data about the transmissibility of the human immunodeficiency virus (HIV), the virus that causes AIDS. In one study of sex partners, one infected with HIV and the other not, research physicians interviewed subjects and collected blood samples over time to determine why the immune system of the uninfected partner remained resistant to the virus. The study was considered vitally important since this information could lead to the development of an AIDS vaccine. In developing countries where antiretroviral drugs were too expensive and complicated to use, and exhortations to practice safe sex had failed, an AIDS vaccine offered the only hope of stemming the epidemic. Recognizing this, researchers needed to know how some people could, in effect, vaccinate themselves by harnessing their immune systems to resist the virus. Haiti was an especially productive place in which to conduct these so-called couples studies. Unprotected sex was common since condom use was not well accepted in the culture. Subjects were counseled by researchers to engage in safe sex practices, but it was known that many would ignore this counseling. Without the use of condoms by subjects, researchers could collect data on a sufficient number of uninfected sex partners who were repeatedly exposed to HIV. Plus, prior research had shown that HIV was transmitted via unprotected sex at twice the rate in Haiti as in the United States or Europe. Consequently, there was a larger population of potential subjects than in countries where AIDS prevention practices were more established. Also, Haitian subjects were fairly easy to recruit since the research was conducted in the only clinic in the country that provided free HIV screening and treatment, not just for AIDS but also for venereal disease and tuberculosis. Subjects who enrolled in the study were given access to these services ahead of other needy people.[6]

Despite the fact that important health data were being collected, the study came under criticism. Some worried that the access to free medical care was too powerful an inducement to impoverished Haitians, most of whom had no such access. Others disapproved of the fact that the U.S. research physicians adhered to local standards when it came to counseling against unprotected sex and providing antiretroviral drugs. It was left up to the Haitian patients to inform their sexual partners of an HIV infection, and researchers estimated that at least 60 percent never did so. Couples studies in other countries, in contrast, required that all subjects be informed that one of them was infected with the virus. Haitian couples were allowed to refuse the use of condoms, whereas couples subjects in other countries would be continuously and vigorously counseled about the dangers of such a decision. In addition, antiretroviral drugs, which had been used very effectively in the United States to combat the AIDS virus, were not available in Haiti and not given to the infected study subjects. Under these conditions, researchers could study the natural course of infection and resistance in a sufficient number of people "uncorrupted" by the influence of safe sex practices and anti-AIDS drugs. However, the disparity between the treatment of Haitian and American study subjects troubled many physicians. Research experts agreed that this study could never be performed in the United States, where standards required that antiretrovirals be prescribed for subjects with AIDS and that effective prevention counseling be offered. Commenting on the Haitian trials, Dr. David Rothman, a professor of social medicine at New York's Columbia College of Physicians and Surgeons, said the following: "If in Malawi, why not Appalachia? You have serious investigators trying to do good, trying to save hundreds of thousands of lives, but I consider it ultimately destructive of the investigator's integrity and the well-being of all of us to have an ethic of human experimentation that changes as it travels."[7]

Reacting to these comments, the head of the Haitian research clinic, Dr. Jean William Pape, acknowledged that "the ethical issues sometimes are torturing me." Pape was an American-trained physician who had been battling the AIDS epidemic in Haiti from its beginning, and he had linked up with his former professors at Cornell to conduct research to discover how HIV was being transmitted in his country in the hope that the data would show how to stop the transmission. Pape pointed out that his couples subjects benefited from the same counseling and free condoms available to everyone who visited the clinic. He thought that offering life-saving antiretroviral drugs to the relatively small number of research subjects would have been an unethical lure to participate in the study. This was the reason that Pape had even refused an offer from the French government to supply antiretroviral drugs to his study subjects. He was also mistrustful of the French commitment to continue to spend $15,000 per subject per year, a commitment that might disappear if the French economy worsened. Ultimately, however, Pape was convinced that if the research succeeded in leading to an AIDS vaccine, the overall benefit would be enormous and worth the sacrifices. Committed to vaccine research, Pape wanted Haitians to be first in line to test vaccines so that they could assert a "moral" claim to an affordable supply of an effective vaccine once one was developed. Dr. Frantz Large, the vice president of the Haitian Medical Association, defended Pape's decisions and reasoning. "He would never do anything unethical," Large said. "But if he had to choose between the survival of 10 people and the survival of a nation, he would probably choose the survival of a nation, and I would, too."[8]

AZT STUDIES IN PREGNANT AFRICAN
AND THAI WOMEN

The debates about human research conducted in developing countries intensified significantly after medical publications revealed that seventeen thousand pregnant AIDS patients, mostly African and Thai, had participated in several studies co-sponsored by U.S., United Nations, and local country health agencies to determine whether a limited course of AZT treatment could prevent perinatal HIV transmission to infants. Years earlier, studies in the United States had shown that a more extensive course (larger doses and longer duration of both oral and intravenous AZT) was effective in preventing HIV transmission, and this treatment had become standard in the United States. However, AZT was unavailable to pregnant AIDS patients in third world countries because of cost and the fact that none of the countries had a sufficient health system infrastructure to administer the complicated treatment regimen. Consequently, researchers wanted to learn if a more affordable, more manageable regimen could be effective. These studies, which are described more extensively in the chapter on placebo use in clinical trials (Chapter 7), caused vociferous debates about the propriety of withholding known effective treatment from the African subjects.

Dr. Marcia Angell, editor of the *New England Journal of Medicine*, was among the physicians actively involved in the third world country trials debate. In one editorial, she wrote about the AZT trials:

> There appears to be a general retreat from the clear principles enunciated in the Nuremberg Code and the Declaration of Helsinki as applied to research in the Third World. Why is that? Is it because the "local standard of care" is different? I don't think so. In my view, that is merely a self-serving justification after the fact. Is it because diseases and their treatments are very different in the Third World, so that information gained in the industrialized world has no relevance and we have to start from scratch? That, too, seems an unlikely explanation, although here again it is often offered as a justification. Sometimes there may be relevant differences between populations, but that cannot be assumed. Unless there are specific indications to the contrary, the safest and most reasonable position is that people everywhere are likely to respond similarly to the same treatment.[9]

Other criticisms of the AZT trials focused on the suspicion that full, informed consent to participate in the studies could not be obtained given the asymmetry in knowledge and authority between AZT researchers and their mostly poor and illiterate subjects.[10] Another bothersome question related to what has been called the "therapeutic misconception," in which the distinction between therapy and research intervention is blurred.[11] For countries that lack adequate health-care services, some researchers and ethicists feared that it could be too easy for local subjects, who might benefit medically from the research intervention, to view the research as medical care. Expectations about continuing access to care, feelings of abandonment, and other problems could flow from such a misconception, making it vital that researchers be clear about their intent. The AZT trials, in which pregnant women may have seen their first and last physician, were considered especially prone to this confusion, fostering fears that the women had been misled.

These concerns seemed justified by reports, such as one by a *New York Times* journalist who had received copies of subjects' interviews by researchers and who also conducted his own interviews of several of the African subjects after they had delivered their babies.[12] The journalist reported that none of the women interviewed, from the illiterate to the best educated, fully understood the implications of the AZT study. Some did not understand that they might have received a placebo, others agreed to participate because they believed that they would receive medical care, and most said that the chance to do anything to save their baby from AIDS was irresistible. Some women became angry when they learned that a different American treatment had previously been found to be effective at preventing AIDS in newborns. Commenting on the *New York Times* article, two members of the Institute for Health Policy Studies at the University of California, San Francisco, stated that it was dangerous to assume that the African women should have been provided the full American AZT treatment. The many differences that existed (for instance, the poorer health status of the Africans combined with a lessened ability to combat AZT side effects) meant that there were greater risks in giving the full American AZT treatment to African women. The academics ended by asking whether Americans would ever extrapolate research data on African women to justify giving the same amounts of AZT to pregnant U.S. women. Their answer? Never.[13] Their view underscored the need to conduct studies so that treatments could be adapted to local circumstances.

HIV TRANSMISSION TRIAL IN UGANDA

Two heterosexual HIV transmission trials conducted in rural villages in Uganda also were considered ethically difficult to justify.[14] Both studies included partners, one of whom was infected with HIV and the other not. One study attempted to learn whether the presence of other sexually transmitted diseases, such as syphilis, increased the transmission of HIV. In this study, half of the subjects were given antibiotics to reduce the prevalence of sexually transmitted diseases and the others were left to seek their own treatment. A second trial studied whether higher levels of HIV in one partner increased the transmission of the virus to the unaffected partner. The studies lasted for up to thirty months, during which time the several hundred subjects were regularly seen at a research clinic for blood drawing and interviews. Subjects were observed in this way but not offered treatment, even in the syphilis study, after other sexually transmitted diseases were detected. Also, according to local custom, researchers left it up to the infected subject to disclose the infection to his or her sexual partner. Again, Uganda's poverty and lack of public health care made it a valuable research site, since research data could be collected without the confounding influence of any AIDS or syphilis treatment. And again, experts stated that such a study could never be performed in the United States, where study subjects with HIV and other infections would be treated and sex partners notified of their exposure to these infections.[15]

Angell continued to voice her earlier objections and thought that the Ugandan subjects were unfairly exploited in order to conduct research that could not be performed in the United States. This was especially unfair, in her view, since the collected data would benefit all AIDS patients. She also wrote that studies such as these should prompt further analysis of the following questions:

Codes of ethics governing research on human subjects require that investigators put the welfare of their subjects above the interests of science and of society, but what does that mean in practical terms? Does it mean only that investigators will not harm their subjects in the course of the research? Or does it mean that investigators undertake a broader responsibility for their subjects' welfare that includes trying to treat illnesses that afflict them, even those under study? If the requirement is simply not to do harm through the research, how can investigators make that limited responsibility clear to their subjects and still ensure their cooperation? Most people, after all, naturally look on doctors primarily as healers, not research scientists.

Does it matter whether the illness studied is difficult or expensive to treat? Treating HIV infection in rural Uganda would indeed be both difficult and expensive, and at best, the treatment would only stave off AIDS for the duration of the study, not prevent it altogether. Treating syphilis, on the other hand, is relatively simple and inexpensive. In the study [of the relationship of sexually transmitted diseases to HIV transmission], should all the other sexually transmitted diseases have been treated by the investigators, but not HIV-1 infection? If the expense of antiretroviral therapy justifies not offering it to subjects in certain parts of the world, should that expense be accepted as immutable? Or should we look more closely at the pricing decisions of the manufacturers of drugs protected by patents and the possibility of competition from generic drugs in developing countries?

The argument that certain subjects are no worse off than if they were not in the study implies that ethical standards governing research should vary with the political and economic conditions of the region. Should they? The answer will depend to some extent on how one sees the limits of the investigators' responsibility. If investigators are responsible for the subjects they enlist in their studies, and only those subjects, then the conditions of the surrounding community are irrelevant. They must do their best for their subjects, regardless. If, however, it is within the purview of investigators to consider the entire population, then perhaps it is inequitable to give research subjects better treatment than their neighbors would receive outside the study.[16]

Although many commentators agreed with Angell's points of view, others did not, and some of these were from the third world countries involved with foreign-sponsored AIDS research. "Things seem so simple in a rich country," Dr. Peter Mugyenyi told one reporter in 1998. Mugyenyi was the director of Uganda's Joint Clinical Research Center, which was to administer Ugandan AIDS vaccine trials in conjunction with a consortium of groups that included the National Institutes of Health and Pasteur-Merieux, the French company that had developed the vaccine and was to provide it for the study. "They sometimes talk about this in America like it's the Tuskegee experiment and we are simple, ignorant dupes," he said, emphasizing that countries facing a health crisis had to make their own determination about what research was in their best interest.[17] Spokespersons from developing countries maintained that if the Americans understood the desperate health needs and the different cultural sensibilities, they would stop insisting that inhibitory Western regulatory and ethical constraints be imposed.

CARDIAC DRUG TRIALS IN ARGENTINA

While many of these contentious research studies involved government and international health organizations and usually an academic partner, pharmaceutical companies also could become embroiled in the difficulties of conducting research in developing countries. In 1997 and 1998, German-based pharmaceutical company Hoechst Marion Roussel conducted Phase II and III clinical trials at a naval hospital in Argentina.[18] The trials were for Cariporide®, a drug expected to reduce cardiac tissue damage after a heart attack, and the naval hospital was one of twenty-six Argentinean study sites and one of two hundred medical centers worldwide that participated in the 11,500-subject trials.[19] In 1998, Hoechst Marion Roussel and its U.S.-based CRO, Quintiles Transnational, noticed some irregularities with the naval hospital trial and notified local authorities. Criminal investigations of the conduct of local researchers led prosecutors to allege that, of the 137 patients given Cariporide at the naval hospital during late 1997 and early 1998, none of them consented to the treatment and signatures on at least 80 consent documents had been forged. Prosecutors also collected evidence that subjects' records contained duplicated electrocardiograms with the characteristic findings needed to justify entering the patient in the trial. At least thirteen subjects enrolled in the study had died, and prosecutors claimed that some of these deaths were attributable to the experimental drug.

While no one thought that the drug company or the CRO had been responsible for these problems, circumstances surrounding the study might have contributed. Some claimed that the money paid the Argentinean physicians ($2,700 for each patient enrolled) was a major incentive to ignore research protocol restrictions about who qualified for the study. Others, such as Luis Zieher, head of a Buenos Aires medical IRB, attributed the problem to an excessive number of medical studies being conducted in his country. Dr. Zieher had seen the monthly number of drug trials sent to his committee for review increase from three to four to twenty in the eight years prior to the Cariporide scandal. At the time, there were an estimated 1,000 or more clinical drug trials being conducted in all of Latin America, and there were reports of physicians struggling to keep up with the supervisory work required for careful research. One oncologist, Dr. Daniel Campos, who located physicians willing to perform clinical drug research, expected the number of trials to increase tenfold in two years. "This is reasonable," Campos said. "We have a huge population, in big cities, so it could be done. But we are also developing countries so we have big inefficiencies, so accidents can occur."[20]

Despite the revelations of this problem, Argentina was considered a sufficiently medically sophisticated and credible country in which to conduct clinical research, and an Aventis spokeswoman stated that her company had found that physicians in developing countries were "no more likely to break the rules than their counterparts anywhere else."[21] However, to promote continuing faith in their reliability, Latin American governments began to create programs to control drug tests, comply with international research standards, and protect patients, and training programs in clinical research procedures were established for physicians.[22]

CONCLUSION

Because of problems with third world country research, various international medical bodies have attempted to create consensus guidelines for acceptable practices. However, it is difficult for many to agree that despite the exigencies created by the AIDS and other epidemics, differences in research practice between first and third world countries should be tolerated. Among those who believe that differences are justifiable, it is difficult to determine where to strike the balance between individual subject, national, international, and (sometimes) corporate interests.

The Nuremberg Code, the Declaration of Helsinki, and the Council for International Organizations of Medical Sciences' "International Ethical Guidelines for Biomedical Research Involving Human Subjects" are authoritative and can be consulted for guidance.[23] However, there are inconsistencies between the guidelines, and some important terms are not specifically defined, nor is there universal agreement about what is needed to satisfy guidelines, for example, that "medical research involving human subjects should only be conducted if the importance of the objective outweighs the inherent risks and burdens to the subject." It is not clear what is to be included in the calculus of "importance" so as to determine what risks are reasonable to impose on subjects. More importantly, these guidelines do not address third world country issues. So, for instance, when the 1996 Declaration of Helsinki states that "in research on man, the interest of science and society should never take precedence over considerations related to the wellbeing of the subject," it is not clear to some if this guideline had been violated when the Haitian AIDS subjects, who would not have received antiretroviral therapy under normal circumstances, did not get the drugs in the American-sponsored couples study.

These and other conundrums prompted an American attempt to clarify ethical requirements for third world research. In April 2001, after extensive work, the President's National Bioethics Advisory Commission (NBAC) published a report entitled *Ethical and Policy Issues in International Research: Clinical Trials in Developing Countries.*[24] In this report, NBAC stated that all of the fundamental principles of the Declaration of Helsinki and the Belmont Report applied to third world country research.[25] NBAC went further and recommended some practices that could be problematic for corporate-sponsored research—for instance, that the existence of less stringent regulatory requirements did not justify doing the research in a developing country. Moreover, the report stated that when an American sponsor proposes to "conduct research in another country when the same research could not be conducted ethically in the sponsoring country, the ethical concerns are more profound, and the research accordingly requires a more rigorous justification." Extrapolating from this view, NBAC recommended that clinical trials conducted in developing countries should be limited to those studies that are responsive to the health needs of the host country, since it might be unethical to conduct a clinical trial for a health condition in a country where that condition was unlikely to be found. NBAC further advised that researchers have a heavy burden to justify why subjects in any control group will not be provided with established effective treatment, whether or not such treatment was available in the host country. Asserting further that the benefits of third world research should extend to the country itself, NBAC also recommended that, "where applicable, U.S. sponsors and researchers should . . . assist in building local capacity for designing, reviewing, and conducting clinical trials in developing countries" and that the American sponsor should "assist in building the capacity of ethics review committees in developing countries to conduct scientific and ethical review of international collaborative research." While the NBAC report contained more explicit guidance for the conduct of third world country research than previous guidelines, it was not clear whether these would become burdensome for companies who continued to engage in this activity.

Determining what constitutes ethical research in one country versus another is a difficult challenge. The standard ethical requirements of independent review and the need for informed, voluntary consent can become ambiguous in the changing contexts of culture and custom, literacy, public health needs, and access to care. All of the studies described above were approved by institutional review boards. All of them were legitimate attempts to collect data on vitally important health questions, and the research data held the promise of markedly improving the health status of future patients. It could be argued that forcing adherence to first world research standards could have prevented or significantly compromised these studies. And it could also be asserted that these studies served a primary ethical obligation to obtain answers to these vital health-care questions as rapidly and unambiguously as possible. And yet, as Angell noted, "With the most altruistic of motives, then, researchers may find themselves slipping across a line that prohibits treating human subjects as means to an end."[26] Her recommendation for this challenge was to encourage others to explore issues honestly, not defensively, and to arrive at solutions that downplay expediency and focus on moral reasoning.[27]

Case Study

VaxGen, Inc., Fighting the AIDS Epidemic[28]

"The AIDS problem is overwhelmingly concentrated in the developing world, where more than 90% of all HIV-infected people now live, and AIDS intelligence and R&D are overwhelmingly concentrated in the industrialized world, where the problem, though serious, is only a small fraction of the global epidemic."[29]

—Peter Piot, Executive Director of UNAIDS

In Spring 1999, Don Francis, president and cofounder of the fledgling vaccine company VaxGen, Inc., let out an immense sigh of relief. Phase III clinical trials for AIDSVAX, an experimental vaccine designed to protect against human immunodeficiency virus, the virus that causes AIDS, were finally approved for a study in Thailand. Francis, having seen firsthand the devastation wrought by infectious diseases, had pledged himself to find an effective vaccine to combat the spread of AIDS in both the developed world and developing countries. Although the disease was a global scourge, AIDS took an unequal toll on victims from developing nations. The go-ahead for the study in Thailand was a triumph, in part, because it was to be conducted using a vaccine developed specifically to combat the strain of HIV that was prevalent there. Over the course of the previous seven years, Francis had negotiated his way through a tremendously complex web of international and national agencies, governments, and social policies to arrive, finally, at the initiation of these trials. In the United States, Francis had achieved the same end less than a year earlier, in June 1998, when VaxGen gained approval from the U.S. Food and Drug Administration for a Phase III study of five thousand homosexual men.

Although similar vaccines were being tested in both trials, the circumstances and policies set up to protect subjects in the U.S. trials were very different from those established for the trials in Thailand. Francis reflected on the possible repercussions of the arrangements. He wondered what, if anything, VaxGen would owe the study subjects in Thailand for their cooperation. He was concerned about VaxGen's responsibilities in the event that subjects became infected with HIV during the study. Finally, if the vaccine was proven to be effective, Francis wondered at what price VaxGen should then sell it to Thailand. The manner in which VaxGen managed the Thai vaccine trials was of great importance: the company was planning to raise the money for the trials via an initial public offering (IPO) in mid-1999. Anti-AIDS vaccine development was expensive, fraught with risk, and very high profile. In addition to Wall Street, the eyes of AIDS research and patient communities around the world would be on VaxGen.

As Francis puzzled over these consequences, he reflected on how the circumstances of the developed and developing areas of the world affected research, funding, health care, and ethics in the battle to develop and implement an effective AIDS vaccine. Despite the differences in the standards under which the trials were regulated, Francis believed that a major milestone on the path toward the eradication of AIDS had been reached, and that progress toward this end was of primary importance.

DON FRANCIS AND THE FIGHT AGAINST AIDS

Donald P. Francis was widely acknowledged as an avid virus hunter, one of the founding fathers of HIV research, and deeply committed to fighting AIDS. Francis's career as a virologist included fighting the cholera virus in Nigeria, smallpox in India, Ebola in the Sudan, and hepatitis B in Phoenix. He had a great deal of experience with vaccine development, and he had seen how effective vaccines could be in eradicating deadly viral diseases. His professional views about the value of vaccines evolved from his firsthand experience of watching countless people die from these diseases, and he was driven by his focus on public health.[30] While working for the U.S. Centers for Disease Control and Prevention (CDC) in the early 1980s, Francis was one of the first to recognize and warn of the dangers of the emerging AIDS epidemic, which was killing gay men within a year or two of the time that symptoms developed. The more he learned about the virus, the more he recognized it as more dangerous than most others he had encountered.[31]

The cases Francis studied convinced him that the virus was spreading from the direct exchange of blood, semen, and other bodily fluids. However, his early warnings that the virus was in the blood pool and was spread by sexual contact were acknowledged slowly. Francis's attempts to institute public health controls to slow the spread of the disease were not initially accepted. He was continually discouraged by the persistent underfunding of anti-AIDS programs, a situation featured in the film adaptation of Randy Shilts's book, *And the Band Played On.* The book portrayed the stormy politics of the early years of the AIDS epidemic, ending with Francis's departure from government service out of a deep frustration with the lack of effort put forth by the Reagan administration to fight the worsening AIDS crisis. Francis also had been disappointed by the early intransigence of the blood banks and sometimes even the gay community in implementing preventive measures. In 1992, having hit dead ends in both the public sector and the communities most affected by the disease, Francis joined Genentech, Inc., a large biotechnology firm in South San Francisco. He was hired to lead a Genentech research team that had been struggling since 1983 with the development of a recombinant AIDS vaccine.[32]

During his years at Genentech, Francis witnessed the growth of the AIDS epidemic. CDC reported in 1997 that approximately one million Americans had been infected with HIV, over half of whom had developed AIDS. More than half of the people diagnosed with AIDS had died from the disease. In addition, between forty and eighty thousand new HIV infections were occurring each year in the United States.[33] UNAIDS, the United Nations agency charged with coordinating all U.N. activities in fighting the AIDS epidemic, reported staggering international statistics on the spread of the disease.[34] Worldwide, twenty-one million people had been infected with HIV, and the number was growing by eighty-five hundred people per day. The vast majority of these people would die of AIDS. The executive director of UNAIDS, Peter Piot, stated, "In heavily affected countries in Africa and Asia, where one out of three urban adults may be infected, AIDS deaths among young and middle-aged adults—workers, managers, political leaders, and military personnel—are threatening health systems, economies, and national stability. With the current scale of global travel, the largely invisible, shifting, and expanding global epidemic of HIV makes the planet a more dangerous place for all." Piot called for a concerted effort among countries, funding sponsors, and those with research and development capability to coordinate research efforts to attack the problem in the third world.

PROMISE OF AN ANTI-AIDS VACCINE
IN THE UNITED STATES

By 1991, after eight years and multiple starts and stops, Genentech's research team had developed what was believed to be an effective anti-AIDS vaccine.[35] The vaccine was developed from an HIV envelope protein called gp120, a protein used by HIV to enter human cells. Genentech scientists, including Francis, had suggested this vaccine approach in 1988, and the early data looked very promising.[36] The vaccine had neutralized HIV in the laboratory and had protected chimpanzees from massive inoculations of virus. Looking at all of the laboratory and animal data, Francis was convinced that the gp120 vaccine was the one to test in humans. Human clinical tests were the only way to learn whether the vaccine was safe, whether it would induce an antibody response, whether that response would prevent HIV infection or lessen its severity, and for how long the vaccine would have an effect. Francis was eager to start clinical trials. But in addition to the need for FDA approvals, VaxGen needed ratification from the National Institute for Allergy and Infectious Diseases (NIAID), the arm of the National Institutes of Health responsible for funding and running the clinical trials of new vaccines entering early human testing in the United States. He also needed World Health Organization (WHO) approval if he wanted to conduct trials globally.

Approvals to begin Phase I and II clinical trials for safety and efficacy were not difficult to achieve. Data from safety studies on twelve hundred volunteers showed that the gp120 vaccine was as safe as any other vaccine and that it caused 99 percent of volunteers to produce anti-HIV antibodies.[37] The next step was to obtain approval to conduct expanded Phase III trials in thousands of volunteer subjects to prove efficacy. In 1994, WHO's Global Programme on AIDS approved expanded trials. After a prolonged meeting discussing the data and the pros and cons of going forward to Phase III, a panel of NIAID scientists also gave its approval. NIAID then scheduled a public meeting to obtain further input about whether to endorse this decision. However, things began to unravel both scientifically and politically before this meeting. The lay press reported that some of the volunteers in the Phase II vaccine trials had become infected with HIV. This information had been reported earlier within the scientific community and, while lamentable, was not disconcerting to most since the gp120 vaccine was not expected to be 100 percent effective. Although some of the volunteers had not had the full course of inoculation and all had contracted HIV through unprotected sex or intravenous (IV) drug use, some of the AIDS activists misconstrued the lay reports and pronounced the vaccine ineffective or even as having caused the infections. Activists came to the NIAID meeting and argued that attempting the trials would be pointless because no one would volunteer to receive an unsafe vaccine. This point of view was reinforced at the meeting by those who understood that volunteering for the gp120 study would exclude a person from most other trials of potentially more beneficial treatments. Others feared that vaccines were unsafe because they gave recipients a false sense of security, prompting them to continue or resume risky behavior— such as unprotected sex among homosexual men and needle sharing between IV drug users. Still others were afraid that any money spent on vaccine research would reduce the amount spent on the sick and dying AIDS patients whose medical care was currently costing about $13 million per day in the United States. Moreover, some believed that company scientists were downplaying the negative aspects of the vaccine in their quest for corporate profits.[38]

The impact of opposition from activists was compounded by scientific opposition to the Phase III trials, which increased before and during the NIAID meeting.[39] Human data from Phase II trials showed that anti-HIV antibodies had been produced, but the significance of this finding was debated since infected patients all developed antibodies but still succumbed to the disease. Scientists argued that if the immune system in HIV-infected people could not destroy the virus, how could a vaccine that activated the same immune response be effective? These scientists believed that the patient's cellular as well as humoral immunity needed to be stimulated to prevent HIV infection, and that the gp120 vaccine could produce only humoral immunity.[40] Other scientists pointed out that not all of the gp120 laboratory data were consistent—the antibodies the vaccine produced could kill laboratory-grown virus but not virus taken from infected patients.[41] While such inconsistent data were not unusual in vaccine development research, opposing scientists thought that too much about the behavior of HIV was unknown, making it premature to expose large numbers of uninfected volunteers to unknown risks from the vaccine. Other scientists thought that gp120 was the most promising of the fourteen experimental vaccines NIAID had tested since 1988 but disagreed about how effective the vaccine needed to be (for example, was 30 percent enough, or should 60 percent be the threshold?) to justify the risk and expense of the expanded trials.[42]

These differing views about the gp120 vaccine were aired at a June 1994 advisory meeting convened by NIAID to consider whether larger vaccine trials should proceed. After hearing from government, academic, and commercial scientists (including Francis) and the AIDS activists, NIAID director Anthony Fauci reversed the earlier recommendation of NIAID's scientific panel and decided that the institute would not fund any expanded clinical research of gp120. It was a controversial decision motivated, some said, by political as much as by scientific factors. However, in justifying the decision, Fauci said:

> Now I am a big advocate, as you probably know, of early availability of drugs for people who are infected. But with a preventive vaccine, you're talking about an otherwise normal person who does not have HIV infection and you're saying you want to inject that person with a product that, as a scientist, you can't in good conscience say there is even a more than reasonable chance of it being effective. And there is the possibility that there could be a deleterious effect.[43]

Although the effects were theoretical at that point, Fauci wanted to wait until NIAID was presented with an AIDS vaccine that had a better chance of success.

To Francis, who was focused on the devastating public health impact of AIDS, this decision was appalling. Francis countered the concerns raised by scientists with historical examples of vaccine development. He was certain that, had all of the unknown questions about smallpox vaccine been answered prior to human testing, no vaccine would ever have been developed to eradicate the disease. The only way to know whether a promising vaccine would work was to do Phase III human trials. Even if the vaccine were only 30 percent effective, that could translate into preventing the loss of hundreds of thousands of lives. And the Phase III trials would also be enormously valuable in understanding how to make a better vaccine. The Salk polio vaccine, which came out in 1955, was only 70 percent effective, but had prevented polio in hundreds of thousands of children before the arguably superior Sabin vaccine was available seven years later. In Francis's view, prolonging inaction until the theoretically perfect vaccine emerged from the laboratory wasted lives and devastated affected societies.

This view was shared by others working on the African AIDS epidemic. Kenrad Nelson, an epidemiologist from Johns Hopkins University, put it this way: "To put up any roadblocks in the face of this kind of data [on the gp120 vaccine] borders on the unethical. This is a plague, and there won't be another vaccine to test for two years, minimum. We should be testing the vaccine we have, if only to calm people down and prime the pump, as AZT did in 1986. You can argue all you want, but if we don't do something, it's a crime."[44] Given the enthusiasm he had seen in the Phase II trial volunteers, Francis was confident that high-risk people would volunteer in sufficient numbers for expanded trials. Finally, even if the gp120 vaccine failed, valuable data on how it failed would advance the state of knowledge. However, none of Francis's arguments prevailed. NIAID's 1994 refusal to fund the gp120 trials effectively stopped research progress on the vaccine at Genentech, after the company had already spent upwards of $50 million on its development.

VAXGEN, INC.

Undaunted by NIAID's decision, Francis was determined to continue the research. In 1995, Genentech's virus research group was spun off into a private company, VaxGen, Inc., with Don Francis as president. Francis retained the vaccine "wizards" from Genentech who had performed the difficult genetic engineering work on the gp120 protein. Bob Nowinski, a Seattle entrepreneur with a Ph.D. in virology, was appointed CEO and chairman, and Genentech kept a 25 percent equity stake in the new company.[45] VaxGen's sole focus was the gp120 approach to developing an effective AIDS vaccine.

The new company had plenty of obstacles to overcome to achieve its goal of a commercially viable, effective AIDS vaccine. The expense and complexity of developing a vaccine that would be effective against various strains of the virus challenged the fledgling company. HIV's ability to mutate meant that multiple strains of the virus had existed within the United States since the epidemic began ten years earlier. One vaccine was not likely to be effective against all strains, which meant that the company might have to make several vaccines. Developing a vaccine to fight any one particular subtype of HIV was an expensive process and ensured that the company was a long way off from profitability even if the company products were effective (see Table 9.1).

Forces that increased the development costs and depressed the amount that the company could charge for the vaccine further raised VaxGen's risks. Vaccines, especially pediatric vaccines, were notorious money losers—expensive to develop, not patentable since most were made from killed virus, tricky to manufacture since live biological organisms are used, often administered only once, prone to liability lawsuits, and sold at low margins with prices controlled by government agencies.[46] These factors had driven many manufacturers out of the market—in 1967, the FDA had licensed twenty-six different vaccine manufacturers, but by 1999, this number had fallen to thirteen. In addition to these factors, Genentech's willingness to let the gp120 vaccine go was attributable to its uncertainty about the AIDS vaccine market: How many people would take the vaccine? Would the government make vaccine use mandatory? and other troublesome uncertainties.

In a January 16, 1987, U.S. Senate committee hearing that focused on AIDS vaccines, Genentech vice president David Martin testified that entering the vaccine market was so risky that he requested government support to guarantee a market (for example, by buying the vaccine and administering it in government-supported programs) and to limit the liability of the vaccine manufacturer.[47] However, VaxGen figured that its vaccine had several commercially promising aspects for a U.S. market. It was likely that an effective AIDS vaccine could obtain premium pricing, and money saved by avoiding costly AIDS treatments would make the vaccine a prime candidate for third-party payer coverage. The company was further encouraged by the passage of the 1986 no-fault National Vaccine Injury Compensation Act, which had radically reduced vaccine-related lawsuits. Finally, the gp120 vaccine was developed with patentable recombinant techniques, which would lessen the likelihood that competitors could easily develop similar vaccines.

Despite these advantages, there were plenty of uncertainties about what would happen to the first AIDS vaccine to hit the U.S. market. Increasingly effective AIDS treatment drugs were eliminating HIV in infected Americans to undetectable levels, turning AIDS from an automatic killer into a chronic disease with manageable consequences. It was conceivable that less anxiety about the disease might lessen demand for a vaccine. These and other imponderables made the U.S. AIDS vaccine market less than sure-fire.

VaxGen's mission, to make HIV vaccines for worldwide use, further complicated the path toward commercialization of the vaccine for the company.[48] Francis had intentionally devoted the company to meeting the needs of the AIDS population for both the developed and the developing worlds. But third world countries with the highest incidence of the disease were also the countries with the highest rates of poverty. This poverty almost ensured that the expensive AIDS treatment drugs available in the United States would never be an option for combatting the disease in the third world. Behavioral prevention (such as encouragement to use condoms or to refrain from risky drug use behavior) had produced only modest results where implemented. As a consequence, Francis and others were convinced that vaccine prevention was the only chance that developing countries had to fight AIDS, but no one was sure how VaxGen could make money selling into such markets.

One avenue was to develop a vaccine for the Western world, sell it at high margins and, once development costs were recouped, sell the vaccine at lower costs to poor nations or strike manufacturing deals with foreign producers. Such a strategy, however, would mean that the vaccine would not reach developing countries for years after it was available in the United States. This had occurred with the hepatitis B vaccine, which had been tested for years in Senegal but, because of cost, was still not routinely available in Africa. Francis rejected this strategy, as did the leaders of developing countries who were desperate for help and did not want to wait. The climate was such that at the Fifth International Congress on AIDS in Asia and the Pacific, Malaysian prime minister Mahathir Mohammad encouraged other developing country leaders to lobby wealthier nations for funding for both preventive and therapeutic AIDS studies. In addition, he urged pharmaceutical companies "not to let profit take precedence over the lives of people infected by HIV."[49]

To overcome the lack of an economic incentive for pharmaceutical companies, a task force of the World Bank was studying the feasibility of creating a guaranteed purchase fund for third world AIDS vaccines.[50] Francis thought a partnership with the World Bank might be an option for VaxGen, but negotiations would be delicate and the outcome far from certain. Dealing with the World Bank and the different third world cultures guaranteed that VaxGen would encounter political difficulties. Throughout all interaction with international bodies, VaxGen knew it would also have to contend with both domestic and international AIDS activists who were increasingly involved in corporate decisions to develop and test AIDS treatments and preventives.

According to Peter Young, CEO of another small AIDS vaccine company, a tough "organizational stomach" was required for the high-cost, high-risk, and high-profile work of commercial AIDS vaccine development. He told one science reporter that "it's an area that's going to knock the participants around a bit."[51] Nonetheless, both American and third world country trials were seen as crucial if VaxGen was to adhere to its overall goal, and Francis was committed to going forward. Despite the potential difficulties, VaxGen raised $27.5 million from private investors and in 1995 began the work of developing two vaccines—one for use in the United States and one for the third world.

In mid-1996, medical information about HIV advanced significantly. Researchers discovered a second strain of HIV in the United States and Europe that was perhaps responsible for more infections than the more commonly known first strain. The eleven infected subjects from the Phase II gp120 vaccine study were tested and found to have become infected with this second strain, the protein of which had not been included in the original gp120 vaccine. Vax-Gen scientists immediately went about reconfiguring the vaccine to include the new strain and performing the testing necessary to show whether the two strains could be incorporated into one vaccine and at what doses. This work led to the creation of AIDSVAX, a gp120 bivalent vaccine that added the outer protein envelope of the second HIV strain. By 1997, and at a cost of an additional $1 million, VaxGen developed another bivalent vaccine for the Asian population. These bivalent vaccines operated with what was called a "sieve" approach—attempting to prevent any breakthrough infections that might sift through the patient's defenses. Said Francis of the new vaccine, "You plug up the holes in the sieve a few at a time. The holes for the second type of HIV were open then. Now we hope they're closed. You keep doing this until nothing can get through."[52]

Francis made the decision to take VaxGen's vaccines into Phase III clinical studies. He reasoned that total efficacy (known as "sterilizing immunity") in preventing HIV infection did not have to be the goal for this vaccine. Rather, Francis believed sterilizing immunity should be a long-term goal that might be achieved with modified versions of AIDSVAX or with combinations of this vaccine with others.[53] Francis reasoned that even if AIDSVAX could not prevent HIV infection in a sufficient number of cases, VaxGen might be able to show that the vaccine was worth marketing if it could offer some protection from the disease. In other words, to be considered effective, the vaccine did not necessarily have to prevent HIV infection if it could prevent the AIDS disease by lowering the level of HIV in the blood or by helping the body eliminate the virus faster. In addition, vaccine production processes had advanced to the degree that Francis believed that the initial vaccine, if it showed some efficacy, could be quickly modified to counteract any emergent HIV variant. This strategy was similar to the current process used for influenza vaccines, which were reconfigured each year.[54]

By the time VaxGen was ready to go into Phase III trials with the new vaccine, the political (if not the economic) climate surrounding AIDS vaccines had improved. In 1997, President Clinton announced a national goal of producing an effective AIDS vaccine within ten years. He called for the creation of a vaccine research center at NIH, which would be housed within NIAID. The NIH budget for vaccine research was increased significantly. Anthony Fauci, the NIAID director who had previously refused to fund the monovalent gp120 Phase III trials, had apparently changed his opinion of the value of this research. "In the past we maybe inappropriately said we'll judge a vaccine primarily on the basis of being able to prevent infection completely," he told one reporter. "Now we're thinking maybe it's enough if you get infection but not disease. Until recently we never considered that." Health officials in the third world were becoming increasingly insistent that vaccine trials needed to begin. Said one physician who headed an AIDS research center in Uganda, "Let's also look at the world and tell the truth. In the history of medicine the only things that have really worked to stop diseases in the third world have been vaccines. Drugs won't work for us. Prevention has obviously failed. Education is almost impossible. Without a vaccine we are going to keep on losing and we are going to lose a lot."[55]

By May 1998, chimpanzee studies showed that the new VaxGen vaccines could protect against HIV infection, and new Phase I and II human studies had shown safety and early evidence of efficacy in inducing an antibody response. Francis continued work on designing the crucial Phase III clinical trials necessary to prove efficacy and to obtain regulatory marketing approval. Despite the promising data and climate, there were still problems in obtaining approval for the Phase III trials. Given the prior gp120 history, some AIDS scientists continued to think the AIDSVAX Phase III trials were premature. In May 1998, 50 scientists wrote to *Science* urging that U.S. Phase III trials be delayed until more was known about HIV immunity.[56] These scientists emphasized that HIV was too different from other viruses for which vaccines had been successfully created, and that the AIDSVAX data were not strong enough to warrant involving (some said "wasting") thousands of volunteers in efficacy trials.[57] David Baltimore, the Nobel laureate who headed the new NIH AIDS Vaccine Research Committee, charged that the Phase III AIDSVAX trial could "seriously dent the reservoir" of people willing to participate in future trials of AIDS vaccines that might be more promising than AIDSVAX.[58]

AIDS activist groups also joined the renewed gp120 debate, but now not all were against further testing. Three major HIV/AIDS activist groups—AIDS Action, the Gay Men's Health Crisis, and the AIDS Coalition to Unleash Power (ACTUP)—had advocated a mix of preventive measures (education about safer sex and needle exchange programs, and research for a vaccine) and therapeutic measures (so-called anti-AIDS drug cocktails and research for a cure) to stop the devastating effects of the disease. However, the prevalent animosity toward big pharmaceutical companies, combined with the earlier failure of the monovalent gp120 vaccine, had colored the activists' reaction to Vax-

Gen's efforts. Opinion editorial pieces by San Francisco AIDS advocates who were wary about the potential success of the Phase III trials appeared in Bay Area newspapers.[59]

Despite the still-mixed opinions about the wisdom of proceeding, VaxGen received FDA approval for the large-scale AIDSVAX trials in May of 1998.[60] In addition, NIAID agreed to collaborate with VaxGen to support the AIDS-VAX Phase III trials. In making the announcement on behalf of NIAID, Fauci stated, "The effort to develop a safe and effective vaccine against HIV/AIDS is a global imperative and the highest priority of the NIH AIDS research program. We expect this collaboration with VaxGen to take us closer to our mutual goal."[61] The U.S. AIDSVAX trials began in June 1998, with the goal of testing the vaccine on fifty-four hundred healthy gay men and heterosexual women at high risk of HIV infection.

COMPETITION

In mid-1998 Vaxgen was the only company with an AIDS vaccine in Phase III clinical trials. Although multiple vaccines had been developed in academic and corporate labs, many candidate vaccines had been abandoned when they failed to show promising early results. Overall, vaccine research was still suffering the impact of NIAID's 1994 refusal to fund the monovalent gp120 research. Funding for AIDS vaccine research was low, representing only 10 percent of the total amount of research dollars spent on developing AIDS treatments.[62] Established pharmaceutical companies had largely shied away from vaccine research, focusing instead on proven money makers—drugs that treated existing AIDS infections or alleviated their devastating effects. Merck & Co., the maker of the anti-AIDS drug Crixivan®, was the only large pharmaceutical company with an AIDS vaccine in early stage development. Chiron, a biotechnology competitor of Genentech's, had developed and was testing its version of a gp120 vaccine, but was behind VaxGen in its efforts.

None of this meant, however, that VaxGen had a clear shot at being the first to enter the market. Pasteur-Meriuex/Connaught (PMC), the vaccine unit of the French drug company Rhone-Poulenc SA, had developed a vaccine consisting of various HIV genes spliced into a live, but harmless, canarypox virus vector. Phase II trials of this vaccine were approved by the NIH in the summer of 1997. Earlier research had shown that this vaccine might provide more complete immunity to HIV—it stimulated both arms of the immune system (producing both antibody and cell-mediated immunity), and it showed laboratory effectiveness against more than one strain of HIV. Other studies showed that the gp120 vaccine boosted the antibody response to the canary-pox vaccine. So, depending on the results of further trials conducted by Vax-Gen and PMC, the canarypox vaccine could supercede, compete with, or complement the AIDSVAX vaccine.[63]

In parallel with VaxGen and PMC's efforts to develop vaccines to combat HIV in developed countries, international agencies were funding small biotechnology companies to develop and test vaccines targeted for the strains of HIV prevalent in Asia and Africa. With the approval of the U.S. trials in hand, Francis also turned his attention to the developing world. He began negotiations with Thailand for trials to combat a different strain of the virus. The company estimated that the cost of the Thai trials would be about $9 million. An IPO was planned for mid-1999 to raise money to cover the costs.

AIDS RESEARCH IN DEVELOPING COUNTRIES

VaxGen's foray into Thailand had been preceded in 1997 by an intense international debate among scientists, physicians, and ethicists about conducting AIDS research in the third world.[64] The debate started in earnest after publication of research sponsored by NIH and CDC, in which low doses of AZT and placebos had been given to HIV-infected pregnant African women to see if the drug in limited (that is, affordable) quantities reduced the transmission of HIV from mothers to infants. The studies were important since, by the year 2000, six million pregnant women in Asia and sub-Saharan Africa were expected to be infected with HIV. The studies were also controversial, since placebos were used despite the fact that AZT had already been shown to reduce the rate of HIV maternal-child transmission and that the drug had been recommended for years in the United States in larger doses for all HIV-infected pregnant women.[65]

Those who criticized the studies claimed that the existence of effective treatment made the use of placebos unethical since researchers were knowingly giving inferior treatment to some participants in the trial. They likened the treatment of these women to the men in the infamous Tuskegee syphilis study, where the same justification for the failure to provide active treatment was used—that the subjects would not have received active treatment under normal circumstances, and the placebo group allowed the investigators to observe what would happen to the African infants if there was no study. In response, those who supported the studies claimed that the realities of economic and medical conditions in the developing world justified treating the human subjects differently.[66]

The CDC and NIH study sponsors argued that it was an unfortunate fact that African women did not receive any HIV prophylactic treatment and the inclusion of placebo study controls would result in the most rapid, accurate, and reliable answer to the question of the value of the low-dose HIV prophylaxis compared to the local standard of care. The director of the Uganda Cancer Institute at Makerere University in Uganda supported the trials and asserted that "the ethics of the design of clinical trials to prevent transmission of HIV-1 from mother to child in developing countries have been criticized. However, a discussion of ethical principles in biomedical research that ignores the socioeconomic heterogeneity of society is not ethical and not worth holding. Policies regarding health management differ within and between industrialized and developing countries because of their different economic capabilities."[67]

Debates about the AZT trials informed the evolving discourse about AIDS vaccine trials. AIDS vaccine trials were contemplated in many African and Asian countries, and members of international medical groups, such as UN-AIDS, were sorting out the pros and cons of various protocols and attempting to develop ethical standards of research conduct.[68] At meetings of health officials, scientists, government leaders, and AIDS representatives, these stakeholders grappled with questions such as: Could a vaccine be tested first in a developing country before being tested in the country where the vaccine was produced? Was it exploitative if a village chief or other representative gave blanket approval to conduct these studies? Could placebo controls be used?

The current standard, whereby testing was required to take place first in the manufacturer's own country,[69] was based on the belief that the risk to subjects would be less where health care was excellent and that studying third world citizens first, especially for vaccines designed to fight Western subtypes, would be exploitative. However, this policy was considered paternalistic by many representatives in African countries, who thought that testing first in America delayed vaccine trials, and therefore prevention, in their countries. In an epidemic, they argued, standards needed to be relaxed, the risk belonged where the people were dying, and countries should be empowered to do what is in their best interest, rather than adhering to paternalistic policies imposed on them by international organizations. In view of the severity of the epidemic, this change was adopted by UNAIDS. It was also agreed that host countries needed to have adequate scientific and administrative capabilities to prevent exploitation and that only individuals, not those in political control, should consent to volunteer. Also, it was considered appropriate to use placebo controls if it was genuinely believed that the efficacy of the vaccine was unknown.[70]

In spite of these advances, two thorny questions remained: First, which standard of medical care—that of the developed or developing country—applied to those subjects who became infected with HIV during trials? And second, how would developing countries get access to successful vaccines that had been tested on their citizens? Both questions challenged stakeholders to find means to bridge the tremendous gaps in economic strength and medical standards between the United States (whose agencies and companies most often conducted the trials) and developing countries in order to find a solution.

On the question of which standard of medical care should be applied to those subjects who became infected with HIV during trials, there were several issues to consider.[71] In the vaccine trials in the United States, any study subject who became infected with HIV would be referred for treatment and would most likely receive three types of antiviral drugs. This triple therapy approach was very expensive (costing $12,000 to $15,000 per year) but had been shown to be so effective in many patients that it reduced the virus in the body to undetectable levels. In addition, for those patients who went on to develop full-blown AIDS and the resultant opportunistic infections, the costs of treatment in the United States could run as high as $200,000 per patient per year.[72] Despite the cost, some advocated that Western agencies and companies conducting the trials were ethically obligated to provide these treatments to third world research subjects. This view was supported by the authoritative Council for International Organizations of Medical Sciences (CIOMS) Guideline 14, which quoted Article II.3 of the Helsinki Declaration: "In any medical study, every patient—including those of a control group, if any—should be assured of the best proven diagnostic and therapeutic method."[73] Others argued that CIOMS had been inconsistent on this point and that the principle should be adaptable to the horrible conditions created by the AIDS epidemic. For instance, since HIV infection was a likely death sentence to a patient in the developing world, provision of triple therapy would be too great an inducement to join the trial and engage in or continue high-risk behavior. In addition, the costs and logistics of supplying these treatments in third world countries with their poor medical infrastructure was daunting, especially if treatment was required for the life of the infected individual.[74] Precedent existed for referring HIV-infected subjects for local (albeit negligible) treatment in studies conducted by U.S. researchers. Dr. Jean William Pape, a native of Haiti and faculty member of the Cornell University Medical School, had performed Haitian

AIDS trials for two decades with funds from U.S. federal grants. The study subjects who became infected with HIV were not provided antiviral therapy since none was available in the country. The vice president of the Haitian Medical Association, which collaborated in the trials, did not regard the practice as exploitative given the probability that the research data would lead to insights about disease transmission. There was another factor to consider regarding the use of Western-standard treatment of infected third world vaccine study subjects. While it was hoped that study vaccines could prevent HIV infection, they were not likely to do so in all cases. If the vaccine failed to prevent infection, it was secondarily hoped that it could trigger enough of an immune response to prevent HIV disease.[75] That made collecting data on the disease prevention ability of the vaccine very important. These so-called secondary endpoints—namely, HIV virus blood levels and viral loads—were valuable predictors of the severity of any HIV disease and of disease progression. A vaccine could still be considered effective if it lowered these secondary endpoints. Providing antiviral drugs, however, decreased both secondary study endpoints—virus blood levels and viral load—making it impossible to sort out whether changes in these endpoints were attributable to the vaccine or the drugs. Triple anti-AIDS therapy, although good for the study subject, significantly limited the value of the study since the full potential of the vaccine could not be tested.

This opportunity to increase the likelihood of an infected person's survival did not exist, however, if study sponsors adhered to the local standards of medical care in developing countries where antiviral drugs were usually beyond reach. In most third world countries, antiviral therapy was too expensive and was available for almost no one. Some pregnant women received single-drug treatment, and very few people received treatment when they became sick with opportunistic infections from AIDS. While this situation was dismal for those who became infected with HIV, those in the vaccine trials who received no antiviral treatment could provide data for the secondary endpoints that would show if the vaccine made AIDS less deadly.[76] Ethicists were invited to comment on this discrepancy between U.S. and third world country trials. Speaking of a vaccine trial contemplated in Uganda, where 20 percent of the people were infected and the country could afford to spend only $6 per person annually on health care, Thomas M. Murray, director of Case Western Reserve University's Center for Biomedical Ethics, said, "The question arises are we basically exporting our risky scientific research, from which we would benefit, to the third world?"[77] The answer to the question of discrepant treatment could determine the ethical, financial, and scientific viability of AIDS vaccine tests. During the summer of 1998, when VaxGen was in negotiations with Thailand, opinions on how to handle this matter were still divided.[78]

Opinions also were split on the second question of ultimate access of vaccines in the third world. According to Dr. Peter Piot, "Everybody is worried that we will use Africa, develop a vaccine there, say thanks and then take it back to Europe and America."[79] Health officials in Africa were voicing the view that third world countries were owed access to AIDS vaccines because the need was so great. According to Dr. Peter Mugyenyi, the director of Uganda's Joint Clinical Research Center, which was about to conduct an AIDS vaccine trial using Pasteur-Merieux's vaccine, "We are participating in the trials not just with our citizens, but with our brains. We have demanded a role in the research and we have sent our best people abroad to help develop the drugs. When this vaccine becomes effective—in a year or 10 years or two generations—we want to be able to say that we have a central interest in this product and you owe us for it."[80] Piot of UNAIDS agreed with this view: "Those taking the risks of HIV vaccine development should be the first to realise the benefit," he said. "So all populations world-wide who have participated in vaccine research should have some form of early and preferential access."[81]

AIDS EPIDEMIC IN THAILAND

The Thai AIDS epidemic was believed to have started in Bangkok in 1988 as a result of the high rate of needle sharing by infected intravenous drug users. The epidemic grew rapidly from there, and the disease became more prevalent in northern Thailand near Chiang Mai, where the most common modes of transmission were sexual intercourse and vertical transmission from infected mother to fetus or infant.[82] By 1998, of all Asian countries, Thailand had the largest percentage of its population infected with HIV—1.6 percent, or an estimated one million HIV-positive people of a total population of sixty million. Despite the fact that early government-sponsored educational programs reduced the increasing infection rates in the general population, the prevalence of HIV was still as high as 30 percent to 40 percent in intravenous drug users and 20 percent to 30 percent in female commercial sex workers.[83] The number of AIDS-related deaths had increased rapidly and was expected to be around seventy thousand cases per year in 2000, and the cumulative number of children under fifteen years of age orphaned by AIDS fatalities was predicted to be about ninety-five thousand. The country, therefore, was heavily burdened by the need to provide health care for the sick and to alleviate the secondary social impacts of AIDS fatalities.

Thailand had only a limited ability to treat citizens infected with HIV. The situation was made worse in 1997 when the national currency—the baht—collapsed, sending the economy into a tailspin. In exchange for promises of strict monetary controls, the International Monetary Fund eventually bailed out the economy with a $17.2 billion loan.[84] As a result, in 1998, the budget of Thailand's national AIDS program was cut by 60 percent.[85] The triple-drug AIDS therapies used in the United States were not feasible for use in Thailand, not only because of cost constraints but also because of issues related to the complexity of the regimen, the necessary follow-up and monitoring of patients, and to some extent, tolerance to the therapies. The official policy in Bangkok was to supply two antiviral drugs to patients infected with HIV only after there was evidence of full-blown AIDS (which at the time in Thailand was a CD4 count below 500) or if the person developed an HIV-related disease.[86] Although Bangkok policy included provision of drugs used to prevent the common opportunistic infections of AIDS, health officials reported in 1998 that the Thai government was able to meet only 18 percent of the potential demand for the treatment of these opportunistic infections.[87] Even though AIDS treatment programs were being cut and drugs were not routinely available, the government increased budgets for HIV research focusing on prevention.

FEASIBILITY OF CONDUCTING CLINICAL TRIALS IN THAILAND

The medical infrastructure and political climate of Thailand made it an opportune country in which to conduct AIDS vaccine trials. Compared to many developing countries, Thailand had a relatively effective medical establishment and the political will to fight the epidemic. Ten years earlier, far in advance of most other countries, the prime minister had chaired a committee to develop a national AIDS strategy. In 1991, the U.S. Army and the Royal Thai Army began a joint study to evaluate the rates of HIV infection among Thai army recruits in order to lay the groundwork for future AIDS vaccine studies.[88] By the time that VaxGen began to make overtures to the government, the Thai strategy included provisions for the testing of a vaccine under a National AIDS Vaccine Plan. Research infrastructure was also in place. The first small-scale vaccine trial had been conducted in 1994. Mahidol University, a respected academic medical institution in Bangkok, had already established a Vaccine Trials Center and an institutional review board whose job it was to review proposed protocols in order to protect the interests of the Thai research subjects. The National Review Committee of the Ministry of Public Health was in place to ensure the welfare of potential trial participants. Furthermore, Mahidol University researchers had clinical research experience, having coordinated studies in accordance with international guidelines for good clinical practices. An ongoing collaboration between UNAIDS, the U.S. Centers for Disease Control, and the Thai Ministry of Public Health had set the stage for a cooperative vaccine research effort in Thailand.[89]

In 1990, CDC had established a permanent field station in Thailand and a collaborative research program with the Thai Ministry of Public Health—the HIV/AIDS Collaboration. Since 1995, this collaboration had involved a range of activities, including measuring the level of new (or *incident*) HIV infections in Thailand, determining the genetic characterization of incident HIV infections, identifying risk factors for infection, identifying a group of individuals who were willing to participate and could be followed over time to evaluate risk behaviors and infection, and working with the community to build the understanding and support necessary to implement vaccine studies.[90]

The conditions in Thailand generally, and in Bangkok specifically, met VaxGen's requirements for conducting studies. VaxGen needed a large population of healthy but at-risk people from which to recruit study volunteers. The Bangkok city government (called the Bangkok Metropolitan Administration) maintained a large drug abuse treatment program with about fifteen clinics serving about eight thousand drug users yearly.[91] VaxGen targeted this group for its studies because the group had a continued high incidence of HIV infection, despite prevention efforts. Prior research had shown that among IV drug users in Bangkok, 6 percent became infected each year despite methadone treatment, education and counseling on HIV prevention, and easy access to sterile needles.[92] It was anticipated that risky behavior in this group would continue and that infections would continue to occur, which would allow VaxGen to determine if its vaccine could reduce the incidence of these infections. Although Bangkok sex workers also had a high prevalence of HIV, the IV drug user population was deemed more appropriate for a long-term study because affiliation with methadone clinics would make these individuals easier to recruit and follow.

In addition to the availability of the study population, there were cultural advantages to conducting trials in Thailand. According to an interview given by a women's health advocate in Thailand, the country operated under a strong hierarchical structure. Deference to authority was prevalent, and trust in the medical establishment specifically had been long-standing. This situation made it more likely that the medical establishment would have the influence to obtain government cooperation in any AIDS research, and also meant that the people recruited into the studies would probably participate. Trust in the medical establishment by the methadone clinic patients who would be recruited was viewed as a key benefit of using this study population. According to the lead Thai researcher who spoke to an American interviewer, "How can we study these people (human beings) if they did not trust us?"[93]

VaxGen's proposal to conduct vaccine trials on Thai citizens involved extensive negotiations with the Thai government. Because of the desperate situation in Thailand, however, the Thai government was in a less-than-powerful position to extract concessions from VaxGen. If the government insisted on the highest standards, no foreign vaccine sponsors would be able to afford to conduct trials on potentially useful vaccines. The Bangkok press, following the issue, had questioned how much compromise was acceptable.[94] Despite the difficulties, the Thai government was more prepared than most to address these questions, since it had previously set up a government committee that focused on the requirements of AIDS vaccine trials conducted in the country by outsiders. The committee was chaired by an AIDS activist who was a member of the Thai senate. Questions such as how much the government would spend on vaccine trials, who would have access to the vaccines, and at what cost, had been addressed. The committee proposed that Thai scientists participate in the research and that the Thai government negotiate rights to a vaccine developed within the country's borders.

Professor Natth Bhamarapravati at the Thai Ministry of Health had been assigned to negotiate first with Genentech and then with VaxGen. He had a strong interest in protecting the rights of potential Thai volunteers and obtaining benefits for the medical community. Natth had lobbied WHO early on to test the gp120 vaccine in Thai volunteers. In 1994, he predicted that AIDS would soon kill one hundred thousand Thai people every year. He sought collaboration with Western researchers to get vaccine research started, since Thailand lacked the money or expertise to conduct the trials.[95] In February of 1995, with WHO's approval, Genentech and researchers at the vaccine testing center at Mahidol University had started Phase I and II trials in recovering Thai IV drug users with the monovalent vaccine containing the viral subtype prevalent in the United States. This early experience made Natth an effective advocate for the volunteers and the public health system. Natth made specific demands of foreign vaccine research sponsors. He wanted the vaccine to contain elements of the HIV strain prevalent in Thailand, to protect the Thai volunteers from exploitation, to involve Thai scientists and laboratories so that no one could say that the volunteers were U.S. "surrogates" for vaccine testing, and to ensure that Thailand would gain the necessary skills to conduct modern vaccine research on its own once VaxGen left. Finally, he wanted access to the vaccine if it proved effective.[96]

In negotiations with VaxGen regarding the AIDSVAX trials, Natth held firm on his demands on the issue of informed consent. Both VaxGen and Natth placed a high importance on informed consent and developed strategies to assure its implementation. A primary concern was whether Thai IV drug users were sufficiently educated to comprehend the VaxGen informed consent process. Clinical trials in the United States required full informed consent from the volunteers in order to ensure that they were aware of all of the potential risks and potential benefits of participating. On this issue, the Thai and VaxGen principals were in accord—both wanted the American standard of full informed consent applied to the Thai volunteers. As a result, VaxGen planned to take many precautions to ensure that the participants understood the important aspects of the trial. There would be trained counselors available to administer not only written materials concerning the trial but also a standardized videotape that all volunteers would be required to watch. A comprehension exam would follow the videotape and would be administered every six months thereafter to ensure that volunteers were retaining the information given to them—essentially, an "ongoing informed consent" process would be used.[97]

A more troublesome question involved whether VaxGen would provide treatment to the study subjects who became infected with HIV.[98] Although the negotiations were not easy, VaxGen and the Thai government agreed that the Thai standard of care would be offered to the trial volunteers. The view prevailed that American-standard therapy was too expensive, too prolonged, often too complicated, and might be an unfair inducement to volunteers.

To ensure skill transfer, Natth made three requests of VaxGen. He asked the company to transfer most of the protocols and skills required to conduct clinical trials—including training of Thai personnel in protocol design, statistical analysis, and data management—to local researchers. Second, Natth asked VaxGen to help Thailand build a national repository to enable the country to store and track samples collected in clinical trials, a task that involved building a facility with generators that would power freezers to store the samples, as well as training scientific personnel to analyze the samples using molecular techniques. Third, Natth asked VaxGen to transfer to Thailand the technology necessary to build a vaccine production facility to produce and distribute the vaccine, if proven effective. VaxGen was willing to assist in the first two requests, but would most likely not be able to provide everything Thailand was asking for. Francis knew that VaxGen would be unable to meet the last request since an appropriate production facility would require hundreds of millions of dollars to build and maintain, would require pristine sanitation that might be impossible to achieve in Thailand, and would keep VaxGen in Thailand much longer than the trials lasted.[99]

The last major issue to be resolved was the cost to the Thai government of the AIDSVAX vaccine, should it prove effective in the trials. Given its financial situation, VaxGen could not afford to give away its vaccine, but anticipated setting a price that was "reasonable" given Thailand's lack of economic resources. But setting this price was not an easy task. Francis had been asked more than once to specify a selling price, and he acknowledged that the price was hard to gauge but believed it would be "more than a few dollars" per vaccination.[100] But even an amount in this range was considered troublesome. Knowing that the Thais could afford very little, VaxGen was lobbying international health organizations like the World Bank to assist developing countries with loans or grants to purchase the vaccine.

AIDSVAX PHASE III PROTOCOL FOR THAILAND[101]

The CDC collaborations and the negotiations with Thailand resulted in a proposal for a double-blind, placebo-controlled trial to test the efficacy of AIDSVAX that incorporated one of the HIV strains prevalent in Thailand in 1999. The study was to be arranged as a collaborative effort between VaxGen, the Mahidol University Faculty of Tropical Medicine in Bangkok, and the HIV/AIDS Collaboration (the research program of the Thai Ministry of Public Health and CDC). The research was expected to cost $9 million. Plans called for the protocol to be reviewed by a number of entities, including the Bangkok Metropolitan Administration, the Faculty of Tropical Medicine of Mahidol University, the Ethical and Scientific Review Committees of the Thailand Ministry of Public Health (MOPH), and the Thailand Food and Drug Administration. The Thailand MOPH also requested independent review and approval from UNAIDS. In the United States, FDA, CDC, and NIH would also review the trial.[102]

From May 1995 to December 1996, VaxGen had conducted a small feasibility study on 1,208 Thai people. This study had demonstrated that the IV drug user population in Bangkok was large enough and was an otherwise feasible study group—IV drug users were well-characterized, had a sufficiently high incidence of HIV infections despite counseling about safe behavior, and had a high willingness to participate. The preliminary studies also showed that the Thai research infrastructure was adequate to manage the studies and the government could provide the necessary individual and political support to carry them out.

The full-scale proposed trial would enroll twenty-five hundred healthy former intravenous drug users who were at risk for acquiring HIV through sexual activity or resumed IV drug use.[103] It was expected to take a year to recruit the subjects from several methadone clinics and three more years to complete the study. Although VaxGen would supervise the studies, researchers from the Bangkok public health administration and Mahidol University would run them. The researchers would be trained on the protocol by VaxGen and would recruit subjects, obtain informed consent, randomly administer the vaccine or a placebo, and collect study data on HIV infection rates and the secondary endpoints of HIV blood levels, viral load, and immune system function. In addition to studying whether the vaccine prevented HIV infection or disease, the researchers would collect data on vaccine side effects and whether immunization resulted in different behaviors among trial participants, such as increased high-risk sexual activity. Because the trial was limited in time, the study would not evaluate complication or death rates from HIV infection or AIDS.

In the informed consent process prior to the study and at each study visit thereafter, the subjects would be counseled about the nature of the study, the unknown level of protection from the vaccine, the fact that administration of the vaccine could cause a transient false-positive HIV test, that such a finding outside of the study could lead to discrimination, and that they may have been assigned to the placebo group. In addition, all subjects would be counseled at every study visit on methods for reducing potential exposure to HIV. The initial educational session, lasting about fifteen to twenty minutes, would be conducted for groups of potential subjects. Using a standardized presentation with audio-visual aids, clinic staff also would provide each subject with a written pamphlet about the study and encourage each potential subject to ask questions. Illiterate subjects would have the written material read to them. This eligibility screening session would take about an hour, for which the participant would be paid 100 baht.[104]

After consenting to participate but before enrolling in the study, each participant would have to pass a test of his or her understanding about study provisions. Participation in the study would be confidential, but subjects would be offered a study identification card that could be useful in explaining a false-positive HIV test in case they were tested when they applied for a job or insurance. The researchers would assist the subject by explaining the study to anyone at the subject's request. If the subject was arrested, as was not uncommon in this population, the researchers would be available to explain the subject's participation and arrange follow-up in jail. Subjects were to be warned that outside discovery of the identification card might subject them to discrimination. Researchers would also ask for permission to contact the subject by letter, phone, or personal visit for study follow-up.

Subjects would be told that there would be no direct benefit to them if they participated, except for free physical exams and blood tests and the free receipt of a Thai medical insurance card if they did not possess one. This card, which cost 100 baht per year, guaranteed Thai subjects the minimum level of health care provided by government hospitals and clinics. Subjects would receive AIDS prevention education, free condoms, and bleach kits to disinfect unclean needles and syringes. If the subject became HIV-infected during the trial, he or she would be referred to local medical clinics for further treatment. The subject would be asked to return to the study clinic at regular intervals to provide all of the follow-up study blood tests for at least twenty-four months, and up to thirty-six months from the date of the confirmed HIV infection. Blood test data would be provided to the subject's physician on request. Subjects were told that VaxGen would not provide any treatment for HIV infection or AIDS, but study researchers would be available to the subjects' physicians for consultations. Subjects would be compensated 350 baht for transportation and time spent at the clinic for each of the fifteen study visits, and an extra 500 baht if they completed all fifteen visits. They would be told that VaxGen would cover any direct medical costs related to medical problems (but not for HIV infection) directly resulting from injection with the vaccine or placebo. Finally, subjects were told that should the vaccine prove effective, the group that received placebo would be offered the full course of vaccine inoculation for free. Signed twelve-page consent forms from each participant were required before the study.

At periodic intervals, data from the study would be monitored by an independent data safety monitoring board, and the study would be stopped if the board found any serious safety problem with the vaccine. The study would also be stopped if the board found statistically significant evidence that the vaccine was greater than 30 percent effective. In such a case, the placebo subjects would be offered the vaccine for free depending on manufacturing capability.

CONCLUSION

Many perplexing questions had been resolved in the negotiations with Thai institutions, although it would be years before VaxGen would have the answer to the most perplexing—the efficacy of the vaccine. Don Francis was gratified to have reached this milestone in the attempt to develop a vaccine that could stem the tide of the AIDS epidemic. He turned his attention to more immediate questions, which were certain to come up during the Thai trials: What, if anything, would VaxGen owe the study subjects in Thailand for their cooperation? If the vaccine was proven to be effective, at what price should VaxGen sell the vaccine to Thailand?

Questions

1. Is it appropriate for VaxGen to use intravenous drug abusers as study subjects for its AIDS vaccine?

2. Is it appropriate for the company to design the AIDS vaccine trials with a placebo control group?

3. What factors should the company take into consideration given that their vaccine studies will take place in Thailand?

4. Has the company appropriately structured the consent and recruitment process for these studies?

5. What if anything does VaxGen owe Thailand for its cooperation with these trials?

6. If the vaccine proves to be sufficiently efficacious for marketing, how should VaxGen market the vaccine in third world countries where AIDS is most prevalent but poverty rates are highest?

Discussion

Conducting medical product research in developing countries raises questions of whether the study country research ethics standards should apply (sometimes called "cultural relativism" and conceptualized by the maxim "when in Rome, do as the Romans do") or whether home country standards are best (sometimes called "cultural imperialism," with the connotation that outside standards are being imposed under the assumption that they are superior). Abiding by concepts of cultural relativism means that appropriate behavior in a country or culture is determined by its laws and customs, and morality is defined by local consensus and practices. Practicing cultural relativism, however, clashes with the notion that ethical principles are meant to be universal rather than culturally determined. Deferring to local standards can also lead a company to exploit locally vulnerable people who lack the means and the institutional structure to avoid the risks and hazards of clinical research. In recruiting volunteers for a drug study, for instance, the differences in education, literacy, poverty, access to medical care, and social mores can mean that people may not be able to exercise the same degree of autonomy and may not be able to make choices that protect their rights and advance their interests. In contrast, imposing home country standards constrains choices that local people and institutions may want to make for themselves and often ignores the local country problems that require different solutions.

Rather than accept one approach over the other, addressing these questions should begin by studying local country conditions so that visiting researchers can obtain a deeper understanding of the social, economic, medical, and political influences on the contemplated trials. Next, researchers should ask whether there are relevant differences between the two countries that can justify different practices. With this understanding and knowledge, firms can evaluate issues of importance using ethical principles and standards. Utilitarian and justice systems are inherently amenable to producing different conclusions in different situations. Rights, however, tend to be more immutable. These differences in ethical systems combined with disparity between countries suggests that some ethical differences in clinical research can be tolerated and others should not be.

TABLE 9.1

VaxGen, Inc., Financial Data

Condensed Statements of Operations, Unaudited
(in thousands of dollars except for per share and footnote data)

Operating Expenses	Quarter Ended 6/30/99	Quarter Ended 6/30/98	Six Months Ended 6/30/99	Six Months Ended 6/30/98
Research and Development	(4,196)	(1,088)	(7,234)	(1,804)
General and Administrative	(3,797)	(1,193)	(4,803)	(1,640)
Loss from operations	(7,993)	(2,281)	(12,037)	(3,444)
Total other income	233	263	517	569
Net loss	(7,760)[a]	(2,018)	(11,520)[a]	(2,875)
Basic and dilute loss per share	(1.10)	(0.33)	(1.51)	(0.47)
Weighted average shares used in computing basic and dilute loss per share	7,685	6,109	7,653	6,109

Condensed Balance Sheets, Unaudited
(in thousands of dollars)

Assets	6/30/99	12/31/98
Cash and investment securities	15,206	19,468
Property and equipment, net	2,496	1,258
Deferred offering costs	1,040	—
Other assets	751	746
Total Assets	19,493	21,472

Liabilities and stockholder's equity	6/30/99	12/31/98
Current liabilities	3,364	2,074
Other liabilities	100	—
Stockholder's equity	16,029	19,398
Total liabilities and stockholder's equity	19,493	21,472

[a] The net loss includes noncash compensation expense of $2,930,000. This expense consists of $2,360,000 related to the issuance of stock options and warrants. The remaining noncash compensation expense of $570,000 is amortization of deferred compensation related to the 1996 Stock Option Plan for the portion of the vesting period lapsed at June 30, 1999.
SOURCE: VaxGen, Inc., financial reports

Washington Post Article— The Body Hunters: Part 6

Life by Luck of the Draw

In Third World Drug Tests, Some Subjects Go Untreated

By Mary Pat Flaherty and Doug Struck
Washington Post Staff Writers. Friday, December 22, 2000; Page A01

LAMPANG, Thailand—In this small city in northern Thailand, a group of pregnant women signed up for an experiment overseen by a U.S. Army doctor who sought to monitor the transfer of HIV infection to newborns.

His passive, observational study offered the women no medicine to prevent HIV transmission in order to give researchers "a more efficient and effective means" of studying them, he wrote in a memorandum. Twenty-two infants were born HIV positive to the unprotected mothers.

At a spartan drug clinic in the heart of Bangkok, heroin addicts lined up on a recent morning to receive an experimental HIV vaccine produced by an American company. Drawn by small payments and offers of free rice, they signed on for a test in which they had a greater chance of receiving a placebo—or dummy shot—than would Americans taking part in the same research in the United States.

In Bangkok's two largest maternity wards, pregnant women infected with HIV, the virus that causes AIDS, enrolled in an American test aimed at reducing AIDS transmission from mothers to children. But half the Thai women were given placebos instead of a proven drug, and 37 babies who might have been spared were born HIV-positive.

Set against a staggering AIDS epidemic, the Thai cases highlight the unequal bargains underlying the recent boom in overseas drug testing by both private and public medical researchers: rich countries have the drugs and hypotheses, while poor countries have vast numbers of patients. Yet the trade-offs made in experiments do not always distribute burdens and benefits evenly.

Medical progress has always depended on some individuals bearing personal risk for society's benefit. Placebos give researchers a clearer view of which experimental therapies work and which do not, many scientists contend. Passive studies that track how a disease moves unimpeded through a population can provide insights into treatment and prevention.

But those long-standing research methods have become more complicated and controversial as scientists from wealthy nations increasingly work amid poverty in developing countries. Such tests have spurred angry debate on review boards of American universities, in the halls of African and Asian health ministries and in chambers of the World Health Organization.

Among the questions: When Western researchers travel to impoverished countries to set up drug experiments, which country's ethical guidelines should apply? While working with poor test subjects, must researchers provide the best treatment available in wealthy countries? Or are they free merely to provide the best local care available—which in some medically deprived settings may mean some test subjects get no treatment at all?

With 800,000 adults of its 61 million residents carrying the virus, Thailand's vast HIV-infected population has spent the last five years on these ethical and scientific frontiers. Open, increasingly democratic and cooperative with the West, Thailand discovered a scourge of AIDS in its midst a decade ago and turned emphatically to its wealthy allies for help.

In 1991, the WHO designated Thailand as a country ripe to test AIDS vaccines, sowing the seeds of research still underway. In 1994, WHO issued a second challenge, encouraging researchers to help developing countries find an affordable, practical alternative to the costly Western method of reducing the transmission of HIV from pregnant women to their infants.

After each appeal, researchers armed with new drugs and theories fanned out through the country. Testing new treatments against placebos, as many did, generated fast answers. But for the men, women and children recruited into such tests, the approach meant the luck of the draw determined who received care and who wound up with nothing.

Many in Thailand tried to "look at the bright side and accept that when you are a poor people you may have the choice between getting some treatment and care in a study or having none," said Vichai Chokevivat, until recently the vice chairman of Thailand's central ethics committee for human research.

Yet others in Thailand chafe at a system that allows Western researchers to present foreign test subjects with choices that provide less care and protection than those same researchers would be obliged to give subjects back in their own countries.

"It seems like every time this is the way things happen to Thailand," said Ratchanee Tunraka, a social worker with Siam Care in Bangkok, a charity that works with needy families, including some who participated in American research projects.

Why, she wondered aloud, are the studies brought to her country set up "to give someone nothing before we all can get a little something?"

A RACE AGAINST AZT

For the past decade, many U.S. researchers working overseas have given test subjects care only as good as the best local care available.

Thailand's experience with this practice has sometimes left a bitter aftermath. Consider, say some Thai doctors, the choices made by Lt. Col. Merlin L. Robb of Maryland's Walter Reed Army Institute of Research.

In late 1994, Robb drafted a proposal for a study of mother-to-child HIV transmission in northern Thailand. He wanted to join with Thai doctors in the city of Lampang to measure HIV characteristics of a mother's blood and cervical fluid for clues about a child's risk of infection. Urgent answers were needed: 10 HIV-positive women a month delivered babies at Lampang Hospital.

From the start, internal memos show, Robb was racing other U.S. researchers vying for access to test subjects in Thailand and racing the march of the anti-viral agent azidothymidine, commonly known as AZT.

Robb had said from the outset that if AZT became available in the area, he would encourage his Thai collaborators to use it. But if AZT did not arrive before his research concluded, he said, it would make for better results—because the drug would not cloud the natural passing of HIV from mother to child.

Robb had barely finished his research proposal before the ethical ground began to shift beneath him. A major study of pregnant, HIV-infected women in the United States and France showed AZT reduced newborn infection rates. The 1994 results were so dramatic—cutting infection rates by two-thirds—that AZT became standard treatment in industrialized countries.

Robb's trial design called for no AZT for mothers or their infected babies. AZT was scarcely available in Thailand, and Robb argued to an Army ethics board that withholding AZT would not deprive women and their children because they had little chance of getting the drug anyway.

On the other hand, giving test volunteers AZT could muddy his research and could, he said, attract "patients from other provinces, consequently increasing the health care burden at [the experiment's hospital] beyond its capabilities."

Two Army ethics board members objected. "We should insist on the use of AZT," wrote Michael Mazaleski, a civilian member of the Army's Human Subjects Research Review Board.

The full panel approved Robb's research, and in 1996 Robb won a grant from a division of the National Institutes of Health that would total $1 million.

Writing to a colleague, Robb said he was "somewhat uncomfortable" with the decision making by bioethicists "since their deliberations seem often devoid of the larger view of advancing medical science for the public good as opposed to the individual."

Less than a year after he enrolled his first mother in the test, Robb learned AZT was making its way to Lampang. A Harvard team was giving AZT to all pregnant women in research it had launched in the area. Meanwhile, Thai health authorities said they planned a pilot study on AZT in local hospitals. With the local standard of care changing, Robb and his team revisited their decision not to use it.

Robb asked NIH in early 1997 if he could redirect $15,000 of his grant to buy AZT and provide it sooner than the Thai government project would. NIH declined, saying the change would require a new, lengthy review of his proposal. It suggested he collaborate with the Harvard team—which also was NIH funded—if he wanted quicker access to AZT.

Robb's team in Lampang did not want to "surrender the site" to Harvard, e-mail messages show, and told him they preferred to wait and get AZT from the Thai government project. In a recent interview, Robb said he never intended for his research to get in the way of women receiving AZT once it was widely available, but he said he also did not want to override his Thai team's decisions.

As a result, the mothers in Robb's study went without AZT for another three months, until July of 1997 when the Thai government project started. The 101 women who got no AZT gave birth to 22 infected infants.

More than four years after his research began, final results have yet to be compiled, but Robb remains convinced the work could eventually prove valuable in the design of an AIDS vaccine. "This was ethical research," he said, that will elucidate "benchmarks for vaccine development."

"It was a disgraceful, shameful study," countered Vallop Thaineua, director of the Ministry of Public Health's regional office in northern Thailand.

But like Robb, his local collaborators take pride in their work. "I do not feel bad about our work. I believe it will be useful," said Vilaiwan Gulgolgarn, a research team member who now treats some of the HIV-infected children born during the study.

"We were ethical," she said, "the drug was not here from the government, and until then we did not need to provide it."

UNEQUAL ODDS

Robb's study was up and running in Lampang when researchers from VaxGen, Inc., a California-based biotechnology firm, arrived in Bangkok.

VaxGen had an AIDS vaccine under development in the United States, where 5,400 subjects, mostly homosexual men, had enlisted in tests. It wanted to add another 2,500 in Thailand, and to meet the need, it turned to drug addicts in Bangkok.

The Bangkok Municipal Authority arranged access to its 17 methadone clinics, where years of trust built up with counselors helped reassure heroin addicts about the experiment. "That's the reason so many agreed," said Kunyarat Maneesinthu, a psychologist at Bang Sue Clinic.

At the heart of negotiations between VaxGen and the Thai government was the question hanging over much of the research shifting to developing countries: How much did VaxGen owe participants or the host country?

VaxGen bargained tough. It risked losing Thai public support when it refused to pledge care for subjects who became HIV positive during the test. Thai health authorities finally stepped in and promised to provide the best local therapy—which was years behind what an American could expect.

VaxGen also refused to guarantee that the vaccine, if proven effective, would be sold to Thais at a reduced price. VaxGen recognizes the "special situation we have with Thailand," company president Donald P. Francis said recently. "They bought in very early to this and we said we would work as hard as we can to reduce the price for them. But we can't give vaccine away and bankrupt the company."

VaxGen also rejected the Thai requests for profit-sharing or a manufacturing plant to be located in the country. A "gentleman's agreement" the company wrote in 1998 to Thai health officials, suggested that if the Thais helped with packaging the vaccine, VaxGen might be able to reduce the country's costs for the vaccine. But "we will have to wait to see what actually happens with the Bangkok study."

The deal seemed the best Thais could get, said Jon Ungphakorn, who reviewed the study and is now a member of the Thai senate. "We were making test subjects available and we were agreeable to that. But on the other hand, we did not have that much bargaining power. Our situation was desperate."

Inside Bangkok's drug clinics, VaxGen used methods that would have been novel in the U.S. to recruit and track volunteers, records and interviews show. The company joined in a clinic program that offered free rice to addicts who brought in five friends. It tracked addicts into jails if they were arrested during the experiment so that shots and blood tests could be administered.

The Thai experiment's structure contrasted with the U.S. tests. In each arm, some volunteers received real vaccine and some dummy medicine, a calculated risk since participants in both studies were at high risk of contracting the virus. But Thais in VaxGen's ongoing study have a one-in-two chance of getting the real medicine. American volunteers have a two-out-of-three chance.

The Thai and American tests were designed differently because "it was thought it might be a motivational factor for American gay groups to participate" if they had a better chance at getting a vaccine, explained John G. Curd, VaxGen's senior vice president for medical affairs. "That may have been part of it," said Francis, adding that there was also a scientific reason involved. With U.S. infection rates so low, a larger pool of subjects receiving the vaccine meant researchers would reach enough people exposed to the virus. That way, researchers could determine more clearly if the vaccine was working.

Debate over designs of the trials was inconsequential to Thai addicts, who in interviews said they signed up for the test out of a mix of motives.

Wivat Chotchatmala, 35 and eight years an addict, said he volunteered "because I want the money"—about $9 for each of 15 visits, about a day's pay for drivers of *tuk-tuk*s, Bangkok's three-wheeled motorcycle taxis. But he also wanted to "do something useful for society and get a chance maybe to protect myself."

The vaccine volunteers "are swept up in the mood that they can do something for their country. That is a powerful and persuasive appeal for Thais," said Supatra Nakapew, director of the Centre for AIDS Rights in Bangkok.

VaxGen has invested $585,000 in equipment and facilities—which will remain in Bangkok when the test is over. But VaxGen's principal Thai investigator, Kachit Choopanya, said his overriding hope is that the vaccine will work. "That is the benefit we want most."

Next fall, a VaxGen committee will examine early results from the American study arm. VaxGen says it will stop both branches of the experiment and seek FDA approval if the vaccine proves 30 percent effective—a low threshold compared with other common vaccines.

If the drug is approved, VaxGen says, the Thais will immediately get one benefit akin to the U.S. side: All volunteers who received placebos will be vaccinated free.

ETHICAL FIRESTORM

The "race to the bottom" is how some medical ethicists have described drug researchers' moves into developing countries. But public health researchers, including some from developing countries, denounce as "ethical imperialism" the notion that Western standards of care always must prevail.

"The easy thing to accuse [international drug testing] of is Yankee exploitation, of taking advantage of disadvantaged populations," said Robert H. Rubin, professor of health sciences and technology at Harvard Medical School and a clinical trial pioneer in the United States. "Frankly, that's nonsense. It has to be done right, and appropriately, [but] if you believe as fervently as I do that there is benefit to society . . . then all society should bear some of the burdens" of developing new drugs.

The opposing viewpoints clashed sharply this fall as the World Medical Association met to revise the 1964 Declaration of Helsinki, the statement of principles that has guided ethical decisions in drug experiments around the world. With representatives from 45 countries, including developing nations that have become hotbeds for drug research, the conference voted to clarify language on the use of placebos, making it unethical to use dummy medicines on some subjects in trials where proven treatments may be available. The declaration does not have the force of law in the United States, but it wields considerable moral clout.

Outrage over American experiments on pregnant women in Thailand and sub-Saharan Africa was a driving force behind the change.

Public and private researchers in the United States are still unsure how they can comply with the strong international mandate while trying to tackle the treatment and prevention of life-threatening disease. The National Bioethics Advisory Commission, a presidentially appointed panel that is drafting ethical guidelines, has struggled with both the placebo issue and questions about what researchers owe local populations once an experiment is completed.

"Clearly, this is an evolving issue," said Helene Gayle, director of the Centers for Disease Control and Prevention's National Center for HIV, STD and TB programs. "Through research, we cannot change the reality that there are inequities and there is poverty in the world. We should, as citizens of the world, attack that reality, but not through constraining research."

But ultimately, the West's anguished ethical debates occur far from the ordinary, struggling families swept along in the global drug testing boom.

So it was for Petprow Madornglang, recruited in November 1997 for an AZT test conducted by the CDC.

Madornglang, who lived in the rural province of Ayutthaya, was one of 397 HIV-infected pregnant women who signed up for the test at Bangkok's Rajavithi Hospital. Once a week until she gave birth, she made the two-hour trip, crowding into the back of a small truck, then transferring to a van that left only when it had a full load.

Under the study launched in 1996, half of the pregnant women in the experiment received AZT, but in a shorter course—for fewer weeks and less frequent doses—than was standard in the U.S. The Thai newborns would get no AZT, unlike American infants who had received AZT for six weeks after birth.

The CDC's decision to use a placebo for half of the Thai study's participants—thus exposing some of their children to HIV, which presumably would have been prevented by AZT—outraged medical ethicists in the United States.

"If you have a safe and effective treatment anywhere in the world for a life-threatening condition, from that point on you cannot ethically conduct a clinical trial that gives some people placebo," said LeRoy Walters, a Georgetown University bioethicist. Researchers had other options. A Harvard team was studying how different doses of AZT worked on the transmission rate, for example.

But dropping the dummy pill from the research, the CDC contended, would have required adding more test subjects to ensure statistical integrity, adding time to the launch of the study and muddling the comparison. The Thai central ethics committee agreed.

"We felt it was not only ethical, but it was essential to conduct" the study, said the CDC's Gayle.

The CDC study tracked Madornglang and the other mother-child pairs for 18 months, and in the end, reported that the short course of AZT could reduce transmission by half. The results helped shape national health policy in Thailand, which early this year pledged to provide the treatment free to pregnant women.

With only half a chance at help, Madornglang wound up with the worst half, said her sister and a Thai doctor. She got the placebo.

In Bangkok, Madornglang's family still replays the "what ifs."

Her sister, Anchalee Soithong, did not want her in the test. Soithong volunteered at the Thai Red Cross, which offered the equivalent of the American-style treatment. She also knew that another Bangkok hospital had a more modest AZT program. She tried to persuade, cajole, and berate her sister into listening on a night when they huddled together in a bedroom, whispering about the infection and the pregnancy, trying to hide the news from their mother.

"I didn't want her to take a chance with her baby," Soithong recalled. But Madornglang wouldn't change her plans.

Madornglang joined the research in November 1997 while showing symptoms of HIV, including fungus in her mouth and skin lesions, according to a summary of her case.

After seven months, researchers referred her for medical care for her HIV symptoms, giving her some antibiotics. Despite that, she withered. And when she returned 10 weeks later, she was not further investigated or treated, according to a summary of her case.

Madornglang died in October 1998. She was 28.

"Placebo or AZT? Which worked better? That was their question and she helped them get the answer," Soithong said. "My question was why did they not take better care of my sister?"

Madornglang left behind her son born in January 1998, one of the 37 infants born with HIV. She called him Kittisak, but nicknamed him "Ice," because it seemed soothing in such a hot climate. And "because it sounded American, like that singer," said Soithong.

The boy received AZT and other treatments as his health deteriorated.

Ice lived long enough to pull himself up along the edge of tables, but not long enough to learn how to walk. He died last December. He was 23 months old.

Notes

1. For a general discussion of the factors involved in the international commercial development of medical products, see Spilker B. International development. In *Multinational pharmaceutical companies: Principles and practice*. New York: Raven Press; 1994. pp. 711–18.

2. Contract research organizations (CROs) were independent businesses that contracted with pharmaceutical companies to conduct or manage research on the company products. Primarily, CROs were used for clinical research and their existence increased rapidly in the 1990s because they offered research expertise, access to potential subjects, and efficiency in getting a product through the regulatory phases of research. They were especially useful for smaller biotechnology companies that lacked in-house staff to conduct late-stage, preapproval clinical research.

3. Latin American fever. *CenterWatch Newsletter* 2000; 7. Available from http://CenterWatch.com/bookstore/backissues/vol7iss5.html.

4. DeYoung K, Nelson D. Latin America is ripe for trials, and fraud; frantic pace could overwhelm controls. *Washington Post* 2000 Dec 21; Sect. A:01; Borger J. Dying for drugs: Volunteers or victims? Concern grows over control of drug trials. *Guardian* (London) 2001 Feb 14;4.

5. Angell M. The ethics of clinical research in the third world. *New England Journal of Medicine* 1997; 337:847–49. Copyright 1997 Massachusetts Medical Society. All rights reserved. Bernstein N. Oversight agencies give program scant review. *New York Times* 1999 June 6; Sect. 1:10.

6. See Note 5, Bernstein.

7. Bernstein N. Strings attached: A special report; for subjects in Haiti study, free AIDS care has a price. *New York Times* 1999 June 6; Sect. 1:1.

8. Ibid.

9. See Note 5, Angell.

10. Lurie P, Wolfe SM. Unethical trials of interventions to reduce perinatal transmission of the human immunodeficiency virus in developing countries. *New England Journal of Medicine* 1997; 337:853–56.

11. Appelbaum PS, Roth LH, Lidz CW, et al. False hopes and best data: Consent to research and the therapeutic misconception. *Hastings Center Report* 1987; 17:20–24.

12. French HW. AIDS research in Africa: juggling risks and hopes. *New York Times* 1997 Oct 9; Sect. A:1.

13. Kahn JG, Marseille E. A false assumption on African AIDS tests. *New York Times* 1997 Oct 11; Sect. A:10.

14. Angell M. Investigators' responsibilities for human subjects in developing countries. *New England Journal of Medicine* 2000; 342:967–69. Copyright 2000 Massachusetts Medical Society. All rights reserved.

15. Ibid.

16. Ibid.

17. Specter M. Urgency tempers ethics concerns in Uganda trial of AIDS vaccine. *New York Times* 1998 Oct 1; Sect. A:1.

18. This company later merged with France's Rhone-Poulenc SA to become Aventis SA.

19. See Note 4, DeYoung, Nelson; Note 4, Borger.

20. See Note 4, Borger.

21. Ibid.

22. See Note 4, DeYoung, Nelson.

23. Council for International Organizations of Medical Sciences. *International ethical guidelines for biomedical research involving human subjects.* Geneva; 1982, rev. 1993.

24. National Bioethics Advisory Commission. *Ethical and policy issues in international research: Clinical trials in developing countries.* Washington, DC; 2001. Available at http://bioethics.georgetown.edu/nbac/pubs.html.

25. The one provision that NBAC disagreed with was the 2000 revision to the Declaration of Helsinki providing that the use of placebos in medical research is always unethical if treatment is available for the condition in question.

26. See Note 5, Angell.

27. See Note 14.

28. The initial case study was prepared by Jennifer Wilds and Betty Pang under the guidance of and with later revisions by Margaret Eaton. The input and assistance of Donald Francis and Marlene Chernow of VaxGen, Inc., is greatly appreciated. The events described in this case study occurred up until spring 1999.

29. Piot P. AIDS: A global response. *Science* 1996; 272:1855–60.

30. Personal interview with Don Francis, 1999 Nov 11.

31. At the time, there was no test to detect infection, and the prolonged latency period before symptoms of the infection appeared meant that there was plenty of time to spread the infection to others. The disease was likened to an iceberg, with only a small number of recognized cases and a huge base of undetected infected people.

32. Recombinant vaccines were made by genetically engineering noninfective portions of the virus that would trick the human immune system into fighting the vaccine as if it were the whole live virus. The goal of such a vaccine was the production of anti-HIV antibodies that would confer immunity against the virus. See www.vaxgen.com.

33. Centers for Disease Control and Prevention. *Morbidity and Mortality Weekly Report* 1997; 46:165–67.

34. All UNAIDS statistics were obtained from www.unaids.org.

35. Stolberg S. Promise, disappointment mark AIDS vaccine quest. *Los Angeles Times* 1994 Aug 9; Sect. A:1.

36. The theory behind the gp120 vaccine was that antibodies to the harmless gp120 protein would develop and attach to the virus's outer envelope, thus preventing the virus from connecting to its usual human receptor and initiating infection. Using the envelope protein would avoid incorporating the infective genetic material that resided in the core of the virus. A similar strategy had been effective with other vaccines such as for hepatitis B. See http://vaxgen.com.

37. Belshe RB, Graham B, Keefer MC, et al. Neutralizing antibodies to HIV-1 in seronegative volunteers immunized with recombinant gp120 from the MN strain of HIV-1. *Journal of the American Medical Association* 1994; 272:475–80.

38. Green J. Who put the lid on gp120? *New York Times* 1995 Mar 26; Sect. 6:50.

39. Snow B. Community perspectives on participating in research, advocacy, and progress. *HIV vaccine handbook.* Published by the AIDS Vaccine Advocacy Coalition, 1999 Apr. Available from www.avac.org.

40. Cellular or cell-mediated immunity marshals immune cells to kill other infected cells. In humoral or antibody immunity, the immune system makes antibodies to neutralize virus in the liquid (noncellular) part of the blood. Theoretically, both are needed since HIV is transmitted by different routes (sexual, intravenous, and perinatal) and by different modes (as cell-free and cell-associated viruses). See Fast P, Snow W. HIV vaccine development; an overview. HIV/AIDS Information Center, *Journal of the American Medical Association*, 1997 Mar 25. Available from www.ama-assn.org/special/hiv/treatmnt/updates/vacessay.htm.

41. Cohen J. US panel votes to delay real-world vaccine trials. *Science* 1994; 264:1839.

42. See Note 38.

43. Ibid.

44. Ibid.

45. At the time, Genentech was majority-owned by Swiss pharmaceutical company Roche Holding AG.

46. Weiss R. Advances inject hope into quest for vaccine. *Washington Post* 1997 Sept 3; Sect. A:1; Goldman B. What vaccines are hot. *Signals Magazine* 1999 Jan 18. Available at www.signalsmag.com/signalsmag.nsf.

47. Cohen J. *Shots in the dark: The wayward search for an AIDS vaccine.* New York: W.W. Norton; 2001. p. 72.

48. VaxGen mission statement. Available from www.vaxgen.com.

49. Tan W. Mahathir to rich states: Bear research costs. *Straits Times* (Singapore) 1999 Oct 25; p. 30.

50. Wright J. Follow the money: The economics of AIDS vaccine development. An interview with the World Bank's Hans Binswanger. *HIV InSite.* Available from www.avac.org/readings/binswanger.html.

51. Dove A. World Bank task force push/pulls AIDS vaccine. *Nature Biotechnology* 1999; 17:846–47.

52. Cha A. First major trial of an AIDS vaccine. *San Jose Mercury News* 1998 Dec 12. Available from www.fc.net/zarathus/aids/company_will_test_aids_vaccine.txt.

53. According to Marlene Chernow at VaxGen, FDA eventually agreed with this view and stated that any vaccine offering more than 30 percent protection from the disease would be considered beneficial enough for market approval.

54. See Note 46, Weiss.

55. Specter M. Uganda AIDS vaccine test: Urgency affects ethics rules. *New York Times* 1998 Oct 1; Sect. A:1.

56. AIDS Vaccine Research Committee. AIDS vaccine development. *Science* 1998; 280:803.

57. These differences included the poor immunogenicity of the HIV envelope glycoproteins and their resistance to neutralizing antibodies, the extensive variation in the viral genome, and the enhanced ability of the virus to become integrated in the host genome of immune cells.

58. King RT. FDA permits testing for AIDS vaccine: VaxGen will launch large-scale trials in U.S. and also in Thailand. *Asian Wall Street Journal* 1998 June 4; p 9.

59. Snow B. VaxGen: Pushing the envelope. *Bay Area Reporter* 1998 Jan 29. Available from www.actupgg.org/BAR/art012998.html.

60. Altman LK. FDA approves full scale tests of AIDS vaccine. *New York Times* 1998 June 4; Sect. A:1.

61. M2Presswire. *U.S. HHS: NIAID collaborates with VaxGen on vaccine studies.* Dow Jones Publications Library 1998 Aug 18.

62. See Note 51.

63. See Note 58.

64. See, e.g., Varmus H, Satcher D. Ethical complexities of conducting research in developing countries. *New England Journal of Medicine* 1997; 337:1003; see also Note 5, Angell; Note 10.

65. The AZT treatment regimen used in Western countries required that women undergo HIV testing and counseling early in pregnancy, comply with a lengthy course of oral AZT, receive intravenous AZT during labor, and refrain from breast-feeding. In addition, the newborn infants were given six weeks of oral AZT, and both mothers and infants were carefully monitored for adverse effects of the drug. This regimen was deemed not feasible for African study women, who often received little or no prenatal care, did not deliver in a hospital, and relied on breast milk to feed their newborns. In addition to these strenuous requirements on mothers and the health-care system, the cost of the AZT regimen for mother and child was too expensive. In Malawi, for instance, the Western AZT treatment regimen cost more than six hundred times the annual per capita allocation for health care. See Note 64, Varmus, Satcher.

66. Bloom BR. The highest attainable standard: Ethical issues in AIDS vaccines. *Science* 1998; 279:186–88.

67. Mbidde E. Bioethics and local circumstances. *Science* 1998 Jan 9; 279:155.

68. UNAIDS. *Ethical considerations in HIV preventive vaccine research.* Proceed-

ings of a meeting held 1997 Sept 23–24; Geneva. Available from www.unaids.org/ publications/documents/vaccines/vaccines/Ethicsresearch.pdf.

69. International ethical guidelines for biomedical research involving human subjects. CIOMS, 1982, rev. 1993; Geneva.

70. UNAIDS. Proceedings of a meeting held 1997 Sept 23–24; Geneva. Available from www.unaids.org/publications/documents/vaccines/vaccines/Ethicsresearch.pdf; see also Note 55.

71. See Note 66.

72. VaxGen mission statement. Available from www.vaxgen.com.

73. International ethical guidelines for biomedical research involving human subjects. CIOMS, 1982, rev. 1993; Geneva.

74. See Note 68.

75. Vaccines that do not prevent infection but do prevent disease (e.g., polio, tetanus, diphtheria, measles, hepatitis B, and influenza) work by reducing the number of invading microorganisms, increasing the rate of clearance of the infection, preventing the secondary consequences of infection, or preventing transmission. See Note 66.

76. See Note 66; Note 68.

77. See Note 55.

78. Altman LK. Ethics panel urges easing of restrictions on AIDS vaccines. *New York Times* 1998 June 28; Sect.1:6; Cohen J. No consensus on rules for AIDS vaccine trials. *Science* 1998; 281:22–23.

79. See Note 55.

80. Ibid.

81. Piot P. New ethical guidelines on HIV vaccine research pave the way for large-scale international trials of HIV vaccines. 1998 June 29, Geneva. Available from www.unaids.org.

82. Sivaraman S. Religion—Thailand: Buddhist monks enlist in fight against HIV/AIDS. Available from www.oneworld.org/ips2/jan98/hiv.html.

83. Phoolcharoen W. HIV/AIDS prevention in Thailand, success and challenges. *Science* 1998; 280:1873–74.

84. Theparat C. IMF gets a drubbing as national plan discussed. *Bangkok Post* 1999 Apr 10. Available from www.bkkpost.samart.co.th/.

85. See Note 83.

86. Bangkok metropolitan administration guidelines for clinical care of HIV-infected patients. 1998 May 27. Described in *Questions and answers on the Thailand Phase III vaccine study and CDC's collaboration.* Centers for Disease Control and Prevention, 1999 Feb. Available from www.cdc.gov/nchstp/hiv_aids/pubs/facts/vaccineqa.htm.

87. Pothisiri P, Tangcharoensathien V, Lertiendumrong J. *Funding priorities for HIV/AIDS crisis in Thailand.* 12th World AIDS Conference. 1998 June; Geneva. Available from www.worldbank.org/aids-econ/thaifund.htm.

88. Cohen, J. *Shots in the dark: The wayward search for an AIDS vaccine.* New York: W.W. Norton; 2001. p. 388.

89. Personal interview with Marlene Chernow, 1999 Nov 23.

90. *Questions and answers on the Thailand Phase III vaccine study and CDC's collaboration.* Centers for Disease Control and Prevention, 1999 Feb. Available from www.cdc.gov/nchstp/hiv_aids/pubs/facts/vaccineqa.htm.

91. Personal interview with Marlene Chernow, 1999 Nov 23.

92. See Note 90.

93. Harris R. AIDS vaccine—Thailand. *All Things Considered.* Broadcast on National Public Radio, 2000 July 13. Available from http://search.npr.org/cf/cmn/cmnpdoifm.cfm?PrgDate=7 percent2F13 percent2F2000&PrgID=2.

94. Thaitawat N. On the right track. *Bangkok Post* 1999 Apr 12. Available from www.bkkpost.samart.co.th/.

95. See Note 38.

96. Personal interview with Marlene Chernow, 1999 Nov 23; see also Note 93.

97. Personal interview with Marlene Chernow, 1999 Nov 23.

98. Rao K. Testing issues: A large HIV-vaccine trial in Thailand presents ethical dilemmas. *Asia Week* 1999 May 7. Available from www.asiaweek.com/asiaweek/99/0507/feat3.html.

99. Personal interview with Don Francis, 1999 Nov 11; personal interview with Marlene Chernow, 1999 Nov 23.

100. See Note 98.

101. Information about the investigational protocol is from interviews with Donald Francis and Marlene Chernow, and from VaxGen's protocol, entitled "A Phase III Trial to Determine the Efficacy of Bivalent AIDSVAX® B/E Vaccine in Intravenous Drug Users in Bangkok, Thailand."

102. See Note 90.

103. Smaller numbers of subjects could be used in Thailand than in the United States because of the higher rates of infection in Thailand (4–8 percent HIV prevalence in the IV drug user population) compared to the United States (1.5 percent in the homosexual male population). Also, some scientists thought that greater viral genetic diversity could make vaccines less effective, and there was a wider genetic diversity (range of HIV strains) in the United States compared to Thailand. In the United States, the prevalent subtype B had been present since the mid to late 1970s and had had over two decades to genetically diverge. By comparison, the Thai epidemic did not begin until 1988, and the subtype E viruses predominant there were not as diverse.

104. According to the Thai National Statistical Office, per capita yearly income in Bangkok in 1998 was about 89,000 baht, making it the wealthiest region in the country. But many of the Bangkok IV drug users were more likely to be closer to the poverty line, set at about 8,800 baht per year. See Per capita debt of Thais up 34 percent due to economic crisis. *Bangkok Post* 1999 Sept 8; Method to calculate poverty revised. *Bangkok Post* 1998 Apr 12. Both available from www.bkkpost.samart.co.th/.

Anticipating and Managing
Postmarket Problems

There are various reasons why medical products do not achieve anticipated acceptance, or sometimes fail and must be pulled from the market. A major reason is that the product turns out to be less efficacious or safe than was originally expected. Another reason is that the product, once on the market, is not used in the manner for which it was intended—resulting in an adverse type of "off label" use. Another reason for product failure, increasingly raised by the commercialization of genetic technologies, is rejection of the product by physicians, patients, or the public. Because premarket testing typically is designed (but can never be guaranteed) to assure a company and the Food and Drug Administration that a regulated product will be reasonably safe and beneficial for the intended claim, these studies rarely shed light on the other reasons that products fail. Hence, there is always some degree of uncertainty in the bioscience product business about how a product will fare once on the market. While some of these difficulties can be anticipated in advance, the one problem that cannot and which is an ever-present reality is that medical and biologic knowledge is continually evolving. This evolution makes it certain that new information will be uncovered about a disease or how a medical product interacts with the disease. New knowledge can be discovered during the R&D phases of product development or after the product has been marketed. In either case, new information sometimes means that a medical product is less efficacious or more toxic than expected. How companies prepare for and manage all of these uncertainties can affect their future and impact physician prescribers and patients, the ultimate consumers of the product.

UNCERTAINTY ABOUT PRODUCT SAFETY AND EFFICACY

The FDA officially recognizes in its regulations that widespread use of drugs, biologics, and medical devices may be necessary to uncover serious but less common or unanticipated problems. Premarket clinical trials are rarely large enough or of sufficient duration to predict the incidence of all adverse effects, or in what circumstances the product will fail to benefit the patient. For example, a rare adverse event occurring in fewer than one in ten thousand persons is not likely to be identified in premarket testing.[1] Considering that some medical products will be used by millions, even a low-incidence side effect means that a large number of patients are likely to suffer from an unexpected adverse event, which can range from minimal harm to death. Once the product is launched, information can be gathered to answer the following questions: (1) will the product have the same effect in the general population as it did in the smaller sample of research subjects? (2) what happens when large numbers of physicians with differing levels and depths of training, experience, and abilities start to use the product? (3) what happens when the product is used outside of the tightly controlled research setting and is given to heterogeneous populations of patients who may be sicker or healthier, have other diseases, are pregnant, younger, or older, take other prescription or over-the-counter drugs, or are noncompliant with instructions? (4) what happens when the product is used for longer periods of time? and (5) does the time of research versus the time of general use (often for decades after the research) make a difference in outcome?[2] The extent to which clinical trials and other premarket research are designed to answer these questions can give the manufacturer added assurance that the product will behave in the general public as it did in premarketing investigations. Also, the more closely the company follows the experiences of postmarket use, the earlier it will learn if there are reasons to doubt the efficacy or safety of the product.

While the FDA requirements for premarket testing and postmarketing surveillance are vital to provide assurances of efficacy and safety, medical products based on genomic information and genetic technology challenge the FDA's abilities to review and monitor products. One reason for this difficulty is the fact that genetic technologies (such as gene therapies, gene tests, xenotransplantation products, and genetically modified foods) are proliferating faster than are generally agreed-upon standards about what constitutes their safety and efficacy.[3] Unlike many traditional pharmaceuticals, biotechnology products are more likely to be novel or intended for entirely new indications, so that the FDA cannot draw on past experience and is sometimes forced to consider whether it can even regulate the product and, if so, how. For other products, FDA jurisdiction is clear but the FDA has inadequate expertise to generate timely approval standards. In comparison, corporate technology and expertise is often much more focused and advanced. To add to the complexity, understanding of interindividual human genetic variation and its implications for product development and use is still in its early stages but is rapidly evolving. Also, postmarketing surveillance depends to a large extent on voluntary reporting by physicians, which can delay discovery of problems. This, coupled with trends to streamline government and shorten regulatory review time for drugs, biologics, and devices, gives companies more discretion to decide which studies to perform and what constitutes adequate pre- and postmarket safety and efficacy data.[4]

The consequences of the inability to predict product behavior after marketing can cause several types of harm for a company—financial (poor product sales), regulatory (FDA product labeling restrictions or product recall), or legal (product liability lawsuits), all of which can lead to further public relations and financial setbacks for any company. The diabetes drug Rezulin (troglitazone) is an example of a drug that caused all of these problems for manufacturer Warner-Lambert.

About fifteen million Americans suffer from adult-onset diabetes, and uncontrolled cases require treatment with injectable insulin. Clinical studies had shown that Rezulin, a drug with a unique mechanism of action compared to other antidiabetic drugs, could eliminate the need for injectable insulin in many diabetic patients. Consequently, there was great enthusiasm in the physician and patient communities and at the FDA about speeding this drug to market. However, animal and human studies had shown that the drug could cause liver problems, and indeed soon after Rezulin's approval, adverse drug reaction reports began to link the drug to incidences of liver toxicity. As these reports came in to FDA, the agency required Warner-Lambert to upgrade its risk warnings three times and to advise physicians to test the liver function of treated patients more frequently. However, as more liver toxicity reports came in, the safety of the drug was questioned by regulators, and Public Citizen's Health Research Group petitioned the FDA to remove Rezulin from the market. When dozens of cases of acute liver failure (some of which required liver transplants) and sixty-three deaths were linked to Rezulin use, the FDA forced a drug recall in March 1999, about two years after initial marketing. By that time, about five hundred thousand U.S. patients had taken Rezulin and the company had grossed $2.1 billion in sales of the drug. During postmarketing review of the problem and after the drug was recalled, the FDA and the company were the subject of widespread public criticism about their handling of the safety problem; critics called the process "fast approval, slow removal." Case reports linking the drug to liver damage kept appearing. As of the end of 2000, the drug was blamed for 391 patient deaths and over four hundred lawsuits had been filed against Warner-Lambert and its successors.[5]

PRODUCT MISUSE

In addition to paying attention to a product's attributes, companies also must anticipate how a product will be used once it is removed from the controlled research environment and placed on the open market. In the case of medical products, physicians and other professionals often require training in order to use the product effectively and safely, and some companies are required, or voluntarily undertake, to educate patients on safe product use.[6] Product training is of greater importance in situations where physicians have little or no experience in the field relevant to the product use. Examples of these situations include the use of noninvasive surgical devices (for example, endoscopic tools and microcameras) by surgeons trained only in open surgical techniques, the use by general practitioners with minimal training in psychiatry of a psychotropic drug newly marketed for a geriatric dementia, or the use of gene tests by physicians with no training in the relatively new field of the genetics of human disease. In addition, once a product is on the market, physicians are legally entitled to prescribe the product "off label" for any use, despite the fact that the company can only market the product for its approved labeled indications. For example, drugs approved and labeled to treat one form of cancer are often effective and are prescribed for other cancers, and the FDA has no legal authority to stop physicians from making the professional decision to offer such treatment. However, such use can lead to problems for companies, since the larger the off-label market, the more the company can be suspected of illegal off-label promotion.

There are also times when companies do run afoul of the off-label marketing prohibition. In these cases, the FDA can issue warning letters to a company to cease off-label marketing, and occasionally the agency has obtained injunctions to stop such marketing. The punishment of last resort lies in the power to seek criminal charges for violation of the Food and Drug Act. One widely publicized instance occurred when Ortho Pharmaceuticals, a subsidiary of Johnson & Johnson, was accused of illegally promoting its prescription acne drug RetinA® for use on facial wrinkles and to prevent premature skin aging. This promotion, which began in 1988 and resulted in a quadrupling of product sales to $115 million the following year, was investigated by the FDA and the Department of Justice following a congressional investigation of the FDA's enforcement of prescription drug promotion laws. In the report of the congressional investigation, Ortho Pharmaceuticals and Johnson & Johnson were accused of illegal off-label promotion, and particular physicians who promoted this off-label use were criticized for failing to disclose their financial ties to the two companies. Eventually, Ortho Pharmaceuticals was not indicted for illegal promotion, but the company did plead guilty to illegal destruction of documents and obstructing justice in a federal investigation, for which it paid $7.5 million in penalties and costs. Ironically, the company sought and subsequently received FDA approval to market Retin-A for use in combating facial wrinkles.[7]

PUBLIC ACCEPTANCE

In addition to the possible negative experiences that can occur in situations like those of Warner-Lambert and Ortho Pharmaceuticals, companies that commercialize genetic technologies might find themselves confronting a relatively new societal skepticism or hesitancy to accept new products. While most larger companies have experienced a variety of expected and common postmarketing difficulties, this last issue is new to the industry. The Monsanto sample case study presented in Chapter 3 of this text is an example of the difficulties companies can face when marketing novel genetic products. Xenotransplantation products and those derived from stem cells are also predicted to generate public acceptance difficulties.

EVOLVING MEDICAL INFORMATION

Disease processes are always imperfectly understood, some more than others. Drugs and biologics designed to target disease will also always create unwanted side effects either as a result of their effect on the disease (an antihypertensive can cause the blood pressure to go too low) or on another bodily system (the same drug can cause liver damage). Because of these two problems, ongoing medical research efforts are attempting to increase disease and treatment understanding to lessen the uncertainty and risk of medical treatment.

There are times when it takes decades for research to uncover fundamental information about a well-established drug. New revelations about diseases and drugs can sometimes have disastrous effects on the markets of medical products. One such instance resulted in the devastation of a strong market for hormone replacement therapy (HRT) for postmenopausal women. Estrogen had been the mainstay of therapy for those women who suffered from hot flashes with accompanying cardiovascular and gastric discomfort, night sweats and sleep disturbances, and urogenital dryness.[8] Estrogen had also been shown to prevent the loss of bone mineralization that led to bone fractures, the sequelae of which were common causes of death in elderly women. Estrogen had also been shown in some studies to lower the risk of cardiovascular disease and death from heart attack and stroke in postmenopausal women. Estrogen alone however was known to increase the risk of breast and endometrial cancer. Many women were prescribed estrogen in combination with a progestogen to eliminate the endometrial cancer risk.

The most popular form of these combined hormones was the product Prempro®, manufactured by the giant pharmaceutical company Wyeth, formerly American Home Products. The market for these products was very large; about fourteen million of the fifty million postmenopausal women in the United States were taking some form of HRT.[9] Despite widespread use of HRT, enough of the studies documenting its benefits and risks were observational in nature without the preferred controls most medical scientists like to see. Over the years, therefore, there had been frequent calls for large-scale prospective controlled studies to establish the risks and benefits of HRT. Such an effort would be so lengthy, costly, and logistically difficult, however, that no controlled studies were done in healthy women until 1991, more than forty years after the lead drug Premarin® had been introduced to the market. The study was the called Women's Health Initiative, a National Institutes of Health randomized, placebo-controlled, double-blind 8.5-year trial to study "the most common causes of death, disability, and impaired quality of life in postmenopausal women." This study involved sixteen thousand women and cost more than $600 million. One part of the study, the one involving an assessment of the risks of Wyeth's Prempro, was stopped early because of evidence that Prempro minimally increased the risks of cardiovascular disease and breast cancer.[10] Another arm of the study using Wyeth's Premarin (estrogen alone) was continued, but the future of this product became uncertain given the Prempro findings.[11]

Although the evidence showed that the risks of Prempro were only minimally higher than placebo, there were other, although less effective, options available to women for the acute symptoms and bone-weakening effects of menopause. As a result, many physicians recommended that women stop taking HRT. Obviously, this had an impact on Wyeth's market for Prempro, which was being prescribed to 77 percent of women receiving combination hormonal therapy. Together, Prempro and Premarin accounted for 15 percent of Wyeth's $14.1 billion sales in the prior year. Sales of Prempro ($732 million in the prior year) fell 40 percent in the quarters after the announcement of the study risks. The fate of Premarin sales also became uncertain. Analysts were figuring that Wyeth's HRT business could drop by 50 percent over the following four years.[12]

Biotech companies were perhaps even more prone to the uncertainties caused by evolving medical knowledge since many biotech companies were focused on developing novel products for disorders that had so far evaded attempts at treatment. Nasty surprises during the clinical trial process were therefore unfortunately common for such cutting-edge products. Genzyme's Phase II trial of NeuroCell-PD (see the case study in Chapter 7) is one example of this kind of problem. NeuroCell-PD was a product intended to insert dopamine producing cells into the brains of Parkinson disease patients. Since the lack of dopamine was responsible for the symptoms of Parkinson disease and since the Phase I trials had been encouraging, there was every reason to believe that this product would be effective in the expanded trials. However, the initial analysis of the data from the Phase II trial showed that NeuroCell-PD was no more effective than placebo. This disappointing result might have been anticipated and controlled for had the Genzyme researches had access to a study published five months after the announcement of the Phase II trial results. In this other study, Canadian researchers were studying the placebo effect in Parkinson disease patients and found that an expectation or anticipation of therapeutic benefit from an intervention was related to an increase in the production of dopamine in the brain.[13] Prior to this study, researchers, including those at Genzyme, knew that the placebo effect in Parkinson disease patients was strong, but they did not know why. This study helped explain the phenomenon. Had Genzyme known about this physiological response, the design of the Phase II trial would undoubtedly have been altered and the results possibly more encouraging.

CONCLUSION

Until recently, it was customary to expect that the main focus of a bioscience company should be on identifying medically promising products and getting them approved by the FDA as quickly and efficiently as possible. However, as illustrated by the examples described above, some companies have come to appreciate that using standard pharmaceutical industry practices and regulatory controls are not sufficient to ensure product success and prevent harm to the company, reassure the physicians prescribing their products, and benefit and instill confidence in the patients who receive them. Consequently, many companies in this industry are exploring ways to reduce regulatory, professional, and public backlash so that market entry is smoother and product sales can be sustained. These approaches include lobbying efforts to forestall harmful legislation, developing public education and public relations programs to explain the benefits of biotechnology, conducting trials to predict how the product will be used and perceived once available to the general public, placing voluntary limitations on target markets, expanding product labeling, instituting rigorous consent processes, and conducting wider postmarketing surveillance to collect data about potential problems created by product use.

The following case study is an example of two companies facing regulatory, medical, and public uncertainty about the relative benefits and risks of a new genetic medical product. The case study raises the question of whether the marketing approaches described above (or other strategies) would have been effective in improving market acceptance of this product.

Case Study

Myriad and OncorMed and the
Marketing of the First Genetic Tests
for Breast Cancer Susceptibility[14]

In December 1995, the CEOs of two companies at opposite ends of the country operating in the uncharted area of commercial genetic testing faced the same dilemma. For the previous two years, Myriad Genetics CEO Peter Meldrum and OncorMed CEO Timothy Triche had led their companies in a competition to develop a genetic test for breast and ovarian cancer susceptibility (see Tables 10.1 and 10.2 for company financial data). Through 1995, both companies had offered genetic testing only to women who participated in their research studies. In 1995, the two companies were considering selling their testing services to physicians generally. Although the market for this testing service looked very promising, some scientists and patient activist groups believed that it was premature to provide testing outside of a carefully controlled research environment where data could be collected on an ongoing basis to answer significant questions about the health consequences of genetic mutations and the potential benefits and risks of testing. Specifically, they argued that commercialization should wait because knowledge about inherited predisposition to breast cancer was still emerging, and medical care options for mutation carriers were limited and not proven to be of benefit. In addition, data on the psychological and social effects on women who were tested were still evolving. Those in favor of restricting such testing to the research setting wanted laws in place to protect individuals from irresponsible testing practices, loss of privacy, and genetic discrimination. In this environment, it was up to Meldrum and Triche to determine whether their companies should begin marketing their tests. If they decided to proceed, they would need to design effective marketing strategies and address the concerns of those outside the company.

BREAST AND OVARIAN CANCER SUSCEPTIBILITY, SCREENING, AND RISK REDUCTION: STATE OF THE ART PRIOR TO GENETIC TESTING

In 1995, it was estimated that one in eight women would develop breast cancer in her lifetime.[15] Breast cancer was the most common cancer in women and the second leading cause of cancer-related death in women. In 1994, an estimated 183,000 women were diagnosed with breast cancer in the United States, and approximately 46,000 died from the disease.[16] Given this high prevalence, breast cancer screening had become an important option to explore in the fight against the disease.

The objective of screening is to detect cancer when it is early and treatable, offering the patient the greatest chance for a cure. On average, 79 percent of women with breast cancer are still alive five years after the cancer is detected. However, the survival rate increases to 93 percent when the tumors are detected early.[17] For years, the recommended screening practices for breast tumors had been physical exams and annual mammograms for women age forty and older. It was recommended that mammograms be performed at younger ages in women considered to be at high risk due to a family history of breast cancer.[18] Suspicious lesions on mammograms were subjected to further imaging studies and, if results were still inconclusive, biopsied to determine if the abnormality was benign or cancerous.

Although a number of technological advances in diagnostic imaging and tissue biopsy had made it possible to detect breast cancer quite early, these methods were not fully utilized, and data on the efficacy of these approaches in high-risk women were considered limited.[19] Some women who had many relatives with breast cancer took prophylactic measures to reduce their risk of cancer by having their breasts removed (mastectomy). This was done to gain some extra assurance that diagnostic tests could not provide. At the Mayo Clinic alone, researcher Lynn C. Hartmann had identified 2,029 women with a family history of breast cancer who had prophylactic mastectomies between 1960 and 1993.[20] While in theory these surgeries would prevent cancers from developing, there was no way to know for sure which women were at high risk, and the efficacy of this strategy in women with strong family histories had yet to be determined.[21] Whether physicians would recommend the surgery seemed to depend on which group of specialists was questioned. Of 742 physicians surveyed in one study, 81 percent of plastic surgeons had recommended the procedure, compared with 38.8 percent of general surgeons and 17.7 percent of gynecologists.[22] The widely ranging practices regarding prophylactic mastectomies left women wondering whether the surgical risks, resulting disfigurement, and social and emotional consequences of the procedure were worth the presumed reduction in risk.

Equally uncertain was the usefulness of cancer screening and prophylactic surgery to reduce the risks of ovarian cancer (the other cancer relevant to the genetic test in question). There was no screening test for ovarian cancer.[23] Prophylactic removal of the ovaries (oophorectomy) caused sterility and the onset of menopause—and, once again, there were no reassuring data in 1995 to indicate that the surgery was worth the traumatic consequences.[24] Early ovarian cancer usually had no symptoms and was difficult to detect. As a result, in two-thirds of cases the cancer was widespread by the time the diagnosis was finally made. With such late discovery, the prognosis for women with ovarian cancer was uniformly grim.[25]

PREDICTING CANCER PREDISPOSITION

The inadequacy of existing screening, prophylactic, and diagnostic measures highlighted the need to discover better ways to *predict* which women were at high risk of developing breast and ovarian cancers. One way to make such a prediction was to look for genetic changes that predisposed a woman to breast cancer. Research had shown that an estimated 5 to 10 percent of all breast cancer was due to inherited genetic mutations in tumor suppressor genes, which meant that some women's chances of developing cancer depended in large part on the genes they inherited.[26] Early in 1994, one of these genes was identified. Mutations in a gene (subsequently called *BRCA1*) appeared to correlate with a much higher than normal risk of developing both breast and ovarian cancer.[27] This finding held the promise that, by testing a woman's DNA for the presence of these mutations, it would be possible to determine her chances of developing these cancers. With this knowledge, women could make more informed choices about the frequency with which they underwent cancer screening tests or whether they would submit to radical and disfiguring surgery. In addition, this information could be useful in making procreative choices. If they knew they were at high genetic risk for breast or ovarian cancer, some women could seek prenatal counseling or might choose not to have children at all in order to prevent passing the genetic mutations on to offspring.

Although the genetic predisposition testing market was new and still evolving, many financial analysts predicted a sizable market for *BRCA*-related cancer susceptibility tests. One estimate placed the demand at one thousand tests per month.[28] Investment analyst David K. Stone of Cowen and Co. in Boston estimated the market potential for the genetic tests at $400–500 million, and other Wall Street researchers predicted the tests would bring in $100 million a year, even if any given individual would only undergo genetic breast cancer testing once in her lifetime.[29] Other analysts agreed that the market potential for gene tests would be large but questioned how rapidly it would grow. "This is a monumental new technology," said Eugene Melnitchenko, an analyst with Legg Mason Wood Walker Inc. in Baltimore. "New technologies are typically incorporated into the medical system very slowly."[30]

THE RACE TO FIND THE BREAST CANCER SUSCEPTIBILITY GENE

The search for the breast cancer susceptibility gene was conducted by forty-five scientists from groups at Myriad Genetics, Eli Lilly, the University of Utah, the Universities of California at Berkeley and San Francisco, Montreal's McGill University, and the National Institutes of Health.[31] This research used genetic linkage techniques and involved studies of the inheritance of genetic differences (polymorphisms) through many generations of more than two hundred families. The goal was to correlate these polymorphisms with the incidence of breast cancer in these families. In October of 1990, Dr. Mary-Claire King, then at the University of California, San Francisco, announced that after nearly twenty years of work, her laboratory had identified a region on chromosome 17 that plays a substantial role in the development of breast cancer.[32] King had found that many women who inherited breast cancer from their relatives also inherited this chromosomal segment. She assumed the presence of a breast cancer susceptibility gene and called it *BRCA1*. One year later, in 1991, *BRCA1* mutations were also found to be associated with an increased lifetime risk of developing ovarian cancer.[33]

Identifying a genetic cause for breast and ovarian cancers, both major killers in women, presented exciting possibilities for future prevention and treatment. An intense effort began to identify the gene. This feat was accomplished in the fall of 1994 when another research group estimated that inheriting the defective segment of chromosome 17 correlated with an 87 percent cumulative risk for developing breast cancer by age eighty and a 40 to 60 percent cumulative risk for developing ovarian cancer.[34] These numbers were much higher than those associated with the general population cumulative lifetime risk of 12 percent for breast cancer and 1.7 percent for ovarian cancer.[35] Also in 1994, a second breast cancer susceptibility gene, called *BRCA2*, was mapped to chromosome 13 and identified and cloned one year later.[36] Together, *BRCA1* and *BRCA2* mutations were believed to account for most of the cases of inherited breast cancer.[37]

Mark Skolnick, a University of Utah geneticist who led the consortium of scientists working on the breast cancer gene discovery project, was initially credited with the final breakthrough on *BRCA1*.[38] Skolnick had hunted for the breast cancer gene but had abandoned his efforts in the late 1980s. He was initially skeptical of King's data, but when a French group announced supporting evidence, Skolnick returned to his mapping project and identified one of the more than one thousand genes on chromosome 17 as the long-sought-after breast cancer gene. Skolnick and his colleagues from Myriad Genetics published their results in the October 7, 1994, issue of *Science*.[39] A year later, the news broke that Patricia Murphy at OncorMed, Inc. had found a common variant of the same gene at around the same time.[40] Patent applications for the *BRCA1* gene were filed by both OncorMed and the University of Utah. The University of Utah then issued an exclusive license to Myriad Genetics. In December 1995, Myriad filed a patent application on the full sequence of a "strong candidate" for *BRCA2*. These patent applications covered all diagnostic and therapeutic uses of the newly discovered genes. Both companies then began the process of developing and commercializing *BRCA* diagnostic gene tests.

THE COMPANIES

Myriad Genetics, Inc.

Mark Skolnick, Walter Gilbert, Ph.D., and Peter Meldrum founded Myriad Genetics in 1991 to make and commercialize gene discoveries. Before becoming the chief scientific officer and executive vice president of research and development at Myriad, Skolnick was the director of the Cancer Epidemiology Center at the University of Utah. Walter Gilbert, who had earned his fame years earlier for developing one of the first gene sequencing techniques, became vice chairman of the board. Peter Meldrum, who had been the president of Native Plants, Inc., a privately held Salt Lake City biotechnology firm that developed genetically engineered agricultural products, was appointed CEO of Myriad.[41]

Myriad's goal was to discover and sequence genes, to ultimately develop tests for genetic contributions to disease, and identify therapeutic uses for genetic discoveries. To fund this work, Myriad raised $10 million in a private placement offer in April 1993. The company's research work on the breast cancer gene was greatly facilitated by an arrangement with the large pharmaceutical company, Eli Lilly, which provided scientific assistance and $4 million to conduct the research. More funds came from the NIH, which provided about $2 million in research grants to Skolnick's group at the University of Utah. To facilitate its disease-related gene hunting, Myriad also collaborated with University of Utah investigators who had extensively studied the genetics of large, multigenerational Utah families with histories of high rates of certain diseases.[42] The medical information gathered from these families, together with genetic analyses of the tens of thousands of their DNA samples, provided Myriad with a competitively advantageous opportunity for accelerating the gene discovery process. Skolnick believed that the *BRCA* gene discoveries would allow for the development of predictive and diagnostic cancer tests and treatments that would save the lives of many women—and that for this reason, Myriad's future seemed bright.

The company remained relatively obscure until 1994 when it gained media attention for cloning the *BRCA1* gene. The announcement demonstrated to the world Myriad's skills at disease-causing-gene discovery. Myriad's success in this area led to lucrative genomics collaborations with several "Big Pharma" companies.[43] Myriad was privately funded through mid-1995 and went public on October 6, 1995, raising a total of almost $54 million through its IPO. In 1995, when Myriad began to contemplate marketing the *BRCA* tests, the company had approximately 190 employees, an accumulated deficit of about $24 million, and was in the development stage with expenditures on research still greater than its revenues.

Oncor, Inc., and OncorMed, Inc.

Oncor, Inc., a biotech company of 150 employees based in Gaithersburg, Maryland, was formed in the 1980s. The company's first diagnostic product, a DNA probe to detect leukemia and lymphoma, was developed in 1989. By 1993, the company was in the process of obtaining federal approval to market genetic test kits to detect cervical, bladder, and breast cancers. In the same year, Oncor created a subsidiary, OncorMed, Inc., to offer what it called "a completely new service"—comprehensive "genetic risk profiles" that combined computer-assisted analysis of familial genetic history with individual genetic testing when the analysis of the first family member indicated increased risk.[44] OncorMed acquired exclusive rights to computer software and a family data base developed by the Hereditary Cancer Institute at Creighton University School of Medicine in Omaha, which had identified more than two hundred forms of inherited cancer.[45]

Timothy Triche, M.D., Ph.D., was appointed OncorMed's CEO. Triche was a professor of pathology and pediatrics at the University of Southern California, Los Angeles, and maintained his academic position when he assumed his managerial role at OncorMed. Patricia Murphy became the company's vice president of genetic services. During her tenure at OncorMed, Murphy also served as an industry representative on the federal NIH-Department of Energy Task Force on Genetic Testing, which was charged with developing genetic testing guidelines.

OncorMed was initially financed with $1 million in capital from Oncor and $3 million in a private placement of convertible preferred stock.[46] In autumn 1994, OncorMed raised approximately $8 million in its first public offering.[47] At the end of 1995, the company had thirty-eight employees and had registered with the Securities and Exchange Commission to conduct a secondary public offering of 2.5 million shares of its common stock. OncorMed was also considered to be still in the development stage, and had an accumulated deficit of about $11.3 million.[48]

One of OncorMed's first services, the Hereditary Cancer Consulting Service, was introduced in May 1994. The service, provided in conjunction with the Hereditary Cancer Institute, assessed an individual's risk of developing inherited cancer and provided guidance concerning appropriate cancer surveillance, testing, and genetic counseling. By early 1996, this service was provided at twenty-two clinical sites. OncorMed trained the physicians and other health professionals who performed the service, and supplied software to assess the cancer "pedigree" of a patient's family, which was used to determine the patient's genetic cancer risk. The company believed that patients identified as being at risk for developing hereditary cancer were potential customers for OncorMed's genetic predisposition testing services.

BRCA GENETIC PREDISPOSITION TESTS

Both OncorMed and Myriad planned to offer their *BRCA* genetic tests as a service. This meant that physicians would order the test, which would then be conducted in the company laboratories. Testing services such as this differed from commonly used diagnostic test kits sold by manufacturers to hospitals and clinic laboratories. Typically, physicians order tests and the tests are performed by technicians in the hospital or clinic lab using materials in a test kit. The testing sequence for *BRCA* mutation analysis, however, required the physician to mail a patient's blood sample to the company laboratory. The company's technicians would then extract the DNA from the white blood cells in the sample and determine whether the DNA sequence contained any *BRCA* mutations. The results of the analysis would then be communicated to the physician.

Myriad's *BRCA1* test sequenced all 16,500 bases of the *BRCA1* gene for the eighty possible mutations that were known at the time. Initially, the test took twenty-eight days to complete (the time was later reduced to ten days), and the company planned to charge $2,400 per individual for the testing service. If a mutation was identified, individual family members could then be tested for that particular mutation for $395.[49] Myriad stated that the risk of test error was negligible, due to a confirmatory resequencing step, and that handling and tracking errors were estimated to be less than 1 percent.[50]

OncorMed planned a three-stage approach to genetic testing. In order to save the consumer time and money, OncorMed labs would screen for the most common mutations first. In the first stage of *BRCA1* testing, the company would perform mutation-specific assays to detect the eight most frequently reported mutations, which accounted for 45 percent of the known *BRCA1* mutations. In the second stage of testing, OncorMed would perform a test to identify a particular deletion in the gene that accounted for an additional 37 percent of all *BRCA1* mutations. If no mutations were discovered in the prior testing, stage 3 testing would involve full sequencing of the gene.[51] Confirmatory resequencing was also done for tests that revealed mutations. OncorMed planned to charge $500 for stage 1 and $800 each for stages 2 and 3.[52] Stages 1 and 2 would take three weeks for completion, and stage 3 would take ten weeks.[53]

REGULATION OF TESTING KITS
AND TESTING SERVICES

In 1993, the Institute of Medicine issued a report that highlighted a disparity between the regulation of genetic testing kits and services.[54] The FDA regulated lab test kits extensively, but not testing services. Given the disparity, there were questions about whether the FDA should extend its authority to regulate genetic testing services.[55] Some commentators felt that the FDA's decision not to regulate testing services was reasonable since the agency lacked the staff and expertise for the task. However, the benefit to be gained, it was argued, was that FDA oversight would provide additional consumer protections that were absent under existing regulatory processes for genetic testing services.

Clinical testing services performed by a laboratory such as Myriad or OncorMed are subject to federal regulation under the Clinical Laboratory Improvement Amendments Act (CLIA) of 1967 and 1988, rather than by the FDA.[56] CLIA regulations focus on the test itself, and CLIA requirements generally govern a test's accuracy and reliability as performed by the laboratory providing the testing service. While CLIA requirements are rigorous and involve the submission of testing data and laboratory inspections by regulators, in 1995 there were no specific federal requirements for or licenses needed for laboratories to perform genetic tests. New York was the only state with such requirements.[57] As a result, the Myriad and OncorMed testing services could be marketed while the companies were still conducting clinical correlation studies designed to determine the clinical utility, reliability, and accuracy of the tests.[58]

FDA regulation, in contrast, focuses on the impact of the test on the person to be tested. If Myriad and OncorMed had chosen to offer their gene tests as finished product test kits, the FDA would regulate the kits as medical devices.[59] In order to market a clinical test kit, manufacturers generally have to demonstrate that the test is safe and effective for use in diagnosing a human condition. The FDA evaluation focuses on whether there are data showing the human benefits and risks of testing. For most genetic predisposition test kits, this would likely require fairly extensive studies showing clinical validity and utility.[60] FDA regulation also takes into account other aspects of testing, such as consent requirements. In addition, the FDA has the authority to regulate medical device advertising, and could require that physicians ordering the test be trained in test interpretation and that patients receive some form of education and counseling to assist in understanding the implications of the test result.[61] Some observers of Myriad's and OncorMed's planned product offerings thought that the FDA should gear up to regulate the marketing of genetic test services, pointing out that the regulation of genetic testing should focus on protecting those who receive the test, a decision that should not be dependent on whether the test itself was conducted using a kit or performed in a company laboratory.[62]

In fact, just prior to OncorMed's and Myriad's marketing of *BRCA* testing services, the Federal Task Force on Genetic Testing composed of physicians, consumers, federal regulatory agency representatives, and diagnostic company representatives—including Patricia Murphy of OncorMed—was formed to study and make recommendations on the regulation of genetic testing, the required education of health professionals, and the criteria to be used to move a genetic test from research into clinical practice use.[63] In March 1996, the task force issued a report, *Interim Principles on Genetic Testing*, in which it took the position that current CLIA regulation of genetic testing services could not assure the clinical validity or utility of the tests, the quality of the informed consent process prior to testing, or the quality of the genetic counseling after testing.[64]

The task force's position was controversial. Gene test corporate executives opposed further regulation. In response to the suggestion that the FDA become involved in the regulation of genetic testing services, Myriad's CEO Mark Skolnick commented:

> There's no difference in my mind or in the government's mind between a lipid assay, a protein assay, an immunoassay, or a DNA assay. If you're performing the assay in your own laboratory, you're a reference laboratory, and you're regulated by CLIA. The testing business is regulated by CLIA, not the FDA, and that's the law. However, if you make and sell a kit, then there's the issue of whether a third party can use it adequately—and that's where the FDA comes in.[65]

OncorMed vice president Patricia Murphy said, "The most efficient way to regulate genetic testing services is to give CLIA more teeth rather than foist the responsibility onto an agency [the FDA] that doesn't want it."[66] Indeed, it was difficult to know what the FDA would require to ensure reasonable efficacy and safety of a gene test. Many in the biotechnology sector were concerned that requirements for large numbers of research subjects to be tested and followed for years—to determine for instance the percentage of people who developed the disease that the test indicated they were at risk for—would fundamentally stifle commercialization for such potentially useful tests.

By the end of 1995, however, the immediate next steps for OncorMed and Myriad were clear: CLIA had certified that both companies had demonstrated that their *BRCA1* sequencing tests accurately and consistently identified *BRCA1* mutations. Commercialization of the tests could begin.

COMMERCIALIZATION OF BRCA TESTING

Benefits of *BRCA* Testing

There were many proponents of making *BRCA* testing widely available to women. Advocates believed that women had the right to decide to avail themselves of important information about their potential health status. Among the many benefits of such testing were:

A negative test result in someone from a family in which affected relatives are known to have a disease-related mutation indicates a low risk of the disease, that is, the same risk as that found in the general population. Having this information can decrease anxiety and reduce the frequency of periodic monitoring for early signs of the disease (for example, mammography). A negative result could enable a woman to purchase health or life insurance at the standard rate.

A positive test result enables a person to prepare for disease. In addition, women who learn before childbearing that they carry a predisposing mutation and therefore risk passing the mutation on to offspring (as well as developing the disease themselves) can make an informed choice about family planning. Knowing that one has inherited a susceptibility to disease provides the opportunity to inform relatives that they also might be at risk.[67]

Test Interpretability

In 1995, genetic tests could clearly identify some mutations in the *BRCA* gene. However, because researchers were continuously reporting newly found mutations—of which only some were correlated to cancer susceptibility, and some of which were of unknown significance—many scientists believed that more research was needed to distinguish cancer-causing mutations from harmless mutations.[68] In late 1995, over one hundred mutations had been identified in *BRCA1*, and it was not clear which of these were responsible for the development of breast and ovarian cancer.[69] It was also becoming apparent that breast cancer susceptibility genes other than *BRCA1* and *BRCA2* would be isolated in the future.[70]

The prediction of cancer risk from the *BRCA* genetic tests was further complicated because knowledge of breast cancer's genetic complexity was still evolving, and research reports continued to appear indicating that factors other than *BRCA* mutations also contributed to breast cancer. Although *BRCA* testing could reveal true inherited breast cancer, this type of inherited cancer was rare and was estimated to account for only 5 to 10 percent of breast cancer cases in the United States.[71] Even if a woman tests negative for *BRCA* mutations, she still has the same cancer risk as the general population—in other words, she could still develop breast cancer due to mutations in other genes; hormones, diet, or environmental factors; or by chance. Therefore, negative results from the *BRCA* tests are not necessarily reassuring. The most reassuring negative test result would occur if the woman being tested found that she lacked the identical genetic mutation that had been found in her relatives who had developed breast or ovarian cancer. The statistical likelihood that there could be two separate genetic mutations linked to breast cancer in the same family is small.

The implications of positive test results also were debated. The major epidemiological study on this question concluded that women with *BRCA* mutations had an 87 percent lifetime risk of developing breast cancer.[72] With further research, however, this figure was questioned as being possibly biased because the study data were obtained from families with an unusually high incidence of cancer. The argument went that even if these families showed an average incidence of *BRCA* mutations the correlation between the mutations and cancer would appear very high due to the bias in the test population. The families might have been highly susceptible to cancer for other reasons. The true correlation between *BRCA* mutations and cancer predisposition in the general population or in other groups of women might be significantly lower than 87 percent.[73] Commenting on this problem, Francis Collins, the director of what was then the National Center for Human Genome Research, stated in a January 1996 editorial in the *New England Journal of Medicine* that "mutational analysis of less biased samples is urgently needed to clarify this issue."[74]

To further complicate matters, the primary cancer-causing mutation could vary from family to family or among different populations.[75] For example, a 1995 study found that a *BRCA1* mutation common in Americans with breast cancer rarely correlated with breast tumors in a Japanese test population.[76] Studies such as this led to the worry that there were ethnic or other variations in the genetic predisposition to breast cancer that would cause physicians who used the *BRCA* test to over- or underpredict the risk of cancer for their patients.

In such a climate it was difficult for physicians to know how to interpret the results of *BRCA* tests. It was generally agreed that the physicians who would order these cancer susceptibility tests needed to be fully educated about test interpretation.[77] However, cancer genetics was a new field about which many physicians had received little, if any, training. In 1995, one-third of medical schools still did not require coursework in genetics. A study in 1993 showed that physicians without genetics training were more likely to order gene tests and less likely to provide in-depth counseling for their patients.[78] According to a press release from the American Society of Clinical Oncology (ASCO):

> "There are not many times in the life of a discipline when a staggering amount of almost entirely new and relevant information floods it," said Dr. Durant, Executive Vice President of the American Society of Clinical Oncologists

(ASCO). In 1996, ASCO recognized the void of current, accessible information on cancer genetics as well as the acute need for all health care professionals to have timely, accurate information in order to help their patients. . . . As a relatively uncharted field, integrating the new frontier of cancer genetics into clinical oncology practice raises a whole host of new responsibilities and challenges for cancer professionals. Medical professionals need to understand the basic concepts and principles of genetics; the role of genetics in diagnosing and managing different cancers; the ethical, legal and social issues surrounding genetic predisposition testing; and how to manage long-term care of patients at high risk for cancer.[79]

For this reason, ASCO began to develop a training curriculum for postgraduate physicians to enable them to interpret breast cancer susceptibility test results and to responsibly manage this testing. But in 1995, that training material was years from completion.

Because of the problems in interpreting the test results, there was widespread agreement that the general female population should not be tested for *BRCA* mutations.[80] Beyond that, however, there was no consensus on how widespread testing should be. Myriad's CEO Mark Skolnick believed that some women would directly benefit initially from having the *BRCA* tests available as soon as possible and that if a larger number of women were tested, it would contribute to the expanding knowledge base about the interpretability of the test. "First, you save lives, especially with closer breast monitoring and prophylactic removal of the ovaries. Then, by testing large numbers of women and collecting information on as many as are willing, we can fine-tune our knowledge," he told one reporter.[81] Some scientists believed that the *BRCA* genetic test results could be satisfactorily interpreted to benefit a select group of women from families with a high incidence of breast and ovarian cancer. Other groups worried that placing strict restrictions on testing might exclude women who would otherwise benefit from receiving the test results. With this in mind, ASCO recommended that a woman be tested if she had at least two first- or second-degree relatives with breast or ovarian cancer.[82] But other scientists believed that the ASCO requirement was too inclusive.[83] The American College of Medical Genetics, American Society of Human Genetics, National Breast Cancer Coalition, and the Advisory Council of the National Center for Human Genome Research recommended that the tests not be commercialized but remain available only through carefully controlled research programs until their accuracy and validity were proved and other questions related to test utility and potential for discrimination were further studied.[84]

Test Utility

Many experts debated whether the results of the *BRCA* tests were helpful, harmful, or irrelevant.[85] With so many questions remaining about the limitations of mammography and of prophylactic mastectomy, professionals in the field began to talk about the "Therapeutic Gap"—referring to the situation in which women learned of their high risk for cancer but had no proven or effective options to prevent it or detect it early. The National Breast Cancer Coalition warned that early mammography might not be informative for young women at high risk for breast cancer. Furthermore, the radiation associated with frequent mammograms might actually increase a woman's risk of developing cancer.[86] Some of those studying the issue had concluded that, so far, the benefits of surgically removing the breasts and ovaries had not been proven, although such surgery would probably delay the onset of cancer.[87] Others worried that some women who tested positive for *BRCA* mutations would be more prone to undergo this disfiguring surgery before data on the efficacy of the procedure were definitive.[88] Until effective options became available to fill the "Gap" between testing and risk reduction, many believed that test commercialization was premature.

A further consideration involved the impact of the *BRCA* test results on a woman's emotional health. Taking the test offered some women peace of mind and the ability to plan for the future by knowing that they either did or did not carry a gene mutation. One study found that some women with family histories of breast cancer requested testing to satisfy curiosity or relieve anxiety.[89] However, the knowledge of the test results and the inherent ambiguities that can ensue can be difficult for some people to handle. In the same study, women who received test results indicating that they had a high risk for breast cancer responded with a range of emotions, including sadness, anger, difficulty with family relations, and guilt about possibly having transmitted the mutations to their children. Some predicted that men would tend not to marry a woman who disclosed that she was at genetic risk for breast cancer. Another possible problem in telling a healthy woman that she has a high risk for developing a potentially lethal disease is the possibility that she will view herself as sick from that point onward.

As a consequence of all of these concerns, there was no consensus on how to address the issue of test utility. Some believed that the tests had potential to save women's lives if they knew they carried the mutations and then acted on that information through vigorous screening or with mastectomies or oophorectomies. Mark Skolnick believed that the tests could not only save lives but was easily cost justifiable. At the Breast Cancer Gene Mutation Testing Conference held on November 23, 1996, in San Francisco, he presented diagnostic cost figures for a woman who tested positive for a *BRCA* mutation and then choose to have an oophorectomy to prevent ovarian cancer. He estimated that, in a population of women with a 20 percent risk for *BRCA* mutation, the cost of testing spread over the twenty years of extra life would amount to $2.00 per day.[90] Dr. Walter Nance, chairman of the department of human genetics at the Medical College of Virginia in Richmond and a past president of the American Society of Human Genetics, expressed his dismay about the delay if the tests were only offered through research. He said, "We have a test here that does have the potential of actually saving lives. That being true, you've got to ask the question, How long can you delay it? How long are you willing to delay it? Are you willing to go through N.I.H. grant cycles and apply for grants? Is that an appropriate way to bring it to the public?"[91] Others, such as Dr. Neil A. Holtzman, a geneticist at the Johns Hopkins Medical Institutions and chairman of the Federal Task Force on Genetic Testing, believed that the tests should be offered only in a carefully controlled research setting until the uncertainties about the tests were resolved. Others went even further and advocated that women in the test studies should not even be told the test results until the benefits and risks of the preventative care strategies were better understood. That opinion sparked indignation from many women, who felt this attitude was overly paternalistic. Joy Simha, a twenty-eight-year-old woman who was denied her test results by New York researchers, protested, "I think [they] need to realize that women have brains. We're not going to just jump on the operating table [for mastectomies]. Who are they to tell me that knowing the results could do me more harm than good?" Simha's interviewer added, "It's also hard to resist concluding that one of the scientists' paramount, if subtly stated, concerns—that women will lose their heads and chop off their breast—might be more muted if breasts weren't the appendages in question."[92]

The Risk of Genetic Discrimination, Employability, and Insurability

Many feared that disclosure of a positive *BRCA* test would result in some women losing, or being unable to obtain, employment or medical or life insurance—since they would likely require expensive and extensive medical treatment in the future and might die prematurely. According to a *Los Angeles Times* article, "[A] spokesman for the Health Insurance Association of America, . . . said it is unfair for consumers to withhold knowledge, even predictive genetic information, of a problem from an insurer. 'The insurance industry needs to be on an equal footing with an applicant,' he said."[93] While the *BRCA* tests were being offered under research protocols, one study conducted at Harvard and Stanford Universities found two hundred individuals who lost jobs, insurance, and educational opportunities because of genetic information indicating a high risk for disease.[94] In 1995, there were no federal laws to protect Americans from genetic discrimination in employment or health insurance eligibility. Neither were there guarantees that the results of cancer risk tests would not be disclosed to employers or insurers.[95] According to one study, the primary reason that women hesitated to undergo genetic testing was that they feared losing their health insurance or having to pay higher premiums if they tested positive for mutations.[96] Because of these concerns, genetic testing was the subject of a U.S. Senate Cancer Coalition hearing, led by senators Dianne Feinstein and Connie Mack, on September 29, 1995. A major issue addressed was whether safeguards against discrimination should be in place prior to the time disease susceptibility gene tests were commercialized. According to Senator Mack, "The scientific data and technology are here, but the social, ethical and legal ramifications have only begun to resonate beyond the scientific community."[97]

The Lack of Policies to Ensure "Informed Consent"

If women were to benefit from genetic testing and avoid the many postulated harms that could occur, scientists, patient activist groups, and professional societies agreed that both the test provider and the recipient should be fully aware of the potential benefits, harms, limitations of, and alternatives to the *BRCA* genetic tests.[98] The consensus, based on widely accepted notions of general medical informed consent, was that both physicians and patients should understand all of the consequences of testing and patients should provide their informed and uncoerced consent to be tested. In addition, before proceeding with testing, it was believed that the test provider and the person to be tested should agree on how the results would be communicated. Following testing, individuals were entitled to receive an appropriate explanation of the test result and counseling about its implications.[99]

At the time, there were no consensus policies in place to ensure that the person to be tested and the test provider received the appropriate education, and there was no standard agreement about what should be included in the informed consent process.[100] Physicians were not required to have had formal training in genetics before ordering genetic tests for their patients. Laboratories were not obligated to provide extensive information to the patient or physician regarding the clinical limitations of their testing services. There was no agreement about whether the responsibility for educating physicians or consumers rested with the physician or with the testing company. In addition, counseling was a time-consuming and expensive process. The number of genetic counselors in the country to whom test candidates would normally be referred for individual counseling was so low that many feared that individuals would not have ready access to this service.[101] In addition, there was great uncertainty about whether counseling would be covered by most medical insurers.

Anticipating this uncertainty, in March of 1994, the National Center for Human Genome Research of the National Institutes of Health issued a "Statement on Use of DNA Testing for Presymptomatic Identification of Cancer Risk," which contained the following recommendations:

> Despite the promise of these discoveries for benefiting humankind, it is premature to offer testing of either high-risk families or the general population as part of general medical practice until a series of crucial questions has been addressed. These questions include, but are not limited to, the following:
>
> - How many different mutations of . . . *BRCA1* will be found, what are their actual frequencies, and what is the risk of cancer associated with each?
>
> - What are the technical and laboratory issues associated with detection of mutations in these genes, what frequency of false-positive and false-negative results will occur, and how can quality control of testing be assured?
>
> - How effective are interventions to prevent cancer morbidity and mortality in high-risk families and in the general population?
>
> - How can education about the complexities of DNA testing be provided to large numbers of potentially at-risk individuals, how can informed consent be ensured, and how can effective, culturally sensitive, nondirective genetic counseling be offered about such profoundly wrenching issues?
>
> - Finally, how will the possibility of genetic discrimination against those found to be at high risk be avoided?[102]

At the time that OncorMed and Myriad were about to launch their *BRCA* genetic tests, the Task Force on Genetic Testing guidelines were in the offing and Francis Collins had this to say about the general use of genetic testing:

> The benefits of presymptomatic testing to determine susceptibility to common cancers such as those of the breast, ovary, colon, and prostate are potentially substantial. Nonetheless, it is critical that we create safeguards to

ensure that the benefits of testing exceed the risks. The technical ability to perform tests for mutations should not be confused with a mandate to offer them. In the long run, the identification of *BRCA1* and other cancer susceptibility genes should permit the development of new and more effective therapies, so that physicians can not only predict future risks but also reduce those risks reliably and safely before disease occurs.[103]

The debates about the use and impact of genetic testing to predict disease continued as Meldrum and Triche worked on their marketing plans for Myriad's and OncorMed's *BRCA* tests. The two CEOs knew that they would be under heavy scrutiny as they decided when and how to market the test and how to address concerns about the risks of *BRCA* testing—that is, whether the underlying data were sufficiently mature to allow for effective test interpretation, and whether and how the test could be marketed so that the benefits of testing outweighed the risks to women.

ONCORMED'S DECISION

OncorMed was the first company to market the *BRCA* test, offering its testing services through physicians beginning in January 1996.[104] In response to the questions surrounding the test, OncorMed decided to offer the testing service only to "patients who will truly derive a clinical benefit."[105] To implement this intent, the company adopted a program for outside review and self-regulation of its marketing plan. An independent institutional review board (IRB) would conduct the outside review. IRB review had been required for years by NIH before any experimental genetic tests were performed at institutions that received government funding. The purpose of such a review was to ensure that the experimental testing minimized risk to persons through full disclosure of and education about the risks of testing, so that individuals could give full informed consent prior to testing. OncorMed's commercial testing was not subject to this NIH requirement, but the company decided to seek the same review and to abide by the recommendations of the outside IRB. The commercial testing protocol submitted by OncorMed to the IRB addressed the issues of test interpretability, risks, informed consent, and education and counseling. This IRB followed the criteria stated in the federal regulatory requirements for the protection of human subjects in research (45 Code of Federal Regulations 46) and overseen by NIH's Office for Protection from Research Risks. The IRB eventually approved OncorMed's commercial testing procedures prior to the time that the test service was first marketed.

APPLICATION FOR TESTING

Women who wanted to be tested by OncorMed had to apply through their own physicians or other health-care providers. OncorMed provided physicians with a packet of professional and consumer information about the *BRCA* testing protocol. Before individuals could obtain access to OncorMed *BRCA* testing services, both they and their physicians had to qualify for testing under the terms of the protocol. Physicians had to go through an elaborate procedure that OncorMed outlined in a testing flowchart. This process required physicians to sign an agreement that would oblige them to:

1. Provide a patient's family cancer history to OncorMed that showed that someone in the family either had a *BRCA* genetic mutation or that there was a clinical or family history suggestive of an inherited form of breast cancer

2. Identify a genetic counselor, a medical and surgical oncologist, and a mental health specialist to whom the patient could be referred

3. Ensure that informed consent was obtained from the patient (as verified by a signed and witnessed six-page consent form) and that the patient received pre- and posttest counseling by one or more professionals knowledgeable about the genetics and management of hereditary breast cancer syndromes

4. Give the test results to the patient in person and develop a management plan with the patient

5. Refer the patient as needed to the specialists that had been identified, provide psychological support, and assist in informing relatives if appropriate

OncorMed verified that the pre- and posttest counseling was provided according to its specification by requiring that the physician complete a signed and dated four-page counseling checklist. Information provided included inheritance data about breast cancer; described the role of *BRCA1* and *BRCA2* in breast cancer and the risk of cancer for someone who tested positive or negative for these mutations; suggested management for those individuals who tested positive or negative; described how testing was conducted; discussed issues regarding informing and testing of relatives; and noted that a positive (and sometimes negative) test result could cause psychological problems, alter family relationships, compromise insurability, lock someone into a job so as to maintain insurance benefits, and pass mutations to children. Candidates for testing were also to be counseled that the test could miss some mutations, that testing results could be ambiguous, and that there was no proven strategy to decrease mortality from a mutation-linked cancer. Finally, patients were told that referrals for psychological support were available if needed.

Regarding the qualifications for women who sought testing, OncorMed wanted to ensure that only women at very high risk of breast cancer were tested for a genetic predisposition. Therefore, the company would test only women who met at least one of the following criteria:

1. Has two or more first- or second-degree blood relatives (related through a single lineage) with either breast or ovarian cancer

2. Has one first- or second-degree blood relative (less than forty-five years) with either breast or ovarian cancer

3. Has breast or ovarian cancer (less than fifty years), or bilateral breast cancer, breast and ovarian cancer; or breast or ovarian cancer plus two relatives with breast or ovarian cancer or one relative with breast or ovarian cancer (less than fifty years)

4. Has relatives with documented mutations in the *BRCA* gene

OncorMed refused to test individuals under the age of eighteen, mentally incapable of providing informed consent, or judged by their physician to be emotionally unable to handle positive or negative test results, and the company reserved the authority to deny testing to ineligible individuals. Following receipt from a physician of all requested materials, including the individual's signed consent, OncorMed would determine whether the person was eligible for testing and, if so, instruct the physician to submit the blood sample to the company laboratory.

Following testing, the results were sent to the health-care provider in writing. If the results were positive, an OncorMed representative called the provider to aid in interpretation. The patient's genetic counselor was required to send OncorMed a signed posttest counseling checklist.[106]

MYRIAD'S DECISION

In October 1996, after premarket evaluation of the test in fourteen U.S. cancer centers, Myriad launched its BRCAnalysis™, a comprehensive *BRCA1* and *BRCA2* gene sequence analysis for determining susceptibility to breast and ovarian cancer. The testing service was marketed to physicians and other health professionals with written information and testing materials. Information about Myriad's testing service was also available to physicians and consumers via the company Web site. According to company financial reports, the service was promoted initially "to women who seek knowledge of their predisposition to breast and ovarian cancer," and for a time, Myriad also marketed its testing service directly to women. Myriad developed its genetic testing criteria in-house without the use of an external review board. The company believed that a wide-ranging group of women could benefit from testing and that decisions made by physicians and women themselves would appropriately control who would be tested and under what circumstances. Myriad also made it known that women who tested positive for a mutation would be contacted to participate in long-term research about the health consequences of having the mutation.

Myriad imposed almost no mandatory requirements for access to its testing services but rather made recommendations and listed guidelines for physicians to follow. Prior to ordering *BRCA* testing, Myriad recommended that physicians obtain a medical and family history to ensure that the patient was an appropriate candidate for testing. Myriad listed the following factors as indicating risks of cancer high enough to justify testing:

1. Those with a diagnosis of breast or ovarian cancer, especially pre-menopausal breast cancer

2. Those with a family history of breast or ovarian cancer

3. Those with a blood relative who is known to have a mutation in *BRCA1* or *BRCA2*[107]

Myriad's literature stated:

If the family history of a woman with breast or ovarian cancer is uncertain or unknown, testing may be appropriate, especially if she developed cancer at an early age or has bilateral breast cancer. Genetic susceptibility mutations have been found in women without a family history (reference given). For example, a woman may have few female relatives, or, since men have a 50% chance of passing a mutation to each of their children, a mutation is frequently passed through the paternal line.[108]

Myriad's literature also included ASCO's genetic susceptibility testing guidelines, which the company endorsed.[109] ASCO's guidelines were more general in nature but consistent with Myriad's and included the recommendation that testing should be performed in conjunction with long-term outcome research, to which Myriad planned to ask women to consent. However, ASCO emphasized that testing should be done only when the test results could be adequately interpreted and the results would influence medical management of the patient or family member. Myriad's material did not contain further information about test interpretation or medical management.

Myriad provided physicians with a pretest checklist of recommendations, paraphrased below:

1. Patients under the age of eighteen or those unable to consent should not be tested.

2. Patients should be given Myriad's education packet (which consisted of the written consent form, the company billing policy, and materials for the physician—pretest checklist, family history from, test order form, and a list of qualified genetic counselors).

3. Physicians were advised to "encourage patients to think about the medical and psychosocial issues associated with testing."

4. Patients should be encouraged to obtain genetic counseling to discuss the medical, psychosocial, and ethical implications of testing. On request, Myriad provided a list of qualified genetic counselors and other professionals willing to provide this service for a fee. The Genetic Counseling Resource Directory from Myriad contained lists of qualified genetic counselors by state. While not purporting to list all available counselors, the list for New York had the highest number of counselors (thirty-four) while twenty-one states had either one or two such counselors listed and seven states were not listed.

5. Physicians were to review the informed consent form with the patient, obtain the patient's signature on the form, and place the form in the patient's medical record. In New York, where there was a legal requirement to do so, physicians were to mail a copy of the signed consent to Myriad.

6. Physicians were to complete Myriad's test request form, sign it, and send it in with the patient's blood sample. The checklist stated that the physician's signature was also an indication that informed consent for testing had been obtained from the patient.

Physicians requesting the test on behalf of a patient completed Myriad's test request form, which contained information about the patient's family medical history, specifically with regard to cancer. The form notified physicians that Myriad would not test anyone under the age of eighteen or test "for purposes of fetal assessment." The physician signature line was preceded with the statement, "I hereby confirm that patient informed consent has been signed and is on file." Unlike OncorMed, Myriad did not refuse to test based on inappropriate patient selection, did not require a copy of the signed consent, and did not require verification of the availability of qualified counselors to assist the patient or that counseling had taken place. While Myriad provided physicians with a list of recommended topics to be included in counseling,[110] the counseling information was less specific than OncorMed's, and there was no requirement that a minimum set of facts and issues must be addressed with the patient before and after testing.

INFORMED CONSENT

The basic differences between OncorMed's mandatory consent form and Myriad's recommended consent form were:

- OncorMed's form stated that the patient was required to be counseled prior to testing, while Myriad's stated that genetic counselors were available.
- OncorMed's form stated that the patient might want to talk to a psychologist to help decide on testing and for support during and after testing.
- OncorMed's form provided more explicit descriptions about the risk that testing posed for insurability, including the possibility that testing could affect insurability or lock the patient into a job to prevent the loss of coverage. OncorMed's consent form suggested that the patient review and adjust insurance coverage prior to testing.
- OncorMed's form warned that the results of the test would be placed in the patient's medical record, thereby disclosing the test result to others when the patient was referred to other health professionals.
- OncorMed's form offered patients access to the company's genetic counselor or oncology nurse through an 800 number. The form also identified an impartial third-party law firm that could be contacted to address patients' complaints.
- Myriad's form stated that laboratory mix-ups could cause errors in results.
- Myriad's form, in a section entitled Financial Responsibility, stated that "because the BRCA1 and BRCA2 analysis is new and expensive and of uncertain value, your health care plan may not cover payment for it." OncorMed's form did warn about noncoverage but did not contain the explicit reasons contained in Myriad's form. Myriad's form also offered patient assistance in obtaining coverage and in appealing denials of coverage.

Myriad offered a financial assistance program for patients who could not afford the $2,400 cost of testing.

Myriad invited patients to enroll in a confidential long-term study that would improve knowledge of the consequences of having a genetic predisposition for breast cancer. The study would look at how many patients with the genetic mutation get cancer, when the cancer develops, and how they respond to treatment.

DEVELOPMENTS AFTER BRCA GENETIC TESTING
SERVICES WERE INTRODUCED TO THE MARKET

New Research on Cancer Risk Associated
with *BRCA* Mutations

Following the marketing of *BRCA* genetic tests by Myriad and OncorMed in 1996, published studies indicated that information about cancer risk and *BRCA* mutation was rapidly changing. In May 1997, the *New England Journal of Medicine* published the results of two studies that showed that the 87 percent breast cancer risk figure initially associated with having a mutation in *BRCA1* or *BRCA2* was not accurate for broader populations of women.[111] Depending on who was tested, the risk of developing breast cancer could be in the mid-50 percent range or even lower. In an editorial published in the same issue, Dr. Bernadine Healy, the first woman to run the NIH, stated:

> The pressure for the immediate application of these [*BRCA* gene] discoveries to clinical care was overwhelming from the outset. The race to discover new genes was visible and competitive, the promise of substantial economic returns from screening tests compelling, and the public hunger for a breakthrough in breast-cancer treatment intense. . . . These reports should alert us to the limitations of the expanding medical practice of making gene-based statistical prophecies. The problem is not that the evolving information is not valuable but, rather, that it holds great potential for misapplication. . . . It is too early to use *BRCA* gene testing in everyday clinical practice, because it violates a common-sense rule of medicine: don't order a test if you lack the facts to know how to interpret the result. When it comes to the care of an individual woman facing many health risks, including the risk of breast cancer, genetic information should become a crucial factor only when woven into the tapestry of her overall health. Physicians and their patients must be wary of overestimating the benefit to the patient or her family if the right information is applied in the wrong way or applied too soon.[112]

New Research on Cancer Risk Reduction Options

In March 1998, data from a large multicenter study, the Breast Cancer Prevention Trial, showed that a drug called tamoxifen produced a 49 percent reduction in the incidence of breast cancer in high-risk women as compared to women taking placebo medication.[113] In 1999, Lynn Hartmann's research at the Mayo Clinic showed that prophylactic mastectomy was 90 percent effective in reducing the risk of breast cancer in women who had a family history of the disease.[114] These two developments gave women more options to lower their risk of breast cancer, thus potentially removing some obstacles to being tested for the breast cancer gene.

Patent Disputes

From the moment the *BRCA1* gene was cloned, several groups began fighting for patent ownership of its sequence. Skolnick and his colleagues at Myriad were the first party to file for a patent on the *BRCA1* sequence (in August 1994), but ownership was immediately disputed. In February 1995, the NIH, the University of Utah, and Myriad agreed to credit investigators from all three institutions as inventors.[115] This agreement left Myriad with the commercial rights to license use of the gene to Eli Lilly pharmaceuticals and to Hybritech, Inc., of San Diego. The NIH abandoned its own patent application as a result of the agreement but was to receive an undisclosed percentage of the royalty profits. OncorMed subsequently challenged Myriad's *BRCA1* patent in a lawsuit that was settled in May 1998. In that settlement, Myriad received exclusive rights for *BRCA* testing, and OncorMed received an undisclosed monetary settlement from Myriad and agreed to discontinue its *BRCA* testing business.[116]

CANCER TESTING BUSINESS OF ONCORMED, ONCOR, AND MYRIAD AS OF 1999

Analyst Predictions and Scientific Commentary

Just before Myriad launched its BRCAnalysis tests, many financial analysts were still upbeat about the prospects for this market. In September 1996, Matthew Murray of Lehman Brothers in New York commented that the breast cancer test would be "the most immediate pathway to cash flow from genomics. . . . We believe that there will be a strong demand for this test."[117] Such predictions were premature, however, since initial sales of the test service lagged significantly behind projections (see following).[118]

In early 1997, one commentator from *Science* described Myriad's market difficulties as follows:

> [The BRCAnalysis test] looked like a sure winner: a test that would give
> women from families in which breast cancer is rife a chance to know whether
> they carry the genetic defect. But instead of reeling in the cash, Myriad has
> run into a series of obstacles—including concern about the need for federal
> regulation of the field—that suggest genetic testing may not lead to the quick
> commercial payoff some had predicted. Myriad's apparent difficulties reflect
> uncertainties facing any company hoping to strike it rich in diagnostics. Many
> tests will involve genes like BRCA1 and BRCA2 which are associated with
> disease in certain families but whose function is poorly understood, so
> patients—and most physicians—will have trouble interpreting the test
> results. Indeed, some professional groups, including the American College
> of Medical Genetics, have recommended that genetic tests be used only in
> research projects until their accuracy and validity are proved.[119]

OncorMed, Inc.

Timothy Triche of OncorMed conceded that "it's not exactly a roaring
market" when he revealed in 1997 that OncorMed performed only one-tenth
the number of tests expected. According to Securities and Exchange Commission filings in calendar year 1997, OncorMed lost $10.7 million on revenue
of $959,000 and had an accumulated deficit of approximately $29.5 million.
Triche summed up the disappointing results in early 1998 by stating, "Everyone misunderstood this field."[120] On July 7, 1998, Gene Logic, Inc., bought
OncorMed for $38.2 million in stock.

Oncor, Inc.

Oncor, Inc., learned what the FDA considered adequate data to support the
marketing of a gene test. In December of 1995, Oncor's attempt to obtain FDA
approval for a test kit to detect a breast cancer gene called *HER-2/neu* was rejected by the FDA advisory panel to which it had been assigned. Oncor had
submitted the marketing application along with gene test data from 244 women.
The test was rejected because Oncor's study group was not considered large
enough to prove that testing for the gene either worked properly or was useful
in deciding how to treat breast cancer. By a 6–1 vote, the advisory panel told Oncor that, to gain approval, it needed to study many more women; one panelist
recommended that data on two thousand women would be needed.[121] During
the company's continuing struggle to get this test kit approved by the FDA, in

January 1997, Oncor, Inc., was listed by the investment analysis firm of Cowen & Co. as one of the top one hundred biotechnology firms based on capitalization. Oncor finally obtained approval for the *HER-2/neu* test in January 1998, but by that time the company was in financial difficulty and began selling off parts of its business (including OncorMed) and cutting its workforce. In February 1999, Oncor and its Condon Pharmaceutical unit filed for Chapter 11 bankruptcy relief. The company then announced that it intended to reorganize.[122]

Myriad Genetics, Inc.

Myriad Genetics' stock price peaked soon after its BRCAnalysis test was first marketed in October of 1996, but then quickly lost value and did not start to recover until fourth quarter 1999. One year after marketing, in the last quarter of 1997, Myriad performed only 262 *BRCA* tests. In the 1997 fiscal year, Myriad's *BRCA* testing revenue was only $504,045, and overall the company lost $9.2 million, or $1.03 per share, on revenue of $15.2 million.[123] For the fiscal year ending June 30, 1998, total revenues increased 52 percent to $23.2 million. During the same time, genetic testing revenue increased 339 percent to $2.2 million. Myriad attributed the growth in genetic testing revenue to its expanded marketing efforts and the increased acceptance of tests by physicians and consumers. Myriad also was diligent in asserting its patent rights to stop other entities, such as university medical schools, from conducting *BRCA* testing for pay, and the company began negotiating with these entities to license access to the *BRCA* tests from Myriad. However, in 1998, Myriad was still losing money, with a net loss for the year of $9.8 million.

For the year ending June 30, 1999, total revenues increased to around $25.3 million. This increase was due primarily to greater genetic testing revenue, which more than doubled for the 1999 fiscal year, increasing 136 percent to $5.2 million. The gross margin on genetic testing also increased, from 37 percent in fiscal 1998 to 41 percent for fiscal 1999. Net loss for fiscal 1999 was essentially flat at $9.99 million.

During this time, breast cancer genetic testing was becoming more acceptable for several reasons. Studies had confirmed that taking two drugs (tamoxifen or forms of birth control hormones) could reduce a woman's chance for developing breast cancer, giving high-risk women who tested positive for *BRCA* mutations another option for risk reduction. Myriad funded a study at the Dana-Farber Cancer Institute to collect data on the incidence of insurance discrimination in 131 individuals who had *BRCA* genetic testing. The study revealed that health insurance rates did not increase for any patients nor were any policies canceled. Myriad reported that more medical insurers (approaching four hundred) had decided to cover the costs of testing, and better than 94 percent of those who sought insurance reimbursement were successful. In addition, some medical associations were publishing breast cancer gene testing guidelines for physicians to use to inform their practice (see Appendix 10.1 for one example). Along the same lines, Myriad funded the American Medical Association to develop medical education material entitled "The Role of Genetic Susceptibility Testing for Breast & Ovarian Cancer," which provided physicians with current information on genetic testing for breast and ovarian cancer. The material included criteria for identifying candidates for testing, the interpretation of test results, and management strategies for individuals found to have *BRCA* gene mutations. Myriad also had discovered a way to decrease the turnaround time to deliver breast cancer genetic test results to seven days. Slowly but surely, Myriad was growing the business of breast cancer genetic testing.[124]

Questions

1. Compare and contrast OncorMed's with Myriad's marketing of their breast cancer genetic tests.

2. Were the breast cancer genetic tests ready for market? Should these companies have marketed these tests when and how they did?

3. What is the responsibility of a company that markets a medical diagnostic product when the underlying accuracy, interpretation, and efficacy data are still evolving?

Discussion

This case study explores the problems companies face when deciding how and when to market their products when the data underlying product efficacy and safety are rapidly evolving. The case also examines two companies that were marketing into a significant amount of skepticism and resistance, and the different marketing approaches taken by these two companies can be used to compare the ethical aspects of their marketing decisions. The utilitarian question focuses on the actions that can be taken to enhance the overall utility of the tests (delayed marketing, cautious or limited marketing, and full-speed-ahead marketing). The outcome of the utilitarian analysis may depend on whether business managers believe that the accountability for responsible testing lies with the company or the physicians and genetic counselors who administer the tests. The rights analysis involves identifying and prioritizing the rights of the company to market an accurate test, the rights of women who want access to the tests, and the position of those who claim that, even if they are fully informed about the psychosocial harms, women's right to informed consent about medical treatments cannot be achieved with tests that generate misinformation, unreliable information, or information with low predictive value. Devising a marketing plan that would balance the risks and benefits and, as much as possible, respect rights for all relevant parties is the ultimate object of such an analysis.

TABLE 10.1

OncorMed, Inc., Financial Data

Five Year Summary						
Year	Revenues	Net Income	Earnings per share	Cash/ Securities	Working Capital	Total Assets
1997	$959,645	$-10,746,329	$-1.39	$1,478,551	—	$3,176,615
1996	627,390	-7,455,973	-1.10	7,498,680	—	9,113,975
1995	311,387	-6,510,547	-1.32	718,844	—	2,451,874
1994	34,303	-3,981,373	-0.90	7,262,010	—	8,372,183
1993	n/a	-838,352	-0.20	3,848,621	—	4,046,366

SOURCE: OncorMed SEC 10k Report, filed 4/1/98.

TABLE 10.2

Myriad Genetics, Inc., Financial Data

Five Year Summary						
Year	Revenues	Net Income	Earnings per share	Cash/ Securities	Working Capital	Total Assets
1999	$25,313,406	$-9,995,453	$-1.06	$38,926,459	$8,348,224	$53,550,940
1998	23,210,581	-9,797,035	-1.05	53,109,493	21,806,290	67,391,972
1997	15,236,099	-9,206,280	-1.03	63,077,439	38,796,960	76,063,331
1996	6,628,624	-5,897,473	-0.78	70,002,780	41,665,513	79,607,497
1995	1,294,500	-5,268,383	-1.19	16,140,935	13,784,051	19,744,451

SOURCE: Myriad Genetics SEC 10k Report, filed 9/28/99.

Genetic Susceptibility to Breast and Ovarian Cancer: Assessment, Counseling and Testing Guidelines, 1999[125]

American College of Medical Genetics Foundation
With support from:
New York State Department of Health

EXECUTIVE SUMMARY

Education and Genetic Counseling

The patient should be encouraged to consider how her or his behavior would change depending on the test result. However, making such decisions in the abstract may not always be predictive of actual behavior when confronted with test results. The patient must be educated as to the potential benefits and burdens of genetic testing in order to make an informed decision about whether or not DNA-based mutation testing would be appropriate for her or him. Mutation testing can confer both benefits and burdens.

Benefits can be conferred whether the test reveals a mutation or not.

Benefits of DETECTING a mutation can include:

the reduction of uncertainty and the often associated anxiety of "not knowing";

the potential for reduced morbidity and mortality due either to enhanced surveillance, or to preventive measures such as chemoprophylaxis regimens and/or prophylactic surgery;

the opportunity to alert relatives to their potential risk and available services;

the opportunity to participate in clinical trials and related research.

Benefits of NOT DETECTING a mutation (when an affected relative has been found to have one) include:

reassurance and reduction of anxiety; and

avoidance of unnecessary intensive monitoring strategies and prophylactic surgical measures and their attendant risks and costs.

Burdens can also be conferred by a positive, negative, or uncertain test result. These are expensive tests, which may or may not be covered by third party payers.

Burdens of DETECTING a mutation can include:

anxiety;

depression;

reduced self-esteem;

frustration associated with the unproven effectiveness of available interventions;

the risks and costs of additional surveillance or prophylaxis, which may or may not be covered by insurance policies;

strained relationships with a partner or with relatives;

guilt about possible transmission to children;

stigmatization;

possible discrimination by health, life or disability insurance companies, by employers, or by others; and

the potential (but as yet unproven) hazards of more frequent and earlier mammograms in *BRCA1* and/or *BRCA2* mutation carriers.

Burdens of NOT DETECTING a mutation include:

potential for neglect of routine surveillance due to the mistaken belief that risk is zero in the absence of a detected mutation;

survivor guilt, i.e., feeling undeserving of negative test results when other family members test positive and are suffering because of present or potential disease.

Burdens of a test result of "uncertain significance" include:

the need to evaluate other family members to determine its significance;

the need to maintain intensive surveillance until the significance of the genetic alteration is known; and

anxiety, frustration, and other adverse psychological sequelae associated with uncertainty.

Notes

1. Center for Drug Evaluation and Research. *CDER report to the nation 2000: Drug safety and quality*. Bethesda, MD: Food and Drug Administration; 2000. Available from www.fda.gov/cder/reports/RTN2000/RTN2000-3.HTM.

2. Spilker B. Extrapolating animal safety data to humans. In *Multinational pharmaceutical companies: Principles and practice*. New York: Raven Press; 1994. pp. 281–82; Brewer T, Colditz GA. Postmarketing surveillance and adverse drug reactions: Current perspectives and future needs. *Journal of the American Medical Association* 1999; 281:824–29.

3. Cuttler SH. The Food and Drug Administration's regulation of genetically engineered human drugs. *Journal of Pharmacy and Law* 1992; 1:191, 204.

4. Klein DF. The report by the Institute of Medicine and postmarketing surveillance. *Archives of General Psychiatry* 1999; 56:353–54.

5. Schwartz J. Is FDA too quick to clear drugs? Growing recalls, side-effect risks raise questions. *Washington Post* 1999 Mar 23; Sect. A:1; Noah BA. Adverse drug reactions: Harnessing experiential data to promote patient welfare. *Catholic University Law Review* 2000; 49:449–504; Willman D. Risk was known as FDA OK's fatal drug study: New documents show Warner-Lambert trivialized liver toxicity of diabetes pill Rezulin while seeking federal approval. *Los Angeles Times* 2001 Mar 11; Sect. A:1.

6. For agricultural products such as genetically modified seeds, farmers need the proper instruction about safe and effective planting, growing, and harvesting.

7. Foreman J. Drawing the fine line on Retin A; U.S. panel slaps doctors for allegedly touting it as a wrinkle smoother. *Boston Globe* 1992 Nov 23; 13; Schwartz J. Ortho Pharmaceutical Corp. will pay $7.5 million to the government after admitting company officials shredded documents during a federal investigation of the promotion of an acne cream as a wrinkle remedy. *Washington Post* 1995 Apr 12; Sect. A:10.

8. The most widely prescribed form of estrogen replacement was Premarin, which was obtained from the urine of pregnant horses. This product was manufactured by Wyeth-Ayerst Laboratories, formerly American Home Products. This product was controversial with animal rights groups who objected to the treatment of the mares from which urine was collected.

9. Brubaker B. Drug firm seeks to revive product; with stock falling, Wyeth says media distorted findings. *Washington Post* 2002 July 24; Sect. E:1.

10. The lead author of the study described the risk data as indicating that the average risk to the individual woman was one tenth of 1 percent per year for breast can-

cer and similarly for heart attacks. This statistic meant that, for every ten thousand women receiving combined estrogen plus progestogen, there would be (projected) no more than seven excess coronary heart disease events, eight more breast cancers, eight more strokes, and eight more pulmonary emboli. The data also indicated that the HRT in the same number of women would cause six fewer colorectal cancers and five fewer hip fractures. No changes in death rates were seen between drugs and placebo.

11. Writing Group for the Women's Health Initiative Investigators. Risks and benefits of estrogen plus progestin in healthy postmenopausal women: Principal results from the Women's Health Initiative Randomized Controlled Trial. *Journal of the American Medical Association* 2002; 288:321–33; Hopkins TJ. Hormone trial for disease prevention stopped early. *British Medical Journal* 2002; 325:61.

12. Barrett A. Why Wyeth still has the sweats. *Business Week Online* 2002 Sept 27. Available from www.businessweek.com/bwdaily/dnflash/sep2002/nf20020926_0907. htm.

13. Fuente-Fernández R, Ruth TJ, Sossi V, et al. Expectation and dopamine release: Mechanism of the placebo effect in Parkinson's Disease. *Science* 2001 Aug 10; 1164–66.

14. The initial case study was prepared by Rebecca Farkas and Daniel Greenwald under the guidance of and with further revisions by Margaret Eaton. The input and assistance of Brian Allen, genetics counselor, University of California, San Francisco, is greatly appreciated. No company executives from OncorMed or Myriad participated in the preparation of this case study. The events described in this case study occurred up until late 1999.

15. National Advisory Council for Human Genome Research. Statement on use of DNA testing for pre-symptomatic identification of cancer risk. *Journal of the American Medical Association* 1994; 271:785.

16. *Cancer facts and figures 1994.* American Cancer Society 1994. Available from www.cancer.org.

Cancer facts and figures, 1995. American Cancer Society, 1995; National Center for Health Statistics, 1994; Public Health Service, 1995. Available from www.cancer.org, www.cdc.gov/nchs/default.htm, and www.cdc.gov/cancer/nbccedp/facts.htm.

17. Landis SH, Murray T, Bolden S, et al. Cancer statistics, 1998. *CA: A Cancer Journal for Clinicians* 1998; 48:6–29.

18. Murphy GP, Lawrence W, Lenhard RE, editors. *American Cancer Society textbook of clinical oncology.* Atlanta, GA: American Cancer Society; 1995.

19. DeVita VT, Rosenberg SA, Hellman S, editors. *Cancer: Principles and practice of oncology.* 5th ed. Philadelphia: Lippincott-Raven; 1997. pp. 1560–61.

20. Hartmann L, Jenkins R, Schaid D, et al. Prophylactic mastectomy (PM): Preliminary retrospective cohort analysis (meeting abstract). *Proceedings of the Annual Meeting of the American Association for Cancer Research* 1997; 38:A1123.

21. See Note 19, pp. 2875–76.

22. Houn F, Helzlsouer K, Friedman NB, et al. The practice of prophylactic mastectomy: A survey of Maryland surgeons. *American Journal of Public Health* 1995; 85:801–5.

23. NIH Consensus Development Panel on Ovarian Cancer. Ovarian cancer:

Screening, treatment, and follow-up. *Journal of the American Medical Association* 1995; 273:491–97.

24. Tobacman JK, Greene M, Tucker MA, et al. Intra-abdominal carcinomatosis after prophylactic oophorectomy in ovarian-cancer-prone families. *Lancet* 1982; 2:795–97.

25. Goldman L, Bennett JC, editors. *Cecil textbook of medicine.* 21st ed. Philadelphia: W.B. Saunders; 2000. p. 1322.

26. It is widely accepted by the medical community that approximately 5 to 10 percent of all cancer cases are hereditary.

27. The acronym stood for *breast cancer gene 1*. Families with a high number of breast cancers also tend to have a higher than normal incidence of ovarian cancer. See Medline Plus, Health Information, Ovarian Cancer, National Library of Medicine. Available from www.nlm.nih.gov/medlineplus/ovariancancer.html.

28. Kolata G. Genetic testing falls short of public embrace. *New York Times* 1998 Mar 27; Sect. A:16.

29. Saltus R. Gene test for cancer risk is offered; some geneticists dispute its value. *Boston Globe* 1996 Oct 25; Sect. A:1.

30. Southerland D. Oncor looks to profit as new diagnostic products reach market. *Washington Post* 1993 Dec 27; p. F8.

31. Marshall E. A showdown over gene fragments; commercial control of genetic data; includes related information on BRCA1 patent. *Science* 1994; 266:2081.

32. King mapped the *BRCA1* gene while at the University of California, Berkeley. Afterwards, she moved to the University of Washington.

Hall JM, Lee MK, Newman B, et al. Linkage of early-onset familial breast cancer to chromosome 17q21. *Science* 1990; 250:1684–89.

33. Ford D, Easton DF, Bishop DT, et al. Risks of cancer in BRCA1–mutation carriers. Breast Cancer Linkage Consortium. *Lancet* 1994; 343:692–95.

34. Easton DF, Bishop DT, Ford D, et al. Genetic linkage analysis in familial breast and ovarian cancer: Results from 214 families. Breast Cancer Linkage Consortium. *American Journal of Human Genetics* 1993; 52:678–701.

35. Cumulative lifetime risk is the risk for developing the disease over the life of the patient.

36. Tavtigian SV, Simard J, Rommens J, et al. The complete BRCA2 gene and mutations in chromosome 13q-linked kindreds. *Nature Genetics* 1996; 12:333–37.

37. Narod SA, Ford D, Devilee P, et al. An evaluation of genetic heterogeneity in 145 breast-ovarian cancer families. Breast Cancer Linkage Consortium. *American Journal of Human Genetics* 1995; 56:254–64.

38. See Note 31.

39. Yoshio M, Swensen J, Shattuck-Eidens D., et al. A strong candidate for the breast and ovarian cancer susceptibility gene BRCA1. *Science* 1994 Oct 7; 266:66–71.

40. Riordan T. A dark horse has scored a victory in the race to commercialize a gene linked to breast cancer. *New York Times* 1997 Aug 18; Sect. D:2.

41. Myriad Web site. Available from www.myriad.com.

42. Myriad relied on an approach called positional cloning, genetic research that is

conducted in large families that suffer from an inherited disease. Scientists search for genetic sequences shared by the family members carrying the disease. When these "markers" are found, it is likely that the disease gene is nearby. Utah was settled by many large families with a dozen or more children each, thereby creating hundreds of grandchildren and thousands of descendants. These families were very useful for disease gene discovery research. As Myriad said in its June 1997 SEC 10k Report, "By using the extensive and detailed genealogical records kept by the families themselves, [Myriad] is better able to resolve the ambiguities caused by interactions between environmental factors and multiple predisposition genes. Although in practice combining data from several multi-generational families is more efficient, [Myriad] can often positionally clone a gene related to a disease by studying DNA from a single large extended family. This type of analysis is not possible using small families because the interactions between environmental factors and multiple causal genes may lead to erroneous conclusions regarding the chromosomal location of a gene."

43. Novartis ($25 million, five-year agreement to discover genes involved in certain types of cardiovascular disease), and Bayer ($25 million, five-year agreement to discover genes involved in obesity, osteoporosis, and asthma). These agreements also included equity investments and provisions for royalties on future products developed from the Myriad research.

44. Business Briefs. *Washington Post* 1993 Dec 20; Sect. F:16.

45. See Note 30.

46. Southerland D. Business Briefs. *Washington Post* 1993 Dec 20; Sect. F:16.

47. Oncor, Inc.'s subsidiary, OncorMed, Inc. commences initial public offering. *PR Newswire* 1994 Sept 28.

48. Zimm A. OncorMed Inc. registers with SEC for secondary public offering. *Daily Record* (Baltimore) 1995 Nov 2; p. 5.

49. Billing Policy; Information on terms of payment and reimbursement procedures for genetic susceptibility analysis. Myriad Genetics Laboratories, Inc., 1996.

50. BRCAnalysis, Comprehensive BRCA1 and BRCA2 sequence analysis for susceptibility to breast and ovarian cancer, Myriad Genetic Laboratories, Inc., 1966.

51. Carter CL, Scott JA, Glauber PM, et al. The OncorMed approach to genetic testing. *Genetic Testing* 1997; 1:137–44.

52. Hilzenrath DD. Md. firm's gene test to intensify bioethics debate; new service from OncorMed designed to detect predisposition to breast, ovarian cancer. *Washington Post* 1996 July 25; Sect. D:14.

53. OncorMed; Genetic testing for hereditary breast and ovarian cancer, shipping and handling guidelines, 1997 Sept 15; supplied by Leslie Alexander, DrPh., former vice president for corporate affairs and marketing, OncorMed.

54. Andrews L, Fullarton JE, Holtzman NA, et al. *Assessing genetic risks: Implications for health and social policy.* Institute of Medicine. Washington, DC: National Academy Press; 1994.

55. Holtzman N, Murphy PD, Watson MS, et al. Predictive genetic testing: From basic research to clinical practice. *Science* 1997; 278:602–05.

56. 42 *United States Code* 201 et seq.

57. Gutman S. The role of Food and Drug Administration regulation of in vitro diagnostic devices—applications to genetic testing. *Clinical Chemistry* 1999; 45:746–749; Stephenson J. Questions on genetic testing services. *Journal of the American Medical Association* 1995; 274:1661–62.

58. OncorMed 10k report filed with the SEC for period ending 12/31/95, p. 20.

59. Medical devices, classification/reclassification; restricted devices; analyte specific reagents. 61 *Federal Register* 10,484; 1996.

60. According to the Task Force on Genetic Testing, "Clinical validation involves establishing several measures of clinical performance including (1) the probability that the test will be positive in people with the disease (clinical sensitivity), (2) the probability that the test will be negative in people without the disease (clinical specificity), and (3) the probability that people with positive test results will get the disease (positive predictive value (PPV)) and that people with negative results will not get the disease (negative predictive value). Predictive value depends on the prevalence of the disease in the group or population being studied, as well as on the clinical sensitivity and specificity of the test." Clinical utility assessments would include such things as the medical, social, financial, and psychological impact of testing on patients of both positive and negative test results. From Promoting safe and effective genetic testing in the United States. *Final report of the Task Force on Genetic Testing*, Chapter 2; 1997 Sept. Available from www.nhgri.nih.gov/ELSI/TFGT_final/.

61. These predictions were based on FDA-imposed requirements for the approval of Oncor's Inform HER-2/neu breast cancer genetic test kit. See Berselli B. Oncor puts its future to the test; a gene screen for recurring breast cancer could determine the firm's profit outlook. *Washington Post* 1998 Jan 26; Sect. F:5. See also Task Force on Genetic Testing, infra.

62. See Note 57, Stephenson.

63. The Task Force on Genetic Testing was created by the National Institutes of Health (NIH)–Department of Energy (DOE) Working Group on Ethical, Legal, and Social Implications of Human Genome Research "to make recommendations to ensure the development of safe and effective genetic tests, their delivery in laboratories of assured quality, and their appropriate use by health care providers and consumers." See www.med.jhu.edu/tfgtelsi/principles.html.

64. Task Force on Genetic Testing of the NIH-DOE Working Group on Ethical, Legal, and Social Implications of Human Genome Research. Draft interim principles. Available from www.med.jhu.edu/tfgtelsi/principles.html.

65. See Note 57, Stephenson.

66. Seachrist L. Panel stymied over role FDA should play in regulating genetic testing. *BioWorld Today* 1997 Apr 7.

67. Promoting safe and effective genetic testing in the United States. *Final report of the Task Force on Genetic Testing*, Chapter 1; 1997 Sept. Available from www.nhgri.nih.gov/ELSI/TFGT_final/.

See also Note 19, pp. 2875–76.

68. Shattuck-Eidens D, Oliphant A, McClure M, et al. BRCA1 sequence analysis in women at high risk for susceptibility mutations: Risk factor analysis and implications for genetic testing. *Journal of the American Medical Association* 1997; 278:1242–50.

69. By early 1999, researchers were predicting that there were upwards of five hundred to seven hundred mutations in the *BRCA1* and *BRCA2* genes.

Summary of meeting. National Cancer Advisory Board meeting, Bethesda, MD; 1996 May 7–8. Summary available at http://deainfo.nci.nih.gov/advisory/ncab/archive/minutes/Ncab0596.htm.

70. Serova OM, Mazoyer S, Puget N, et al. Mutations in BRCA1 and BRCA2 in breast cancer families: Are there more breast cancer-susceptibility genes? *American Journal of Human Genetics* 1997; 60:486–95.

71. Task Force on Genetic Testing of the NIH-DOE Working Group on Ethical, Legal, and Social Implications of Human Genome Research. Draft interim principles. Available from www.med.jhu.edu/tfgtelsi/principles.html.

Weber B, Garber J. Familial breast cancer. In Harris JR, Lippman ME, Morrow M, et al., editors, *Diseases of the breast*. Philadelphia: Lippincott-Raven; 1996. p. 168.

72. See Note 34.

73. Ponder B. Genetic testing for cancer risk. *Science* 1997; 278:1050–54.

74. Collins FS. BRCA1: Lots of mutations, lots of dilemmas. *New England Journal of Medicine* 1996; 334:186–88.

75. Task Force on Genetic Testing of the NIH-DOE Working Group on Ethical, Legal, and Social Implications of Human Genome Research. Draft interim principles. Available from www.med.jhu.edu/tfgtelsi/principles.html.

76. Inoue R, Rukutomi T, Ushijimi T, et al. Germline mutation of BRCA1 in Japanese breast cancer families. *Cancer Research* 1995; 55:3521–24.

77. Parker LS, Majeske, RA. Standards of care and ethical concerns in genetic testing and screening. *Clinical Obstetrics & Gynecology* 1996; 39:873–84; Bombard AT, Fields AL, Aufox S, et al. The genetics of ovarian cancer: An assessment of current screening protocols and recommendations for counseling families at risk. *Clinical Obstetrics & Gynecology* 1996; 39:860–82.

78. Hofman KJ, Tambor ES, Chase GA, et al. Physicians' knowledge of genetics and genetic tests. *Academic Medicine* 1993; 68:625–32.

79. American Society of Clinical Oncology. Inaugural curriculum on genetic testing for cancer equips doctors with knowledge to counsel and care for patients with family history of disease. Press release, 1998 Dec 11.

80. See Note 57, Stephenson.

81. Kahn P. Coming to grips with genes and risk. *Science* 1996 Oct 25; 274:496–98.

82. American Society of Clinical Oncology. Statement of the American Society of Clinical Oncology: Genetic testing for cancer susceptibility, adopted on February 20, 1996. *Journal of Clinical Oncology* 1996; 14:1730–36.

83. See Note 73.

84. American Society of Human Genetics. Statement of the American Society of Human Genetics, Ad Hoc Committee on Genetic Testing for Breast and Ovarian

Cancer. Genetic testing for breast and ovarian cancer predisposition. *American Journal of Human Genetics* 1994; 55:ii–iv; see also Note 15; Note 74.

85. CLIA did not require that companies prove their tests were useful for patients.

86. Statement of the National Breast Cancer Coalition. Presymptomatic genetic testing for heritable breast cancer risk, 1995.

87. Task Force on Genetic Testing of the NIH-DOE Working Group on Ethical, Legal, and Social Implications of Human Genome Research. Draft interim principles. Available from www.med.jhu.edu/tfgtelsi/principles.html.

88. Wadman M. Women need not apply; the DNA test that doctors don't want to share. *Washington Post* 1996 May 5; Sect. C:3.

89. Summary of meeting. National Cancer Advisory Board meeting; 1996 May 7–8. From the National Cancer Institute, National Institutes of Health.

90. This figure was the result of adding the cost of testing five women to identify one positive ($12,000) to the cost of testing 7.5 of the woman's relatives to identify three positives ($3,000). These diagnostic costs were applied to the one woman who elected oophorectomy and gained twenty extra years of life (7,500 days).

91. Kolata G. Breaking ranks: Lab offers to assess risk of breast cancer. *New York Times* 1996 Apr 1; Sect. A:1.

92. See Note 88.

93. MonManey T. Many don't want to know genetic risk of cancer; study: Despite history of disease in families, just 43 percent choose to take gene test. Many fear jeopardizing insurance. *Los Angeles Times* 1996 June 26; Sect. A:1.

94. Billings PR, Kohn MA, de Cuevas M, et al. Discrimination as a consequence of genetic testing. *American Journal of Human Genetics* 1992; 50:476–82.

95. Ostrer H, Allen W, Crandall LA, et al. Insurance and genetic testing: Where are we now? *American Journal of Human Genetics* 1993; 52:565–77.

96. Summary of meeting. National Cancer Advisory Board meeting; 1996 May 7–8. From the National Cancer Institute, National Institutes of Health.

97. Press Release, Senator Connie Mack, 1995 Sept 29. Available from www.senate.gov/mack/.

98. Summary of meeting. National Cancer Advisory Board meeting; 1996 May 7–8. From the National Cancer Institute, National Institutes of Health; American Society of Clinical Oncology. Statement of the American Society of Clinical Oncology: Genetic testing for cancer susceptibility, adopted on February 20, 1996. *Journal of Clinical Oncology* 1996; 14:1730–36; Statement of the National Breast Cancer Coalition. Presymptomatic genetic testing for heritable breast cancer risk, 1995; National Institutes of Health–Department of Energy Working Group on Ethical, Legal, and Social Implications of Human Genome Research. Interim principles of the Task Force on Genetic Testing; 1996. Available from www.nhgri.nih.gov/ELSI/TFGT.

Commentary on the ASCO statement on genetic testing for cancer susceptibility (National Action Plan on Breast Cancer position paper). *Journal of Clinical Oncology* 1996; 14:1737–40.

99. National Institutes of Health–Department of Energy Working Group on Eth-

ical, Legal, and Social Implications of Human Genome Research. Interim principles of the Task Force on Genetic Testing, 1996. Available from www.nhgri.nih.gov/ELSI/TFGT.

100. Many researchers required a rigorous informed consent process to ensure that women fully understood the consequences of being tested. For instance, the University of Pennsylvania required that patients read and sign a seven-page, double-sided written consent, watch an educational video, and spend two to three hours with genetic counselors over two pretesting visits and one posttest visit. Such a rigorous research practice was not likely to be followed in clinical practice.

101. American Society of Clinical Oncology. Statement of the American Society of Clinical Oncology: Genetic testing for cancer susceptibility, adopted on February 20, 1996. *Journal of Clinical Oncology* 1996; 14:1730–36; National Institutes of Health–Department of Energy Working Group on Ethical, Legal, and Social Implications of Human Genome Research. Interim principles of the Task Force on Genetic Testing, 1996. Available from www.nhgri.nih.gov/ELSI/TFGT.

102. See Note 15.

103. See Note 74.

104. At that time, the company had also introduced genetic predisposition testing services for hereditary nonpolyposis colon cancer, familial melanoma, medullary thyroid cancer, and Li-Fraumeni Syndrome.

105. This and the following information is from OncorMed's "Hereditary Breast and Ovarian Cancer Education and Testing Packet," 1996 and 1997.

106. See Note 51.

107. Testing recommendations for Ashkenazi Jewish women, who were believed to be at higher risk for certain mutations, were omitted from this case study.

108. BRCAnalysis, a reference guide for health care professionals. Myriad Genetic Laboratories, Inc., 1996.

109. American Society of Clinical Oncology. Statement of the American Society of Clinical Oncology: Genetic testing for cancer susceptibility, adopted on February 20, 1996. *Journal of Clinical Oncology* 1996; 14:1730–36.

110. The categories of these recommendations were: the risks, benefits, and efficacy of genetic testing; the implications and limitations of the testing procedure and results, including how a positive or negative test result would change the management of an individual already diagnosed with breast or ovarian cancer; education regarding interventions and risk management, including surveillance; the possible psychosocial responses of the patient and family and the availability of psychosocial support; the availability of qualified professionals to provide counseling and to offer follow-up medical services; the fact that genetic susceptibility testing is voluntary; confidentiality of results and the possibility of insurance and/or work-related discrimination based on positive results; and cost of testing and counseling.

Myriad warned doctors about the risks of genetic discrimination in its BRCAnalysis promotional kit, but the company was criticized for providing misleading information. The Myriad kit assured doctors that the Equal Employment Opportunity Commission "has included language in the Americans With Disabilities Act making it unlawful to discriminate" against patients who tested positive for BRCA1 mutations. However, in 1996, the application of this law to genetic testing had not yet been tested in the courts. See Wadman M. The DNA hard sell. *New York Times* 1996 Dec 16; Sect. A:15.

Breast, ovarian cancer genetic testing introduced by Myriad. *Medical Industry Today* 1996 Oct 25.

See also Note 29.

111. Struewing JP, Hartge P, Wacholder S, et al. The risk of cancer associated with specific mutations of BRCA1 and BRCA2 among Ashkenazi Jews. *New England Journal of Medicine* 1997; 336:1401-08; Couch FJ, DeShano ML, Blackwood MA, et al. BRCA1 mutations in women attending clinics that evaluate the risk of breast cancer. *New England Journal of Medicine* 1997; 336:1409-15.

112. Healy B. BRCA genes: Bookmaking, fortunetelling, and medical care [editorial]. *New England Journal of Medicine* 1997; 336:1448-49. Copyright 1997 Massachusetts Medical Society. All rights reserved.

113. Fisher B, Costantino JP, Wickerham DL, et al. Tamoxifen for prevention of breast cancer: Report of the National Surgical Adjuvant Breast and Bowel Project P-1 Study. *Journal of the National Cancer Institute* 1998; 90:1371-88.

114. Hartmann LC, Schaid DJ, Woods JE, et al. Efficacy of bilateral prophylactic mastectomy in women with a family history of breast cancer. *New England Journal of Medicine* 1999; 340:77-84.

115. Skolnick AA. Cancer gene patent dispute settled. *Journal of the American Medical Association* 1995; 273:833.

116. Settlement gives Myriad rights to genetic testing. *Drug and Biotechnology News* 1998 May 20.

117. Marshall E, Gene tests get tested. *Science* 1997 Feb 7; 275:782. Used with permission from the American Association for the Advancement of Science.

118. See Note 28.

119. See Note 117.

120. See Note 28.

121. AP. Panel rejects cancer gene test kit. *Los Angeles Times* 1995 Dec 1; Sect. A:39.

122. Goldreich S. Gaithersburg, Md., biotechnology firm files for bankruptcy. *Washington Times* 1999 Feb 27.

123. Gillis J. Cancer discovery could provide boost to gene test market; predisposition may proceed prevention. *Washington Post* 1998 Apr 7; Sect. C:2.

124. Information in this paragraph was obtained from Myriad Genetics press releases.

125. American College of Medical Genetics and New York State Department of Health. Available from www.health.state.ny.us/nysdoh/cancer/obcancer/contents.htm. Used with permission.

Access to Medical Products

Drug and medical products companies produce valuable, sometimes life-saving commodities that cannot always be accessed by the neediest patients. Reasons for lack of access include: the drug is experimental and the patient does not meet the eligibility criteria for the study; the patient is eligible for the study but is randomized into a placebo control group; the drug is not approved for marketing in the patient's country; the supply of the marketed drug is insufficient to meet demand; or the patient cannot afford the drug, either because it is not covered by insurance or the patient is too poor to pay out of pocket. Lack of access can also be perceived but not real, as when a physician refuses to prescribe a drug that the patient is convinced he or she needs. Reasons for physician refusal to prescribe range from determinations that the drug lacks efficacy or would be too toxic for a particular patient to the belief that the patient is too unreliable to adhere to a complicated administration regimen.

Lack of access to medical products by some individuals has always existed. However, not until the AIDS crisis in the early 1980s were drug companies or the Food and Drug Administration forced to deal directly with patients on this issue. In the face of a deadly disease, with no available treatments that attacked the AIDS virus directly, desperate patients organized for the purposes of forcing FDA to speed drug approvals, forcing companies to allow early access to experimental treatments, and making treatments affordable for all who needed them. The fact that the AIDS activists were the first to make access to experimental drugs a national issue makes their interactions with FDA and drug manufacturers an instructive lesson on how distributive justice issues can influence corporate activity.

AIDS ACTIVISTS AND THE FOOD AND DRUG ADMINISTRATION

Until the early 1980s, FDA drug approval was based largely on considerations of sufficient safety and efficacy to promote the general public good and protect the public health. FDA's approach has always been risk-adverse, based on the impetus for its initial creation—to prevent deaths and injuries from unsafe medicinals. Over the years, and especially with the regulatory changes in the 1960s following the thalidomide scare, the FDA procedures for drug approval became the most scientifically rigorous and complicated in the world, resulting in approval times as long as ten years from the date of investigational new drug (IND) application submission.[1] However, this regulatory mind-set was altered when the AIDS crisis surfaced in the early 1980s. Because there were no treatments to halt the progression of AIDS and prevent an early death, many AIDS patients did not care if a particular drug candidate was experimental or if it could be unsafe—they wanted access to any drug with the potential for benefit, no matter how slim, and were even willing to try drugs when there was little or even no data to support efficacy. Using slogans such as "trials are treatment," AIDS activists demanded access to clinical trials.[2] This movement began to alter the notion that the sole purpose of clinical trials was to collect research data on an investigational drug.[3] But, since access to AIDS drugs was initially limited to research, black markets sprang up for drugs available only in other countries, and home remedies for substances rumored to help the disease were sought and self-administered. In addition, AIDS patients were suspicious that discrimination against gays had stifled progress in the search for AIDS treatments, and they were frustrated by the indifference of the Reagan administration to their plight. In this environment, the slow review and approval processes at FDA were considered unresponsive to the needs of the rapidly growing number of dying patients. AIDS activist groups began to accuse FDA of exacerbating a health-care crisis.[4]

Numerous political activist groups began to organize in the 1980s to prompt FDA to expedite its review and approval processes for new AIDS drugs, both those that attacked HIV directly and those intended to treat the deadly collection of cancers and infectious diseases caused by HIV's immune system destruction.[5] These activists were highly motivated and started using political and legal means to achieve their goals. However, their initial efforts were thwarted since courts tended to give deference to FDA's mandate to exercise its discretion to control the drug approval process. This, combined with prior FDA actions concerning the legal rights of the terminally ill to access unapproved drugs, worked against the goals of the AIDS activists.

In the 1970s, some cancer patients attempted to obtain Laetrile, an unapproved drug derived from peach or apricot pits intended for use in treating cancers for which there were no other treatment alternatives. Since the substance was not available in the United States and it was illegal to import unapproved drugs, cancer patients had attempted to obtain a legally recognized exception for Laetrile. After FDA refusal to grant an exception, patients sued in federal court to enjoin the government from preventing the importation of Laetrile. In this suit, the plaintiffs used two arguments—that terminally ill patients had a constitutionally protected privacy right to decide to use Laetrile, and that the Federal Food and Drug Act definitions of "safe" and "efficacious" as interpreted by the FDA should be liberalized when the drugs in question were intended to be used in terminally ill patients.[6] The California state courts were also used to test a privacy theory, since the state's constitution contained an explicit right to privacy (unlike the federal constitution). But the California Supreme Court, in a split decision, rejected the argument that cancer patients and their doctors had a constitutionally protected privacy right to use Laetrile. In her dissenting opinion, however, the liberal chief justice Rose Bird believed that this was the wrong result:

> Cancer is a disease with potentially fatal consequences; this makes the choice of treatment one of the more important decisions a person may ever make, touching intimately on his or her being. For this reason, I believe the right to privacy . . . prevents the state from interfering with a person's choice of treatment on the sole grounds that the person has chosen a treatment which the state considers "ineffective."[7]

The federal court lawsuit was appealed to the U.S. Supreme Court, and the outcome was consistent with the California case; the justices ruled that FDA could not be required by the courts to give terminally ill patients special consideration when it came to determining whether a drug was safe or effective enough to be approved for sale in the United States.[8]

Despite the fact that the courts were not likely to reverse established precedent and allow dying AIDS patients early access to experimental anti-HIV drugs, activists sued the FDA anyway. This suit took years to process and then failed on an early motion for summary judgment.[9] Because legal redress was not available, it was clear to the activists that different measures were needed to change the status quo. The most effective methods chosen by the activists to obtain government concessions involved acts of civil unrest. Openly critical of the FDA's slowness, activists picketed FDA headquarters, making headlines each time. The biggest protest occurred in 1988 when activists staged a large demonstration in front of the FDA headquarters that resulted in a shutdown of the agency. Over one thousand protestors marched, drew the outlines of dead bodies on the sidewalks, and carried tombstone replicas to emphasize how many patients had died of AIDS. These and other protests caused FDA to develop new regulatory procedures that allowed for both early access to experimental drugs and faster drug approvals for use in desperately ill patients.[10]

EARLY ACCESS: COMPASSIONATE USE, TREATMENT INDS, AND PARALLEL TRACK PROGRAMS

Prior to the emergence of the AIDS epidemic, on a case-by-case basis FDA had occasionally permitted early access to experimental drugs for severely ill patients who might die before a potentially life-saving drug was approved. These allowances were considered "compassionate" exceptions to the IND regulations that forbid the use of an experimental drug outside of FDA-authorized clinical research protocols. To obtain the exemption, the sick patient would have to convince his or her physician to apply for a compassionate use IND, a process that required extensive paperwork and took a significant amount of time. Once the IND was approved by FDA allowing human research to commence, the drug company had to agree to divert its research supply of the drug for this purpose and give it to the physician free of charge, since FDA regulations also forbid the selling of experimental drugs. Because not all companies were willing to meet these conditions and because of the cumbersome procedures used by FDA, compassionate use INDs were not widely useful as a means to get very sick patients treated with experimental drugs.[11]

In 1987, FDA generated more liberal regulations that allowed AIDS patients to obtain early access to investigational drugs.[12] These so-called treatment IND regulations were not patient- and doctor-specific. Rather, for investigational drugs intended for use in serious or life-threatening diseases for which no other treatments were available, access depended on whether the experimental drug showed enough promise in IND clinical trials to make it reasonable for use by seriously ill or dying patients. In order for such a drug to qualify for treatment IND status, the company had to be actively pursuing marketing approval and data had to be collected on the patients who received the drug similar to the data collected under the formal, more routine clinical trials. Drug companies were also allowed to charge for drugs used under treatment INDs. Either a physician or the drug company could apply for treatment IND status for a drug, and FDA would govern when the drug was qualified to be categorized as such. For immediately life-threatening conditions, for which the threat of unknown risk was considered subordinate to the desperate need of patients for a drug with even limited evidence of efficacy, access could be obtained as early as during Phase II trials.

For many AIDS patients, these new regulations were viewed as life saving, but critics of the new program quickly surfaced. Many physicians and others were concerned that the use of untested drugs on desperately ill patients could constitute financial exploitation of dying patients and expose these patients to potentially lethal side effects that had not yet surfaced in limited testing. FDA also left itself open to continued challenges by AIDS activists to allow for treatment IND use more frequently and earlier in the clinical trial process. Finally, since most medical insurance programs would not cover the costs of experimental drug treatment, many patients complained that the revised regulatory policy regarding access was unavailable to all but the wealthiest patients, unless controls were placed on drug prices.[13]

Later in 1992, FDA made further concessions to the AIDS patients when it instituted the AIDS drug "parallel track" program.[14] Like treatment INDs, this program allowed for expanded access to promising experimental drugs for AIDS and HIV-related conditions, but parallel track added two new features. Requirements for providing evidence of drug effectiveness were less stringent than those generally required for a treatment IND, and AIDS patients and activists were included among a group of experts on the AIDS Research Advisory Committee that advised FDA about which drugs qualified for parallel track designation. This new program met some of the AIDS patient demands, but it was unclear at the start how often FDA would use this new program to grant expanded access and also how many patients would be able to afford these early experimental drugs. Parallel track made medical professionals even more anxious. With earlier access, even less would be known about the effects of the drugs, and some physicians deplored this added risk and the further degradation of the drug evaluation process.[15]

Expanded access programs were difficult for pharmaceutical companies to manage. They diverted drug supplies from clinical trials and complicated the already difficult clinical trial processes. John Curd, a medical director at Genentech who worked on the clinical trials of the breast cancer biologic Herceptin®, said this about working with breast cancer activists who protested and demanded compassionate access to the drug prior to FDA approval:

> We didn't want to do this. It costs money. It takes time. It's a diversion. It slows the progress of our clinical trials. But we began to understand something that we heard from one of the women . . . in one of the first meetings, that it is not all just an intellectual argument: "Some of this is an emotional argument, and for those of us who are dealing with breast cancer or people who we know and love and have breast cancer, it's an emotional issue. We need to know that you are going to do something—not everything, but something."[16]

PERSONAL USE IMPORT EXEMPTION

In 1982, after the Laetrile lawsuit, FDA proposed that it could permit an exception to the restrictions on the importation of unapproved drugs for a "reasonable" quantity of drug for personal use.[17] In making the proposal, the agency stated that these exemptions from the import restrictions represented a reasonable exercise of its enforcement discretion so long as personal use was the sole reason for import. Therefore, to avoid legal sanctions, a personal use importer could not distribute the drug commercially, could not import an excessive quantity (typically, no more than three months supply at a time), needed to provide to FDA the name and address of his or her treating physician, and affirm in writing that the drug was for the patient's own use. FDA had the ability to inspect incoming drugs and confiscate them if it determined that the drug was dangerous or was being illegally commercialized within the United States. If so, FDA would issue an "import alert," which removed the drug from the personal use exception and forbade any further importation. While never officially made a regulation, this new legal exemption proposal was immediately exercised by AIDS patients, who could now turn what was a black market operation into something that was at least ambiguously legal. AIDS patients soon banded together into buyers' clubs to coordinate the importation of foreign drugs, while still publicly insisting that the FDA approval process for domestic AIDS drugs was too slow to help them. Initially unsure about how buyers' clubs fit within the new importation proposal, one club invited FDA and the press to Manhattan to witness the unloading of a truck filled with foreign drugs for hundreds of local patients. When FDA did not appear to arrest the participants, the buyers' clubs began to import in earnest. Both approved and unapproved drugs were imported, and the clubs even funded manufacturing plants to make copies of both foreign drugs and home remedy products. In 1992, it was estimated that five thousand individuals bought an estimated $1.25 million worth of AIDS drugs from just one buyers' club in New York, the People With AIDS (PWA) Health Group. There were similar buyers' clubs in most large U.S. cities conducting a similar amount of business, some operating at cost and others for a profit, some scrupulous about what they imported and some not.[18]

It did not take long, however, for the realization to emerge that the buyers' club solution was a poor substitute for the FDA's albeit lengthy processes to ensure rigorous scientific analysis of a drug's safety, efficacy, purity, and consistency. For instance, most buyers' clubs stopped importing one antiviral drug when FDA laboratories found it to have potentially serious variations in potency and quality. Patients who no longer had access to the drug were left confused and worried. "It was a scary thing," said one patient. "It just adds to the uncertainty of all of this. . . . I have to take drugs before I have data establishing that they're doing what they're supposed to do, and then I can't even have the security of knowing they're being made properly."[19] Many physicians thought that numerous drugs obtained through buyers' clubs were at best exploitative and ineffective quackery, and at worst would make patients sicker than they already were. Some of these physicians would refuse to treat patients unless they stopped using imported drugs. Those physicians who did agree to treat patients using imported drugs often had difficulty managing overall treatment, since they had little information about how the drug affected the disease or influenced the other approved drugs the patients were taking. Medical researchers worried that if too many AIDS patients took the imported drugs, they would not be available to enroll in the domestic studies, thereby delaying U.S. AIDS drug research. Study results could also be compromised by the surreptitious use of the unapproved imports. Pharmaceutical companies were opposed to the personal use exemption when it was employed to obtain cheaper or "counterfeit" versions of the company's approved drugs. It was feared that commercial R&D efforts would be stifled if a drug's market was significantly undercut by foreign imports. Even the buyers' clubs felt conflicted, since most were organized as temporary efforts primarily to provoke the more effective industry-FDA system to quickly approve treatments so that the clubs could go out of business. "This is not an appropriate place for anyone to come for health care," said a spokesperson from the buyers' club PWA

Health Group.[20] In the long run, it was clear that the personal use import exemption and the altruism of the buyers' clubs could not successfully serve the purpose of increasing access to safe and effective experimental AIDS drugs.

ACCELERATED DRUG APPROVAL

The problems with expanded access and personal use import exemptions served to highlight the need to get more effective AIDS drugs quickly to market. Because the long-term risks for future patients were difficult to predict, FDA was initially unwilling to agree that its review and approval process should be less rigorous for patients who were currently dying. However, activism in the AIDS communities escalated to make the point that, for those who faced certain death, the certain risk of delay outweighed the uncertain risk of drug side effects. Also, AIDS patients would gladly accept a drug with even minimal efficacy on the chance that it would delay death until a better drug was approved. The activists railed against what they considered to be the paternalistic and bureaucratically unresponsive attitude of FDA to their critical need for treatments. These were difficult arguments to counter, and FDA began to consider how it could balance the need to keep the drug supply safe and effective yet speed up the process of getting drugs approved and on the market. Ten days after the large AIDS activist protest in 1988, the agency announced plans for an expedited approval process for drugs intended for use in previously untreatable, life-threatening diseases. These regulations focused on early approval rather than research access.

Two sets of regulations were proposed in the late 1980s and subsequently adopted in the early 1990s. Called "Subpart E" and "Accelerated Approval" regulations, these liberalized the review and approval processes for drugs intended to treat serious and life-threatening diseases.[21] Included in these so-called fast-track regulations were provisions to reduce the time for the clinical investigation phase of drug review, the amount of reduction tailored to the severity of the disease threat, and the availability of alternative treatments. Fast-track regulations also provided for early consultation between FDA and the drug company about the process to obtain approval, closer FDA monitoring of clinical trials, use of so-called surrogate endpoints to qualify as evidence of drug efficacy,[22] and consolidated and shortened clinical trials. The regulations allowed drugs to be marketed with less than full evidence of safety and efficacy so long as the company agreed to continue to collect data after marketing (called Phase IV postmarketing research). Together, these provisions allowed for greater regulatory flexibility that could truncate the clinical trial process and get promising products on the market while data were still being collected.[23]

These regulations succeeded in reducing the regulatory review time for new drug applications (NDAs) for AIDS drugs to less than five months rather than the fifteen months that was typical of other drugs. The total review and approval period for all drugs went from an average of over 10 years to 3.3 years for drugs on a fast-track program. The speed, however, bothered some who believed that drugs would be prematurely marketed only to be recalled later for lack of efficacy or greater-than-expected toxicity. For example, surrogate markers later might be found to be problematic if no clear relationship was eventually established linking their presence to the drugs effect on the course of the disease. Or patients might start to die from drug side effects sooner than from the disease. Indeed, it was only after the marketing of AZT (the first approved anti-AIDS drug) that defects surfaced about the clinical trials testing its safety and efficacy. Postmarketing analysis showed that the Phase II AZT studies were stopped too soon, that only a small portion of the subjects had completed the required six months of treatment, that there were gaps in the data collected, that there might have been bias in the way that data were reported, and that subjects were not racially or otherwise diverse enough to accurately predict the effects in patients who lacked the characteristics of the mostly Caucasian study subjects.[24] Initially hailed as a godsend to AIDS patients, AZT came to be known as a highly toxic drug with limited abilities to control the disease. One clinical investigator, disappointed in the way another AIDS drug was fast-tracked, commented, "Until our society places greater value on the knowledge of whether a new therapeutic agent is safe and effective than [it does] on personal choice based on little or no information . . . research results will not meet the expectations of patients or society."[25] Yet another view persisted that considered the risk tolerance of AIDS patients and held that AZT, while certainly not as good a drug as those that were subsequently approved, gave patients something very important—some degree of efficacy and the hope that by living longer, they would be around to benefit from improvements that would follow.

As with any program that attempts to balance opposing positions, FDA was both praised and criticized for its efforts and decisions to allow access to experimental AIDS drugs and to expedite their approval. Some said that the FDA actions were justified to meet the desperate health crisis, and others maintained that FDA had seriously eroded its principles and processes to meet short-term demands while risking potentially serious long-term negative consequences.[26] The goal of ensuring the safety of drugs and the goal of making drugs available to help individuals with diseases would continue to be difficult to balance. The FDA regulatory improvements went a long way toward appeasing the AIDS activists' demands, but the access issues continued to escalate when AIDS patients learned what these newly approved drugs would cost. The activists' focus turned to the pharmaceutical companies as drug price became their new concern.

PHARMACEUTICAL COMPANIES AND DRUG PRICING

Pharmaceutical companies traditionally operate with a focus on identifying a market for a particular product and engaging in research and development to bring the product to market, concentrating thereafter on protecting and growing that market. In this process, outside constituencies include FDA regulators, medical scientists, prescribing physicians, and the business community. Dealing with patient activists and the media attention they received was not something most drug companies were prepared to handle. This lack of preparation hit one pharmaceutical company particularly hard when it became the first to develop a drug that directly attacked the virus that causes AIDS. Early in the AIDS crisis, the activists and the companies shared a common goal—shortening the drug approval time. For many years, pharmaceutical companies had complained that the FDA approval processes caused costly delays in getting needed drugs to market. For the first time, the companies had a powerful ally when the AIDS activists enhanced a political climate increasingly sympathetic to liberalizing regulation. However, any alliance of views disappeared when the pharmaceutical companies announced their AIDS drug prices. Burroughs Wellcome, the first company to market an anti-AIDS drug, has since been credited with catalyzing the existence of the most militant AIDS activists group, the AIDS Coalition to Unleash Power, or ACT-UP.[27] The story of how this came about is also instructive, since Burroughs Wellcome's experience became a well-known cautionary tale for the industry.

Burroughs Wellcome Co. was the American subsidiary of the British pharmaceutical company Wellcome PLC, which on the death of the founders was left to a medical research trust. Consequently, although Wellcome grew to become the twentieth largest pharmaceutical company in the world by the mid-1980s, much of the company's history was heavily focused on research and development. In 1986, the Wellcome Trust sold just over 25 percent of the company to raise money to fight disease in the third world.[28] Prior to that, the U.S.-

based Burroughs Wellcome began to target its formidable R&D talent to developing an anti-AIDS drug. There was little enthusiasm from other pharmaceutical companies to get involved with the disease at the time: HIV was considered very dangerous to work with since there was no certainty about how it was transmitted, little was known about how it caused AIDS (and therefore how to design a drug to interfere with this process), and the market for AIDS drugs was still small. But Burroughs Wellcome had the fourth largest corporate drug research staff in the world, with specific antiviral research expertise, and their vice president of research, Dr. David Barry, was a physician who specialized in viral diseases.

In 1984, Barry ignited company interest in developing a drug to fight AIDS. In a few months, a screening program of available molecules within the company laboratories showed that AZT looked promising.[29] From then on, early testing of AZT was assisted by scientists at FDA, Duke University, and branches of the National Institutes of Health. Burroughs Wellcome's IND application was approved by the FDA in June 1985. Human safety studies were then conducted, which were notable for their swiftness and for the fact that FDA granted many exemptions from the usual research processes—a testament to the urgency felt to find any treatment options for what was beginning to look like an AIDS epidemic. Phase I safety studies were performed, not in healthy individuals as was usual, but in patients sick with AIDS. Phase III trials were skipped entirely after larger-than-usual Phase II trials showed that, even though AZT produced some serious side effects, it appeared to slow the immune system destruction that was the hallmark of AIDS. In March 1987, FDA granted Burroughs Wellcome its NDA and ultimate marketing approval in record time, two years and four months from preclinical testing to approval for marketing, compared to the more typical time period of seven to ten years. The regulatory portion of this timeframe was five working days to review and approve the IND application and 3.5 months to review and approve the NDA.[30]

At the news of Burroughs Wellcome's impressive achievement and of AZT's approval, company stock soared in anticipation of the income that this drug could produce. However, when Burroughs Wellcome set the wholesale market price for the drug at $8,200 per patient per year (which after the retail mark-up would rise to about $9,500 per year), all hell broke loose in the AIDS communities. The activists and many health professionals found the amount to be unconscionably high for a drug that dying patients needed so badly. It was clear that a significant number of AIDS patients would not be able to afford the drug since patients were typically paying for several other medications, many insurance programs covered no prescription drugs, and AIDS patients were at risk for loss of employment due to illness or discrimination. The outrage among patients with AIDS about what they believed to be corporate price gouging led to a series of troublesome events for Burroughs Wellcome. The first was that the militant AIDS activist group, ACT-UP, was formed specifically to protest the price of AZT. ACT-UP members engaged in multiple acts of civil unrest, such as demonstrations on Wall Street that shut down rush-hour traffic and, on another occasion, storming into the New York Stock Exchange and chaining themselves to the balcony railing. During these events, the protesters waved banners and posters that condemned Burroughs Wellcome for its AZT price. After a failed attempt in 1989 to obtain price cuts during a face-to-face meeting with Burroughs Wellcome executives, activists later surreptitiously gained access to company headquarters in North Carolina, barricaded themselves in a conference room, and held a press conference via telephone with the Associated Press until police removed them from the building.[31]

The activists were also successful in getting Congress to investigate Burroughs Wellcome's decisions on the cost and availability of AZT. Burroughs Wellcome's president, Theodore Haigler, and Barry were called to testify before Congress in March 1987 and were challenged by Representative Henry Waxman, a California Democrat, to justify AZT's price. The congressman stressed that there were factors that should have allowed Burroughs Wellcome to set the price lower—the short screening time, the assistance given the company by scientists in federal laboratories, the smaller clinical trials, and the large tax subsidies and market protections the company obtained by getting the drug classified under the Orphan Drug Act.[32] Haigler was asked point blank several times how much, after taxes, it cost the company to get AZT to the point of manufacture. Given the fact that corporate costs and price-setting strategies are usually closely guarded proprietary information, it is not surprising that Haigler responded that he did not have these figures.[33] However, Representative Waxman had done his homework and estimated that income from the sale of AZT would be $45 million per year if only the current forty-five hundred AIDS patients remained on the drug, and that income would rise to $250 million if all of the twenty-five thousand AIDS patients took the drug. Waxman concluded from these figures that Burroughs Wellcome would easily recoup its development costs many times over. After these hearings, Waxman wrote to Burroughs Wellcome and made it clear that the AZT price was deemed excessive, and he threatened to reopen hearings on the matter. Burroughs Wellcome then heard that the government was considering instituting drug price controls, taking over the manufacture of AZT, or revoking the AZT patent.

It was also clear that pressure by the activists to get any price break would continue, since the number of AIDS cases was increasing, and, according to the U.S. Department of Health and Human Services Centers for Disease Control and Prevention (CDC), 90 percent of these patients would die from the disease within five years of diagnosis.[34]

Never before had any pharmaceutical company been subjected to such intense consumer protests, nor had a company been called to Congress and publicly grilled about its internal product pricing strategies. Burroughs Wellcome was not prepared to handle these intrusions into its business and was widely seen as poorly managing these problems. Company executives disagreed that the AZT price was too high. Managers met the criticism by pointing out that, without the ability to recoup their expenses and make a profit selling the drug, Burroughs Wellcome would not have developed Retrovir® and AIDS patients would not have access to it. Commercial involvement was necessary: although government research funds were used in the drug's development, no public agency had the capability to do what was necessary to get the drug on the market. As Burroughs Wellcome president Haigler attempted to explain to Representative Waxman, drug pricing took into account the standard cost of development, production, and distribution calculations but also needed to account for uncertainties, which in the case of the first AIDS drug were considerable. These uncertainties included whether AZT would remain beneficial, the prospect of competition, whether the company could achieve manufacturing efficiencies, and the future of the AIDS crisis. Because of these market conditions, price reductions would only occur if the company could achieve manufacturing efficiencies. Burroughs Wellcome's decision and the rationale it used were not satisfactory to the activists, who claimed that Burroughs Wellcome was taking a free ride on the large amounts of public money that went into AZT's discovery and development, and that the company efforts and expenditures did not justify the high price. They argued that AIDS patients were paying twice for the drug—once as taxpayers who funded the public agencies that assisted with AZT research and then again as patients who paid the high prices for the drug.[35] This battle between Burroughs Wellcome and the AIDS activists continued for many years and spilled over to affect each company that subsequently entered the AIDS drug market.

CONCLUSION

As highlighted by the turmoil surrounding the AIDS crisis and Burroughs Wellcome's experience, access to valuable medical products involves disagreements about the influences and importance of scientific testing, administrative control, personal autonomy, and free market commerce. The optimal balance among these competing social interests will always be difficult to achieve.[36] The imperfect information about diseases and the drugs used to treat them makes such balancing even more difficult. The AIDS crisis showed pharmaceutical companies that these issues would influence drug development efforts from that point on.

Case Study

Merck's U.S. Managed Distribution Program for the HIV Drug Crixivan[37]

"We would not trade it for anything in the world."
—A member of the U.S. Managed Distribution
Team for Crixivan on the experience

One afternoon in the spring of 1996, the members of Merck's U.S. Managed Distribution Team for the drug Crixivan gathered around a table at Merck's West Point facility in Pennsylvania. The team members included representatives from marketing, business development, customer relations, public affairs, and the order management center for prescription drugs. The team had been created to handle a unique problem faced by Merck. In March, the U.S. Food and Drug Administration had approved Merck's new drug application for Crixivan, a novel antiviral drug to fight AIDS. Driven by positive early data from the clinical studies, a tremendous medical need for new HIV treatments, and the demands of AIDS activists to make new medicines available as quickly as possible, FDA had approved Merck's application in a record-setting forty-two days from submission. It was also at least a full six months before Merck's manufacturing facilities would be ready to produce the drug at capacity. Until then, a small pilot plant facility would supply Crixivan for an estimated twenty-five thousand to thirty thousand patients—far less than the nine hundred thousand people living with HIV in the United States and the millions more worldwide who could benefit from the medicine. Propelled by the need to make Crixivan quickly available but concerned about ensuring a continuous supply to individual patients so that immune resistance to the drug would not develop as a result of insufficient dosage, the team had grappled with the issue of how to distribute a drug in limited supply so that all patients who began treatment would have a continuous supply of the medication. Dr. Bradley Sheares, head of the U.S. marketing group for Crixivan, had warned that the worst situation would be to start patients on therapy only to discontinue treatment because Merck could not continue to supply the drug. Such a situation was a set-up for the emergence of viral resistance, which would markedly exacerbate the AIDS epidemic. Members of the U.S. Managed Distribution Team had never before faced such a challenge. After much consideration, they decided to abandon traditional distribution channels, manage distribution from one source, and track all patients starting on therapy with Crixivan. The team had gathered in West Point to review its progress and success in this unique undertaking.

MERCK & CO., INC.

Founded in 1891, by 1995 Merck & Co., Inc., was the largest provider of prescription medicines in the United States as well as in the world. In that year its sales totaled almost $17 billion and net income amounted to $3.3 billion.[38] Pharmaceutical research and drug development was a business that involved solid scientific data, proper timing, a receptive market, and a fair share of calculated risks. The average cost of developing a new drug in the 1990s could be as high as $500 million to $600 million and could take as long as nine to ten years. On average, only three out of ten medicines developed ever covered their development costs through sales. Although recognized for its world-class marketing and sales organization, Merck's core strength was its pharmaceutical research capability, for which it had consistently maintained a solid reputation over the years. Merck's R&D expenditures in 1995 were $1.331 billion, an increase of $100 million from the prior year.[39] In 1994, Merck's research program accounted for 5 percent of total research conducted by pharmaceutical companies worldwide.

In its almost one hundred years of existence, Merck's research laboratories had pursued such diseases as cancer, high blood pressure, and asthma, and had successfully handled these costs and risks. Merck introduced its first formal research program in the 1930s, and soon thereafter, the company's researchers became known for regularly developing novel beneficial medicines and therapies. Among Merck's numerous innovations were the syntheses of vitamin B-6 and hydrocortisone; vaccines against mumps, measles, hepatitis B, and pneumo-coccal pneumonia; penicillin production techniques; a medicine to fight river blindness; and various medications to treat cardiovascular diseases.[40] The com-pany also owned a subsidiary, Merck-Medco, which marketed pharmaceutical benefit management services to managed-care organizations and health bene-fit sponsors in the United States.

Besides its excellence in the field of research, Merck prided itself on being socially responsible and for adhering to the highest ethical standards. The company regularly committed a large part of its profits and resources to phil-anthropic causes, believing that contributing to communities in which it had a presence was an essential component of its corporate responsibility.[41] Merck's philanthropic activities were subject to strict guidelines that focused on two major efforts: advancing scientific knowledge and education, and improving health care.

For example, Merck's Mectizan® Donation Program had pledged to pro-vide Mectizan, a medicine to treat river blindness, free of charge to people in Central and South America, Africa, and Yemen for as many years as necessary. By 1997, nearly eighteen million people around the world had been treated.[42] In addition, the company also supported environmental, artistic, and cultural activities as well as civic institutions, and provided help when disasters or medical emergencies occurred. Merck's corporate philanthropy was an essen-tial element of its self-perception: Merck saw itself not only as a company that excelled in pharmaceutical research, marketing and sales, manufacturing, and distribution, but also as one that strove to make the world a healthier and bet-ter place. The corporate philosophy was summed up in a statement by founder George W. Merck: "We try never to forget that medicine is for the people. It is not for the profits. The profits follow, and if we have remembered that, they have never failed to appear. The better we have remembered that, the larger they have been."[43]

HIV AND AIDS

By the mid-1990s, AIDS was becoming an epidemic that could potentially af-fect anyone, regardless of gender, age, or race. The disease resulted from infec-tion with the human immunodeficiency virus, which was transmitted through exchange of body fluids (for example, blood transfusions, sexual transmission, shared intravenous needle use). Once in the body, the virus attacked the im-mune system, eventually leaving the affected person unable to fight infections or cancers. As the immune system became more damaged, secondary infections and cancers occurred with greater frequency and severity, leading eventually to an AIDS diagnosis.[44] For about the first decade of the epidemic, this diagnosis meant that death would soon follow. From January 1981 to June 1995, nearly half a million Americans had been diagnosed with AIDS and about half of these people had died. By 1995, about one million people in the United States were believed to be infected with HIV. Death rates had increased to the point that, from 1994 to 1996, AIDS was the leading cause of death in Americans twenty-five to forty-four years of age.[45]

This infectious scourge was believed to have started in 1980; it took until 1983 to discover that HIV was the cause and until 1985 to develop a blood test to determine who was infected. By 1985, the virus had established a devastating foothold; however, its identification provided scientists with the opportunity to learn how it worked to destroy the immune system. HIV preferentially infected and entered CD4 cells, the cells primarily responsible for directing the body's immune response. Once the virus started to replicate, it could do so rapidly and kill its host CD4 cell, thereby progressively weakening the immune system. People with healthy immune systems had about 800–1,000 CD4 cells per milliliter of blood. AIDS was diagnosed when CD4 counts fell below 200 per milliliter of blood.[46] At that point, patients would begin to succumb to lethal secondary infections (called "opportunistic infections") and cancers that the body's immune system was too compromised to fight. Scientists also learned that the virus was difficult to kill. A major problem associated with HIV was its ability to mutate rapidly and develop resistance to adverse environments, including drugs, which made it very difficult to develop effective antiviral drugs.[47]

AIDS THERAPIES AND THE MARKET

At the beginning of the epidemic, treatments for AIDS patients were limited and ineffective, meaning that an AIDS diagnosis was a virtual death sentence. Patients died from multiple opportunistic infections and cancers, many of which were rarely found in people with a functioning immune system. As a consequence, current drugs were often useless in combatting them. Many pharmaceutical companies, therefore, were developing drugs to prevent and treat these unusual infections and patients often were taking several of these drugs simultaneously. These new therapies were extending the life span of AIDS patients, but the drugs did not attack the virus itself. At the time, no drugs had been able to eliminate HIV from the body, and the market was immense for any company that could develop a truly effective anti-HIV drug.

As more scientists uncovered information about the life cycle of HIV, some attractive options for drug intervention were revealed. It was discovered that once the virus entered the host cell, it began to replicate its genetic material and package it into virions (newly synthesized viral shells). These virions would then burst from the host cell and infect neighboring cells, killing the host cell in the process. HIV employed a handful of enzymes to carry out this life cycle, three of which were eventually targeted for drug intervention: reverse transcriptase, integrase, and protease.

Reverse Transcriptase

Upon entry to the cell, HIV needs to convert its genetic material into a form compatible with that of the host. The reverse transcriptase (RT) enzyme carries out this task, and RT inhibitor drugs were the first to be developed as potent anti-AIDS drugs. In 1987, Burroughs Wellcome's AZT was the first such drug to be marketed. Although RT inhibitor drugs were effective in increasing CD4 counts and decreasing viral levels, viral resistance developed rapidly. It quickly became clear that HIV mutated soon after starting therapy with AZT or other drugs in this category, resulting in the evolution of strains that were resistant against RT inhibitors.

Integrase

Once HIV has converted its genetic material, the enzyme integrase facilitates the integration of the viral genetic material into the host's genetic material. Pharmaceutical companies, including Merck, had created basic research programs to screen integrase inhibitors for those that showed promising early results in halting the integration of the viral DNA into the host DNA.

Protease

Once the viral genetic material has replicated, proteins are produced in long chains. Before packaging the new virions, the long chains have to be cut into smaller parts. The protease enzyme is responsible for this task.

ESTIMATING MARKET SIZE

Several pharmaceutical companies were developing and testing drugs designed to inhibit these HIV enzymes, and successful efforts were expected to bring substantial profits. However, the size of the anti-AIDS drug market in the mid-1990s was quite difficult to predict. According to the CDC, there were about 225,000 people in the United States living with AIDS, but this number did not provide clear information about the potential U.S. market.[48] One reason for this uncertainty was the rapidly changing information about the virus and advances in treatment options. In 1995, the potential market had expanded greatly because new studies had shown that it made sense to treat HIV infection early rather than wait for the symptoms of full-blown AIDS.[49] However, because HIV infection was not a reportable condition in half of the states, the number of people with this infection was not accurately known, although CDC estimated that the U.S. rate of infection was about forty thousand people per year.[50] Beyond the United States, the market would be restricted to those countries wealthy enough to afford the drugs, and these countries were the ones with the lowest incidence of the disease. And even if the worldwide market for AIDS drugs totaled the predicted $1 billion to $2 billion a year, that market would probably be shared by the twelve to fifteen drugs already released or expected to be released in the following two to three years. It was expected to take years of research (much of it being conducted by the pharmaceutical companies making the drugs) to determine which drug or combination of drugs was the most effective and whether viral resistance could be conquered. Until these data were obtained, the market would be unpredictable and shared by the dozen or so companies conducting research in this area.[51] There were so many different scenarios for the future market that one Merck marketing employee told the Johns Hopkins Business History Group that in her first year on the Crixivan project, her group produced sixteen market forecasts.[52]

MERCK'S ANTI-AIDS PROGRAM AND THE DEVELOPMENT OF CRIXIVAN[53]

In December 1986, the president of Merck Research Laboratories (MRL), Dr. Edward M. Scolnick, made an announcement that Merck would launch an AIDS research program. Scolnick was trained in virology and molecular genetics and had made significant contributions to understanding of the viral causes of cancer. He was particularly drawn to the HIV research effort, not only because the medical need was great but also because HIV resembled the viruses that caused some cancers. To begin tackling AIDS, Scolnick started to assemble a group of scientists to spearhead the research efforts. He brought together

Irving Sigal (who had extensive experience in the area of antiviral therapies and inhibition of enzymes), Emilio A. Emini (who had worked for many years with highly infectious viruses), and Joel Huff (a medicinal chemist interested in the inhibition of enzymes). A collection of intellect, however, was not sufficient. Many other resources were required to move forward with the proposed program. Merck's chief executive officer and Scolnick's predecessor at MRL, P. Roy Vagelos, was enthusiastic about mounting a full-scale research program targeting HIV/AIDS, even though this might be the most costly research program ever conducted at Merck. Fortunately, the capital necessary for the endeavor could be drawn from the successes of Merck's recent blockbuster drugs.

The AIDS research program was pushed ahead on several fronts. Sigal and Huff led the effort in antiviral drug studies while Emini initially looked for a potential vaccine. Though a vaccine was developed in the late 1980s, Merck did not move it into clinical trials. Early enthusiasm faded as those involved realized that, because of HIV's rapid mutation rate, the technical challenges of pursuing an optimal vaccine would be extremely difficult.

Sigal and his group members were investigating antiviral agents, looking for a therapy that would prevent the virus from replicating. They worked to understand the basic nature of the HIV protease enzyme and how to inhibit its activity. In parallel, Huff and his colleagues in medicinal chemistry started the search for a protease inhibitor. They invested much of their time screening candidates from an already existing arsenal of inhibitors that Merck had built up in a previous research program. Between 1987 and 1988, Merck researchers proved and published in scientific journals that the HIV protease was a necessary viral enzyme for the life cycle of the virus, and that they had solved its three-dimensional structure.[54] In December 1988, however, Merck's HIV/AIDS program suffered a demoralizing setback. Sigal, who was thirty-five at the time, had traveled to London to give a lecture and took an early flight home because he missed his wife. That flight was Pan Am Flight 103, which was blown up in an act of terrorism over Lockerbie, Scotland. There were no survivors. Though Sigal had been Merck's main proponent of attacking HIV with a protease inhibitor and progress was difficult without him, the program was pushed forward, deriving energy in part from the momentum of discoveries made in 1988.[55]

The screening of protease inhibitor candidates continued, and by early 1989 a candidate protease inhibitor appeared promising. Early in animal trials, however, it was clear that the compound was extremely toxic. Other researchers were exploring a class of reverse transcriptase inhibitors different from those already on the market. After two years and the screening of twenty-three thousand compounds, only four looked hopeful. Though these passed laboratory and animal safety and efficacy studies, it was clear from early human clinical trials that the HIV virus rapidly developed resistance to all of the compounds.

After four years and the failure of five promising candidates at different stages of clinical testing (four reverse transcriptase inhibitors and one protease inhibitor), Merck pushed on with modifications of the failed candidates. Studies showed that small changes in the structure could result in reduced toxicity and increased effectiveness. These efforts resulted in the development of indinavir sulfate in 1991. This protease inhibitor candidate, which was eventually given the trade name Crixivan, was generally well tolerated and potent against the HIV virus in laboratory tests and in animals. The hope for this new candidate was tempered by its primary shortcoming—an exceedingly difficult and unparalleled synthesis procedure that made it difficult to manufacture. It took one year to make the first one hundred pounds of the drug, enough only for fifty patients at the expected doses needed.[56]

After Merck presented its indinavir research results at scientific meetings, pressure from public health officials and AIDS activists began to mount to get this promising drug into clinical trials. Press reports about Merck's research progress with Crixivan were followed closely by the AIDS community, which was eagerly anticipating access to the drug.[57] The entire Merck research team —scientists, chemists, and engineers—related that they began to squeeze more hours out of the day and more days out of the week to meet the growing demand. This work pace was eventually called "Crixivan Time."

By mid-1992, the drug had passed the necessary safety screens. The Phase I (early human) trials started in late 1992 with just over seventy subjects, first with healthy volunteers and then with AIDS patients. These trials demonstrated that the drug was generally well tolerated and easily absorbed, and also helped to determine optimal dosages. The larger Phase II trials, conducted in 1993 and 1994, helped to evaluate the efficacy of the compound, first with eight AIDS patients and then, when the data started looking very good, with an increasing number of patients. On December 15, 1993, one of Merck's principal investigators presented study data at the First National Conference on Human Retroviruses and Related Infections, and reported that the subjects getting Crixivan experienced a 42 percent drop in HIV levels after two days of treatment compared with subjects on AZT, whose viral levels dropped less than 1 percent. After twelve days on Crixivan or AZT, virus levels had dropped 70 percent and 58 percent respectively, and in three Crixivan subjects, virus levels were undetectable.[58] On the surface, these results were phenomenal. Merck's Edward Scolnick told one reporter, "We were beside ourselves. We thought we had a cure for AIDS."[59] Others were cautiously optimistic, since the history of anti-AIDS drug development was filled with stories of failed candidates.

Sure enough, five weeks later, Merck's scientists found the demoralizing evidence that the HIV in their subjects on Crixivan was showing signs of resistance. By this time, the competitive pressure on Merck was mounting, since there were at least ten other companies who had protease inhibitors in various stages of development. Merck executives discussed the wisdom of cutting their losses and killing the drug. AIDS activists were worried that the negative data would cause Merck to pull out of AIDS drug research altogether. "We were very concerned the company might pull out," said Martin Delaney, an AIDS activist in San Francisco. "We thought they were obsessed with a home-run drug."[60] However, Merck saw some small but potentially promising differences in the Crixivan data and decided to give the drug one last chance. This second chance was designed as an all-out war against the virus.

The strategy for the attack would come from new knowledge about how patients were responding to anti-AIDS drugs. Researchers and physicians had started using what they called combination or "cocktail" therapy as the choice antiviral therapy for AIDS. Theoretically, the use of different drugs would be more powerful because HIV could be disrupted at different stages in its replication cycle, and the virus would have less of a tendency to mutate to a resistant form if faced with multiple drugs rather than one. However, there were some substantial downfalls to the use of combination therapy. Using multiple drugs would be significantly more expensive and require a complicated treatment regimen and dosing schedule. AIDS patients would need to take the antiviral agents as many as six to eight times throughout the day and night, in addition to other anti-infective agents. It was also reasonable to assume that, as with monotherapy, unless the prescribed regimen for the antiviral agents was followed rigorously, resistant HIV strains could appear. Finally, all of these drugs produced side effects that would be exacerbated when the drugs were combined.[61]

Recognizing the risks but also realizing that Crixivan alone in the doses used to date could not produce lasting effectiveness, Merck scientists decided to start new Crixivan studies with significantly higher doses and to test the drug in combination with other anti-AIDS drugs. Merck was determined not to let Crixivan go until it learned if it could be a significant component of an AIDS cocktail therapy. By early 1995, Merck learned that its gamble had paid off. One study showed that, after twenty-four weeks of high-dose Crixivan and AZT, 40 percent of patients had viral levels below the level of detection and no resistance was seen. The Crixivan team members were elated. Such promising results in the middle of a Phase II trial, however, meant that Merck needed to make some critical decisions about whether to spend the large amounts of money it would take to expand to the large-scale Phase III human trials, commit to submitting Crixivan for FDA approval, and start building the manufacturing plant.

Traditionally, pharmaceutical companies waited until receiving encouraging results from Phase III trials before committing to building full-scale manufacturing facilities. However, in the mid-1990s, companies had started considering manufacturing requirements earlier in the human trials process, especially with complicated drugs. Choosing a date to commit to full-scale manufacturing so early in the approval process was a risky proposition and successful timing depended on a number of different factors. Among these factors were the strength of the Phase III study data, the always uncertain FDA approval date, whether new facilities needed to be built and land purchased, the availability of raw materials, the complexity of the manufacturing process (the more complex the procedure, the more time needed to correct batch-to-batch uniformity problems and to reformulate), the shelf life of the drug (in case FDA approval occurred after first production), the difficulty of labor recruitment and training, hazardous waste management, and whether other companies were competing for the same new market.[62]

From the time that the company had focused on Crixivan as a promising candidate, Merck's manufacturing chemists had been wrestling with ways to simplify and shorten the production of the chemical. J. Paul Reider, of Merck Process Research, and Mauricio Futran, Chemical Engineering R&D, were key members of the team that devised and kept revising the production process. Initially, the task looked daunting. "My initial reaction when I saw the molecule was to say there was no way to produce the drug in an affordable manner; it just looked way, way too complex," Dr. Reider told one reporter.[63] But with diligent effort, he and his team went on "Crixivan Time" to develop a feasible production solution.

In January 1995, with the Phase II human trials still ongoing, the members of Merck's senior management for Crixivan and the company's new chief executive officer, Raymond V. Gilmartin, held a "go/no-go" meeting to decide the future of Crixivan. Although the human trial results to date had been promising, concerns remained. The trials had been conducted with a relatively small number of patients, and everyone knew that there was always a high risk that any drug would "wash out" in Phase III trials. In addition, there were no data to provide insight on the potential problem of long-term resistance. Finally, manufacturing the drug would require major innovations and a huge expansion of Merck's production facilities. However, preliminary data from the clinical studies provided extremely promising evidence of the drug's potential benefit to patients. Merck also had early data indicating that Crixivan was more potent than its two closest protease inhibitor rivals from Roche and Abbott (Invirase® and Norvir®).[64] Weighing the risks and benefits, the group decided to start Phase III trials (forty-eight hundred patients in eleven countries) and initiate manufacturing facility expansion. The decision was unprecedented in Merck's history. Never before had the company committed to building full-scale production facilities at such an early stage of product testing. However, all involved thought that the complex manufacturing process for Crixivan required an early commitment.

The production team members knew what they had to do. Patients would need almost 1 kilogram (2.2 lbs.) of Crixivan per year—more than one hundred times greater than the annual dose of most other Merck drugs. Building production facilities that would cover the estimated demand for Crixivan meant that Merck would need to expand its total physical production capacity by 33 percent. The production team decided that it would create Crixivan manufacturing facilities by retrofitting existing U.S. plants.[65] This meant, among other things, that new roads had to be built for the Virginia plant and for the Georgia plant for which Reider had to "beg" for construction workers, most of whom were in Atlanta working to construct facilities for the upcoming Olympics. By the spring of 1995, the production team had made progress and hoped it could be fully operational in eighteen months, six to eight months earlier than initially thought.

By late spring of 1995, Merck initiated Phase III clinical trials—large studies of patients designed to firmly establish the safety and efficacy of drugs under investigation. By late 1995, early trial results were remaining consistent with the Phase II data. At a major scientific meeting in January 1996, Merck's Dr. Emini presented the results from its most promising Phase III study, known as Protocol #035. For the first time, there were indications that the effects of triple combination therapy with Crixivan, AZT, and 3TC in HIV-infected subjects had the potential of turning HIV infection from a death warrant to a manageable chronic disease. Not only did the CD4 counts rise appreciably in study subjects, but also after twenty-four weeks on the triple therapy, 91 percent of patients had HIV levels in their blood below the limit of detection and there were no signs of resistance.[66] No AIDS treatment data had ever been this good. The news was sensational and was reported in the newspapers, on television, and on radio news shows across the country. These findings were so positive that the development cost to date (in the high hundreds of millions of dollars) was looking like it might have been worth the risks.[67]

According to Sheares, "This study revolutionized the treatment of HIV. As a result, the goal of antiretroviral therapy became to reduce the level of virus as low as possible for as long as possible."[68] When the findings from Protocol #035 became widely known, AIDS activists, regulators, people living with HIV, and physicians alike urged Merck to file its NDA for Crixivan marketing approval as quickly as possible so that the drug could be made available without delay. The rapid and profound Crixivan effects seen in this study meant that the drug was a potential life-saver for critically ill AIDS patients. For this reason, AIDS activists were demanding a say in how Merck would make its new drug available.

INVOLVEMENT OF AIDS ACTIVISTS IN THE DEVELOPMENT OF CRIXIVAN

In the late 1980s, as public attention began to focus heavily on HIV and AIDS, Merck was faced with the unfamiliar question of whether to discuss its business plans with patient activists. For much of its history, Merck had had relations primarily with customers (mostly health-care professionals), regulatory and federal agencies, and scientific and academic institutions. But in the late 1980s, special interest groups like AIDS activist groups began to demand, and ultimately receive, attention from Merck and its Public Affairs Department. The driving force behind this change was the rapid increase in public information regarding the AIDS epidemic being supplied by scientific and public health organizations. At the same time, independent AIDS activist groups were banding together, publicly voicing their opinions, and making it impossible for the media and large corporations to ignore the issue of the need for anti-AIDS drugs.

By 1990, the National AIDS Network had over five hundred member organizations.[69] One of the most proactive groups was the AIDS Coalition to Unleash Power, ACT-UP.[70] This organization, which was started specifically to lobby for rapid approval and affordable access to Burroughs Wellcome's AZT, was motivated by the belief that discrimination against gays had stifled

AIDS research progress.[71] The group's public protests and their accusatory and strident demands of pharmaceutical companies had dissuaded some large companies from directly engaging with ACT-UP. Later, however, more moderate groups, such as the Treatment Action Group (TAG), appeared that were even more powerful in some ways, because they became technically and scientifically knowledgeable and could debate with scientists and regulators on all aspects of AIDS effects and treatment. In combination, these groups were emotionally charged, demanding, well organized, politically savvy, knowledgeable, and deeply committed. AIDS activists also had influence with potential drug test subjects, and discouraging words from activists could hinder enrollment in clinical trials. AIDS activists groups were demanding, and often getting, a seat at corporate and government tables where HIV/AIDS treatment and policy decisions were made.[72]

Recognizing the need for caution in this atmosphere, Merck attempted to learn from the negative experience of its competitor pharmaceutical giant Burroughs Wellcome. In 1987, the testing, distribution, and pricing of Burroughs Wellcome's anti-AIDS drug, AZT, had become a public relations disaster. Because it had developed the first anti-AIDS drug, Burroughs Wellcome had become entangled in the emotionally charged debate about HIV/AIDS and the politics of responding to the epidemic. Desperately in need of treatments, AIDS activists and patient advocates were following Burroughs Wellcome's every move and were often publicly critical of the company's decisions. For example, during the human testing phase, after initial data indicated that AZT was effective, the company was harshly criticized for requiring further placebo-controlled trials before seeking marketing approval. Activists were objecting to the fact that very sick study patients would not be getting active treatment and that these placebo studies would delay getting the drug on the market. It was only much later that the AIDS activists admitted that placebo-controlled trials had been required to ensure that AZT was truly effective. Once AZT was approved by FDA, the pressure on Burroughs Wellcome only mounted. The company set the price so that the retail cost for an annual dosage of AZT was close to $10,000. By doing so, Burroughs Wellcome followed the general practice of pharmaceutical companies of recouping the costs of unsuccessful past research as well as accumulating funds for future research through revenues from successful drugs. Critics charged that this pricing policy failed to recognize AIDS as a major public health problem and that the high cost of treatment would limit access to the drug. On the whole, the entire process of AZT development was characterized by antagonism and distrust between the company and the AIDS activists.[73] For an expanded discussion of these events, see the introduction to this chapter.

Merck viewed Burroughs Wellcome's negative experience as a cautionary tale, and the Merck managers decided to take a different approach to avoid a similar public relations debacle. Knowing that Crixivan might be as much in demand as AZT had been initially, Merck managers decided early on to develop relationships with the AIDS community based on open and honest communication. Starting in March 1991, Merck's Public Affairs Department initiated discussions with such AIDS groups as TAG, Gay Men's Health Crisis, Project Inform, ACT-UP, National AIDS Treatment Advocacy Project, and the National Minority AIDS Council.[74] These meetings were sometimes contentious, but all participants viewed them as necessary and valuable, even if general agreement was not always obtained. Overall, the parties shared the common goal of getting useful drugs to AIDS patients as soon as possible.

EARLY ACCESS TO CRIXIVAN

In early 1995, while the Crixivan team at Merck worked feverishly to shorten the time for getting the drug to market, the activist community questioned whether Merck was doing everything it could to get the drug into production. Some committed AIDS activists even went so far as to attempt to manufacture the drug on their own. They began gathering technical information, raising money, and hiring chemists to manufacture Crixivan.[75] The AIDS Project Los Angeles newsletter was soon reporting that the underground price might be $10,000 a year.[76] At the same time, activists were pressuring Merck to hasten access to the drug.

To alleviate pressure from the outside, Merck published substantial information on its manufacturing process. However, critics and activists insisted that Merck, given its financial resources and scientific capabilities, could do better. Because they did not want to wait until Crixivan had FDA marketing approval, several activists demanded that Merck make Crixivan available sooner on a "compassionate use" basis to patients with advanced AIDS. The terms "compassionate use" or, alternatively, "expanded access" referred to the early availability of a drug while it was still in experimental trials and before marketing approval.[77] Such access was often limited to patients in very advanced stages of disease that had few, if any, treatment options left before death. Expanded access programs were specifically designed to make promising drugs available early in the clinical investigation process. These programs were closely monitored by regulatory agencies to ensure, for one thing, that the company was not side-stepping restrictions on marketing experimental drugs. The decision to develop such a program was not an easy one for any company.

Early in the clinical trial phase of any drug testing, a great deal of uncertainty exists with respect to whether the benefits of a drug outweigh the risks from dangerous side effects. Therefore, despite the fact that some very ill patients want the drug, it may not be prudent to provide it. Expanded access patients are not under strict control, as are study subjects, and potential noncompliance and other variations from the prescribed regimen can produce poor results and, in the case of an anti-AIDS drug, HIV resistance. Also, expanded access programs require enormous resources in both financial and human terms. In Merck's case, the limited supply of available drug was a major factor in the decision. Merck already needed to produce much more drug to meet the requirements of its Phase III trials, which would take place in the United States, Brazil, Canada, and Europe. Given the large quantities needed per subject and the need for an uninterrupted supply, Merck was not sure it could handle the burden of producing even more drug for an expanded access program.[78] Moreover, expanded access programs can be complex to administer, and treatment outcomes are highly uncertain. Because expanded access patients are often sicker and have more medical problems than subjects in controlled clinical trials, expanded access outcome data are often of inferior quality and therefore difficult to evaluate. Did the patient not respond because he or she was too close to death or because the drug was ineffective? In addition, FDA had a history of requesting that this data be submitted as part of an NDA, along with other clinical trial data, thereby potentially compromising the ability to get the drug approved. Finally, drug distribution under an expanded access program can lead to difficult and emotional encounters, as company employees and medical advisors interact with patients who might not live to see the drug approved for marketing.

Despite these difficulties, activist and government officials, including the U.S. Department of Health and Human Services secretary Donna Shalala, pressed for early access to life-saving drugs for people with advanced AIDS. Hoffmann-La Roche responded to these demands in early 1995 when it developed a limited compassionate use program for its protease inhibitor, Invirase.[79] Faced with these combined pressures, Merck executives, notably Paul Reider, met with AIDS activists in February 1995. In an emotional meeting (the partner of one of the activists was dying), the activists pleaded for early access to Merck's experimental drug. The activists brought with them some advisors who were experts in drug manufacturing processes. Upon signing confidentiality agreements, the advisors conducted a review of Merck's production facilities, designs, and plans. At the conclusion of this meeting, the advisors agreed that Merck was indeed doing all that it could in the production realm. However, Reider offered at the meeting that enough Crixivan might be spared to supply four hundred patients. Although it was a disappointingly low number, the activists felt that it was a start. Back at the company, Reider pressed hard to explore ways in which they could further overcome production limitations and speed up drug availability. Again, a critical factor in the discussion was ensuring that there would be enough drug to provide continuous treatment for all people starting treatment with Crixivan. In the meantime, activists pressed even harder for more access, jamming Merck's fax machines and sending in thousands of postcard requests.[80] In March 1995, Merck announced that, beginning in July, it could commit to an expanded access program for 2,150 AIDS patients worldwide. The commitment reflected advances in the production facilities at Merck's pilot plant. Although the final number eligible to enroll in the program was still small relative to the estimated nine hundred thousand people living with HIV in the United States, the activists accepted Merck's solution. Merck's unprecedented disclosures of its manufacturing processes helped to quell many of the doubts and concerns that the AIDS community had posed, but did little to decrease the urgency they felt.

In July 1995, Merck launched the Crixivan Program for People with Advanced HIV Disease, which would provide Crixivan at no cost to fourteen hundred people with advanced AIDS in the United States and to seven hundred and fifty people abroad. In the United States, three hundred slots in the program were specifically reserved for patients who for various reasons were rejected from participating in the clinical studies. The other eleven hundred participants were to be chosen by what Merck referred to as a "random selection process" and which others dubbed a "lottery" system.[81] The lottery was to be organized by an outside entity. The condition for participation was that a patient's immune system be extremely compromised: a CD4 cell count below 50 per milliliter (normal range being 800 to 1,000 per milliliter; AIDS was being diagnosed at levels of 200 per milliliter or below). Merck sent a letter to 130,000 doctors nationwide notifying them of the program.[82] Phone registration for the program was then made available seven days a week, from 8 A.M. to 11 P.M., for one month. The company set up an 800 number system and trained one hundred operators to assist patients with registration and with processing the forms for physicians to certify that the patient met medical criteria. Each registered applicant was then assigned a number. When the registration period ended, more than 11,100 people had applied for the program, which had just 1,100 openings. To select from the registrants, Merck hired an outside auditing firm, which used a random number computer program. The patients with the first 1,100 numbers on the list received an offer to participate in the compassionate use program. These letters were sent first-class in a plain white envelope with no indication that the letter came from Merck.[83]

FDA APPROVAL OF CRIXIVAN

FDA was under political pressure to speed the approval of anti-AIDS drugs. During the beginning of President Clinton's 1992 term, DHHS secretary Shalala announced that "the Clinton Administration is committed to the fight against AIDS, including the President's ultimate goal of a cure for this disease. Rapid FDA action on important new drugs is one important part in reaching the long-term goal."[84] Traditionally, FDA's Center for Drug Evaluation and Research (CDER) required that any company seeking marketing approval of an investigational drug complete three increasingly large phases of human studies to test the safety and efficacy of the drug. Following collection and analysis of all study data, the company would then submit an NDA requesting approval to market the drug.

In 1987, in response to the growing demand by AIDS activists and health professionals for anti-AIDS drugs, FDA created a new drug category, the "AA" priority category, to classify all applications for potential AIDS therapies.[85] Drugs in this category would receive high priority and expedited review. In 1992, FDA revised its accelerated approval process for new drugs to include all drugs (those that provide treatment beyond those already on the market) intended for life-threatening and severely debilitating diseases.[86] Under this expedited process, the company and FDA would work together so that market approval could occur before completion of all phases of the clinical trials. However, any accelerated approval was contingent on the completion of the ongoing human trials and ultimate confirmation of the clinical benefits.[87] In addition, the Prescription Drug User Fee Act, passed by Congress in 1992, led to further reduction in FDA approval time because extra money paid by the companies allowed FDA to hire more personnel to process new drug applications.[88] Under this act, the corporate sponsor paid a fee of $225,000 when submitting an NDA for review, with additional fees for each amendment made to the original application. With these laws in place, efforts were being made on multiple fronts to speed the approval process of anti-AIDS drugs.

In September 1995, Roche was the first company to submit an application for the approval of a protease inhibitor (saquinavir, brand name Invirase). After seeing the Roche application and its supporting data, FDA commissioner David Kessler took an unprecedented step to send a signal to Merck and Abbott that he wanted to see their protease applications as well. Kessler, recounting his appearance on ABC's news show *Nightline*, said he "basically came as close to saying these drugs are safe and effective as I could. I almost sent them the approval letter [over the air]. I figured that was the best incentive. I wanted them to know we were ready, and there should be nothing holding them back." Never in the history of FDA had a commissioner made such a public invitation.[89]

Roche received its FDA marketing approval for Invirase in December 1995, about the time that Abbott submitted an application for its protease inhibitor ritonavir, trade-named Norvir. Before the Crixivan Phase III trials were complete, Merck submitted an NDA for Crixivan on January 31, 1996. By that time, Merck had already reviewed a large portion of the data on Crixivan with the FDA. On March 3, 1996, Abbott received FDA approval for Norvir. Ten days later on March 13, 1996, in a record forty-two days, FDA also approved Merck's Crixivan.[90] Between March 1987 and March 1996, when Crixivan was approved, seven anti-AIDS drugs had been approved by FDA. The review-to-approval time for these drugs ranged from 2.5 months to 6 months. These approval times were extremely fast compared to the more usual drug approval times, often measured in years.

Crixivan had obtained accelerated approval for use alone or in combination with reverse transcriptase inhibitors such as AZT and 3TC. At the time of approval, the drug had been shown to reduce viral levels and increase CD_4 counts, but there were no results from controlled clinical trials evaluating Crixivan's ability to halt the progression of HIV infection, increase probability of survival, or reduce the incidence of opportunistic infections. FDA reserved the right to withdraw the granted approval at a later date if the Merck researchers could not eventually demonstrate that Crixivan provided true benefit, such as an extended life span or a slower disease progression.[91] The FDA approval was also dependent on the company's ability to manufacture the drug. As with other approvals, FDA needed to approve manufacturing facilities and processes before a new drug could be cleared for marketing. In the case of Crixivan, however, because of the tremendous medical need to make the drug available as quickly as possible, the agency approved the NDA with only the pilot manufacturing plant fully functional at the time.

The rapid approvals of Crixivan and other AIDS therapies were applauded by the political and medical communities. FDA commissioner Kessler commented: "The pharmaceutical companies that have led the development of protease inhibitors deserve a lot of credit. It's been a historic period in the fight against AIDS. This accelerated approval, a new record for the agency, is further confirmation of our commitment in the fight."[92]

CHALLENGES FACED BY MERCK UPON THE APPROVAL OF CRIXIVAN

While it was extremely fortunate to have a drug approved in such a short time, marketing approval of Crixivan created new challenges for Merck. Everyone working on the development of Crixivan shared Sheares's view that waiting six months for full-scale manufacturing capability simply was not an option. Still on "Crixivan Time," the production team worked to overcome the obstacles and make the drug available as quickly as possible. Some of the challenges they faced included medical need, supply and demand, suboptimal dosing, manufacturing complexity, volume, and scale-up.

Medical Need

The medical demand for a new treatment and the pressures from the activist community intensified once the data from Merck's landmark study, Protocol #035, was revealed. In the previous year about 53,100 adults and adolescents and 450 children had died of AIDS, and there were an estimated 225,000 Americans living with AIDS.[93] Given these numbers, Merck managers knew they had to make the drug available as quickly as possible to patients in need, regardless of the manufacturing production challenges.

Supply and Demand

It was apparent that demand for the drug would outstrip supply. Until the full-scale production facilities were built, Merck's pilot plant could supply Crixivan for only twenty-five thousand to thirty thousand patients with either HIV infection or AIDS, compared to a patient population of nearly one million in the United States.

Suboptimal Dosing

Merck was concerned that under a limited supply scenario, the drug might be hoarded by patients (thereby reducing availability to others) or that low doses of the drug would be used as a way of extending supply (thereby encouraging viral resistance). Researchers knew that suboptimal dosing, even for short periods of time, could provide opportunities for the virus to replicate and become resistant to therapy, not only with Crixivan but also potentially for all other protease inhibitors. If this happened, patient treatment options would be severely constrained.

Manufacturing Complexity

The manufacturing process for Crixivan remained a highly intricate process. This was the most difficult drug synthesis Merck had ever carried out in a production setting. The protocol for synthesis involved fourteen to sixteen steps, and it now took six weeks to produce one batch. The typical Merck drug only involved four or five steps and required two weeks to produce. The most complicated drug Merck had produced before Crixivan involved twelve manufacturing steps.[94] The complexity of the process demanded the construction of equally complex manufacturing facilities. By the time Crixivan was approved, Merck was working with more than one thousand contractors and paying large premiums for overtime work. Merck had convinced the workers of the urgent need for these facilities, and workers were wearing stickers on their hard hats saying, "Crixivan: it must be built." Plant managers and engineering crews at the plant sites were innovating to increase capacity and shorten process times.

Volume

The volume and dose of drug required for treatment was two orders of magnitude greater than the dosage for any other drug made by Merck. Patients were required to take 2.4 grams of Crixivan per day. This was unusually high, as many of Merck's other medicines required daily doses on the order of 5 milligrams.[95] Another difficulty concerned the unpredictability of the market and how Crixivan would fit into the overall treatment strategy for AIDS. Both of these could influence how much of the drug would need to be manufactured.

Scale-up

Merck was supplying the drug for its trials and for compassionate use entirely from its pilot plant, where production had been maximized. The engineers running the plant were experienced only with the production of these relatively small quantities for trials. Merck needed to train a multitude of other employees in the intricacies of manufacturing scale-up for the novel Crixivan manufacturing processes. The company still did not know how long it would take to achieve the large and consistent volume of production required.

U.S. MANAGED DISTRIBUTION TEAM FOR CRIXIVAN

Despite these problems, the Merck managers quickly made the decision to develop a limited Crixivan distribution program to supply as many patients as possible while the company worked to achieve full manufacturing capability. The U.S. Distribution Team for Crixivan was created to make this happen.

Early Thoughts on Managed Distribution

The Crixivan Program for People with Advanced HIV Disease and its lottery selection process, where patients were chosen based on eligibility, had been difficult and uncomfortable to manage. Merck managers were required to choose the patients who could receive the drug and reject others; not an easy task when patients were so desperate. The company wanted a better distribution system. A Merck spokesperson told the *Wall Street Journal*, "We agonized over how we were going to distribute the product, and we looked at a whole host of alternative ways, including holding back the drug until it was in full-scale production."[96] After sorting out the pros and cons, one of the first decisions made by the team was that the limited supplies of Crixivan would be made available to all patients who requested it on a first-come, first-serve basis. Merck would also count and track patients so that people starting therapy with Crixivan could be ensured a continuous, uninterrupted supply of drug. To accurately determine the number of patients it could supply, the team needed to depend on the pilot plant. Communication between all members of the team was crucial. Any shortages needed to be managed immediately so that the team could stop new patients from starting therapy. Merck also decided that if a selected patient's insurance payer did not cover the cost of the drug, Merck would subsidize the cost of the drug under the company's low-income assistance program.[97] After these decisions had been made, the team had to decide how to create a system to distribute the limited drug supply.

Led by Sheares, the team believed strongly that using the conventional drug distribution channels of wholesalers and retail pharmacies would not be prudent in this situation. Usually wholesalers and pharmacies hold about 50 percent of the stock of a popular drug "in the pipeline" at any given time. The team did not want Crixivan sitting on shelves in some parts of the United States and inaccessible in other parts of the country. Also, patients who were fearful of running out of the drug would tend to stock up on supplies. The team feared this sort of misallocation and hoarding, and decided that it had to manage a much larger part of the drug distribution process than was usual. As a result, the team formulated a plan for a centralized and managed distribution in which Merck would track the number of patients taking Crixivan and be constantly aware of and in control of the balance between supply and demand for the drug.

Selection of Stadtlanders as the Sole Distributor

The team members felt that they had a number of options for centralized distribution. They could choose a mail-order pharmacy, a pharmaceutical wholesaler, or a retail pharmacy. Led by Jerry Wisler, of Pharmacy Affairs, a subteam approached a number of such distributors, explained the situation and their skeleton plan for managed distribution, and invited them to submit bids for the contract.

Choosing the "right" distributor required an in-depth look at the candidates. The examination included on-site studies of the candidates' operations (for example, ability to track, coordinate, and fill prescriptions and also manage reimbursements, which required solid relationships with state Medicare, Medicaid, and other payer programs), as well as their financial health (for example, profitability, growth). Since the problem was unique, both conceptually and from the point of view of its sheer magnitude, no bidder had all of the necessary requirements in place. However, the team took this into account and, coordinated by Mary Dermody and Carol Esch of Merck's business development group, searched for a distributor that displayed the most promising potential to scale up existing capabilities. In the final analysis, there were only a few candidates in the running for this major undertaking, and Merck decided to join its forces with Stadtlanders, a mail-order pharmacy based in Pittsburgh, Pennsylvania.

Stadtlanders was chosen because it had a number of crucial capabilities. According to Carol Esch, Stadtlanders was a well-regarded pharmacy with a successful reimbursement management record. Merck believed that Stadtlanders had the ability to track and count patients. Stadtlanders was also familiar with and had relationships with the HIV patient population, since it specialized in supplying drugs for AIDS treatment. It also knew how to preserve the privacy of its customers. Since a large percentage of anti-AIDS treatments were paid for by private and government insurers and medical programs, it was important that Stadtlanders had relationships with these payers and had been reimbursed by them as a supplier of anti-HIV drugs.

Notwithstanding Stadtlanders's capabilities, the establishment of the infrastructure for the managed distribution program required a major build-up effort by Merck and Stadtlanders. After the launch of Crixivan, Stadtlanders had to be able to handle the addition of several thousand new patients a month, which meant that the mail-order pharmacy had to expand its capacity. It rented additional office space and leased computers, telecommunication equipment, and office furniture.[98] Lisa Fettig, a marketing manager for Crixivan at Merck, and her counterpart at Stadtlanders set up the infrastructure. During this time, Merck continued its dialogue with the AIDS community and sought its feedback on the distribution plans. In the final version of the managed distribution program, it was Stadtlanders who kept track of the particulars for each patient who was dispensed Crixivan. One of Lisa Fettig's jobs was to receive new patient counts on a daily basis and, together with the team, make the daily decision of whether to allow additional patients to start therapy. Given the importance of a constant supply, everyone was aware that any slight miscalculation could have grave consequences for the patients. For the team and its partners at Stadtlanders, this was a tension-filled period that required concentrated cooperation, especially for the meticulous exchange of data. In weekly Monday meetings, the team assessed the current developments and planned the balance of supply and demand for the week to come. In addition, Stadtlanders set up a comprehensive system to remind patients sufficiently in advance that a refill was due. Stadtlanders also introduced a patient newsletter on different aspects of HIV/AIDS that it sent out to its customers on a regular basis.

Response to Merck's Managed Distribution by Stadtlanders

Although Merck and Stadtlanders had worked hard at and had a record of established communication with customers and AIDS activists, the Crixivan distribution program was criticized and attacked on two specific fronts. The retail pharmacists claimed that Stadtlanders's exclusive distribution right precluded any competition and disrupted the solid relationships that existed between patients and their local pharmacists, relationships that were necessary given the large numbers of drugs needed by most AIDS patients. Pharmacists were worried that patients would send all of their prescriptions to Stadtlanders. "It's a way for them to obtain names and addresses of people who are HIV-positive," said Edward Bubar, owner of Eddie's Pharmacy in West Hollywood, California. "Telling a patient to go to one pharmacy across the country is absolutely archaic and really breaks the patient-pharmacy relationship." A pharmacy trade group began a letter-writing campaign to federal regulators and lobbied Congress to forbid drug companies to restrict distribution of their drugs.[99]

The other criticism about the distribution program related to the price charged the patient. The total drug costs for some AIDS patients on protease cocktail therapy and other preventive drugs could be as high as $1,000 to $2,000 per month. Merck had set its Crixivan price at $12.00 a day, which was approximately 30 to 40 percent lower than the other protease inhibitors placed on the market by Roche and Abbott.[100] Merck had been praised by many leaders in the HIV treatment community for pricing Crixivan reasonably and responsibly, according to Mike Doodson, executive director in Merck's economic affairs department, who with his staff developed the pricing recommendations for Crixivan. Jules Levin, who ran the National AIDS Treatment Advocacy Project in New York, said that "Merck has done a very humane thing with the price it's charging."[101] Levin's group instead asked Merck's competitors to lower their prices. Other activists were unhappy about the Crixivan price especially since it added to the already high cost of total drug treatment. "I'm not sure what Merck can do to make some people happy," said Levin, who believed that Merck was "trying to be responsible."[102] Stadtlanders marked the price up 37 percent, which the activists attacked as "outrageous."[103] Despite the fact that only 10 percent of patients paid full price, because most were covered by insurance plans that negotiated lower prices, several AIDS activist groups threatened a boycott and staged protests at Stadtlanders's New York facility. Responding to these demands a month after the launch of Crixivan, Stadtlanders introduced a discount card that offered Crixivan at a reduced price to patients not covered by a health plan.[104]

CONCLUSION: U.S. MANAGED DISTRIBUTION TEAM MEETING, SPRING 1996

At Merck's West Point facility, talk at a 1996 meeting turned to assessing the team's success in meeting the challenges it had faced in implementing the managed distribution program. According to Brad Sheares, Mike Doodson, and team members Lisa Fettig, Carol Esch, Mary Dermody, and Jerry Wisler, the managed distribution program for Crixivan had been a first-of-a kind challenge for Merck. Taking control and tracking patients so that continuous, uninterrupted therapy could be guaranteed was difficult, but all felt that it was the right thing to do since their efforts made a difference in the lives of many people living with AIDS. (See Appendix 11.1.) In addition to improving the lives of individuals, it appeared that protease inhibitors, such as Crixivan, in triple combination therapy with reverse transcriptase inhibitors were making significant inroads in arresting AIDS-related deaths. CDC had just reported the first decline in the rates of AIDS-related deaths, by as much as 33 percent in males.[105]

Overall, the team believed it had met the expectations of the many stakeholders concerned about the distribution of the drug, implemented an effective tracking system to catch all patients and refills, managed the supply of the drug to meet the demand, and met the criticisms of retail pharmacies that had been bypassed and activists concerned about the central distribution process. Getting Crixivan to market had taken four hundred people almost ten years and over $700 million. The effort would be remembered at Merck as one of the company's longest and most expensive drug development projects, its most complex manufacturing process, and its biggest production effort.[106] Merck credited Stadtlanders for its professional management and staff, organizational flexibility, ability to reach patients wherever they were located, and relationships with payers. These attributes were critical to the success of the distribution program. There were still many unanswered questions about how Crixivan and the other protease inhibitors were best used to treat HIV infection and AIDS. Sorting through these questions would take years of research.[107] But the drug had been launched. Merck was optimistic that its production obstacles would soon be overcome if they could just continue to match drug supply with the needs of their first patients. The team members left the meeting with an intense conviction that if they could continue their success in managing the distribution of this important drug until full manufacturing capacity was available, it would be the highlight of their professional careers. They had made a difference.

Questions

1. Did Merck handle the "lottery" program for investigational Crixivan appropriately? Compare this program to the one developed to manage the limited postapproval supplies. What distributive justice elements were served or ignored?

2. What are the benefits and risks to companies that allow compassionate use access to clinical research trials?

3. Did Merck appropriately handle the AIDS activists and pharmacists who protested the manner in which the company handled the drug distribution and Merck's and Stadtlanders's drug pricing?

Discussion

This case focuses on a classic distributive justice issue of how to allocate important resources when the demand outstrips supply. Attempting to decide what is fair and reasonable is always difficult when these scarce resources are potentially life saving. In the case of Crixivan, Merck used components of several different distribution systems, all of which had their pluses and minuses. A random selection or a lottery, by itself, can seem arbitrary and cruel. All of the needy patients do not exist at the same time, and with a "first come, first served" program, the rewards go to better-informed, better-connected patients, such as the activists who can get to the front of the line faster. Patients who can pay for the drug also get ahead of those who cannot. However, these are not always the neediest patients. Any distribution system that does not include need as a criterion invites petitions for compassionate exception. In a need-based program, the definition of who is neediest is also tricky. Sicker patients may be most in need but may be so sick as to be beyond help, thereby creating the prospect that the resource will be wasted and that the drug will be denied to someone whose life it could have saved. Patients who can benefit the most may often be the less sick. Worthiness is also suspect as a distribution criterion since denying the drug to an IV drug abuser because of the fear that the risky behavior would resume and obliterate the benefits of the drug can raise the specter of disfavored social worth criteria, which were used when kidney dialysis was new and scarce. Limiting worthiness to medical criteria, a distribution scheme can be set up where patients' physicians must petition Merck and qualify for the drug by showing, for instance, that their physicians certify that they are medically appropriate, will benefit from the drug, are compliant, and so on. Patients who do not have ready access to a motivated physician would be left out of this program. To resolve the disparities inherent in classic distribution schemes, a Rawls's approach with its elements of rights and justice, fair equality of opportunity, and giving greatest advantage to the worst-off patients may provide insights about the fairest approach.

Appendix 11.1

Testimonials from Patients Taking Protease Inhibitors

DAVID SANFORD

This fifty-two-year-old page one features editor of the *Wall Street Journal* was dying of AIDS, had written his own obituary and handed it in to his superiors at the newspaper, and started saying his good-byes. He was then started on a protease inhibitor and, writing of his experience one year later, said:

> What has happened in the past year, at least for me, is a miracle that couldn't have taken place at any other moment. The year 1996 is when everything changed, and very quickly, for people with AIDS. I have been grappling with this disease for nearly a decade and a half, almost since the beginning, when it was called Gay Related Immune Deficiency, or GRID. I've outlived friends and peers, and now I find myself in the unusual position of telling people how I've survived this scourge, something I never thought would happen. My condition could change for the worse tomorrow. But today I feel well again. Thanks to the arrival of the new drugs called protease inhibitors, I am probably more likely to be hit by a truck than to die of AIDS.[108]

STEVE SCHALCHLIN

Steve Schalchlin, a singer and songwriter, started keeping an on-line diary when he was in his thirties, dying of AIDS. He wanted to let other people know about his experience so that others could understand and have compassion for those in his situation. At the time that Crixivan was approved by FDA in March 1996, Schalchlin had fought off multiple infections, but his health was beginning to deteriorate further. He was dangerously underweight, had severe diarrhea from his HIV drugs and an intestinal parasite for which there was no treatment, and he had an ear infection. His physicians started him on intravenous feeding to gain weight and enrolled him in the Crixivan distribution program on April 6, 1996. Because of delays attributed to a loss of insurance coverage and having to switch to Medicaid, he started taking the drug on May 22, 1996. On July 2, 1996, he wrote in his on-line diary:

> Here's the incredible news: my viral load test results, the first test I've had since starting last month on the new protease inhibitor, Crixivan, is beyond my wildest dreams. My viral load—the amount of virus in my blood—has dropped from the dangerous 60,000 parts to—I can't believe it:
>
> Under 100.
>
> That's right. Under 100. From 60,000 to under 100. That means that the drug has, for the moment, stopped the virus dead in its tracks and my body now has a chance to rebuild its immune system because it doesn't have to spend all its time fighting the virus and losing!
>
> This is a miracle and it means I have a new lease on life. Again, remember at the end of last month, we thought it was all over. Now, it's as if God Himself just took a magic wand and cleaned them out of my body. It means the virus is virtually undetectable in my blood!!
>
> Now my t-cells can grow again and if all goes well, we can get me out of the danger zone for most of the worst opportunistic infections. My t-cell count has been around 40. This means I am open to CMV retinitus (which causes blindness), MAC—a disease of the intestinal tract that causes death, MAI, cancer, PCP (pneumonia, which I've already had once and am very susceptible to again), and more.
>
> But now my t-cells have a real chance to go up above 100, maybe close to 200! (800 to 1200 is normal, so I won't be out of the woods as far as life threatening infections go), but this is probably why my diarrhea has stopped too. I should get the new t-cell count today so when I do, you'll be the first to know.

Gradually, Schalchlin regained his weight and his health. He began to call his life at that stage "Living in the Bonus Round." On August 2, 1996, after completing the production of a play and its last performance to a standing ovation, he wrote:

> Right now, I'm basking in a glow that many people can only dream about, but one which I am actually living out. I shall remember this night for a very long time and I will thank God and whomever else wants credit for it. Even though my health is amazing right now, I still intend to live one day at a time to savor every single moment. Tomorrow will take care of tomorrow. None of us are guaranteed anything beyond this moment right now. And I've said it before, but I'll say it again.
>
> I'm just so very, very happy to be alive.[109]

Notes

1. Thalidomide was a drug approved in Europe and Canada in the 1950s and 1960s and used to combat nausea in pregnancy. It was discovered too late that the drug caused severe limb malformations and other birth defects in ten thousand children born of women who took the drug. Thalidomide was never legally approved in the United States, a fact that was widely attributed to the FDA's more conservative approval requirements.

2. Activists also knew that, in addition to receiving access to potentially life-saving drugs, they would also receive excellent and free medical care that, especially for indigent patients, would not otherwise be available. Brotman B. Any volunteers? Being a guinea pig has its risks and its rewards. *Chicago Tribune* 1992 May 19; Sect C:1.

3. This traditional view of research meant that researchers should not proceed with any study unless they were in a state of "clinical equipoise"; that is, the research was justified because the investigators were equally uncertain about whether the drug would or would not prove to be beneficial. If there was a genuine belief that the drug was beneficial, it was considered unethical to continue research; the drug should be administered as treatment.

4. Epstein S. *Impure science: AIDS, activism, and the politics of knowledge.* Berkeley, CA: University of California Press; 1996.

5. Hilts PJ. How the AIDS crisis made drug regulators speed up. *New York Times* 1989 Sept 24; Sect. D:5.

6. Power SH. The right of privacy in choosing medical treatment: Should terminally ill persons have access to drugs not yet approved by the Food and Drug Administration? *John Marshall Law Review* 1987; 20:693–714.

7. People v. Privitera, 23 Cal. 3d 697 at 711, (Bird, CJ, dissenting), cert. denied, 444 U.S. 949 (1979).

8. U.S. v. Rutherford, 442 U.S. 554 (1979).

9. National Gay Rights Advocates v. United States Department of Health & Human Services. No. 87-CV-1735 Civ. (D.D.C. April 26, 1988).

10. See Note 4.

11. Greenberg MD. AIDS experimental drug approval, and the FDA new drug screening process. *New York University Journal of Legislation and Public Policy* 1999–2000; 3:295–350.

12. See 52 *Federal Register* 19,466 and 21 *Code of Federal Regulations* 312.35, 1994.

13. Batterman JS. Brother can you spare a drug: Should the experimental drug dis-

tribution standards be modified in response to the needs of persons with AIDS? *Hofstra Law Review* 1990; 19:191.

14. Announced at 57 *Federal Register* 13,250, 1992. The parallel track program allows promising new drugs for treating AIDS and other HIV-related diseases to be made more widely available to people unable to take standard therapy, and who are not able to participate in controlled studies.

15. See Note 11.

16. Bazell R. *Her-2: The making of Herceptin, a revolutionary treatment for breast cancer.* New York: Random House; 1998. p. 131.

17. In 1989, the personal use import exemption, while not made a formal regulation, was included in the FDA Regulatory Procedures Manual, ch. 9-71-30(C), at pp. 4–5.

18. Span P. Pharmacy for the desperate; AIDS buyers' clubs dispensing untested hope. *Washington Post* 1992 Apr 8:Sect. D:1.

19. Ibid.

20. Ibid.

21. Described in 53 *Federal Register* 41,516, 41,523, 1998, these regulations are 21 *Code of Federal Regulations* 312.80–97 and 21 *Code of Federal Regulations* 314.500, and 21 *Code of Federal Regulations* 601.4. Subpart E states: "The Food and Drug Administration (FDA) has determined that it is appropriate to exercise the broadest flexibility in applying the statutory standards, while preserving appropriate guarantees for safety and effectiveness. These procedures reflect the recognition that physicians and patients are generally willing to accept greater risks or side effects from products that treat life-threatening and severely debilitating illnesses, than they would accept from products that treat less serious illnesses. These procedures also reflect the recognition that the benefits of the drug need to be evaluated in light of the severity of the disease being treated."

22. An example of a surrogate endpoint could be blood tests showing reduction in immune system damage rather than requiring the longer time it would take to show that a drug delayed disease-related death.

23. See Note 11.

24. Ibid.

25. Ibid.

26. Dillman JP. Prescription drug approval and terminal diseases: Desperate times require desperate measures. *Vanderbilt Law Review* 1991; 44:925–51.

27. See Note 4.

28. Wellcome; the dead hand of charity. *Economist* 1990 Dec 22:94.

29. AZT stood for azidothymidine, which Burroughs Wellcome eventually marketed as Retrovir.

30. Emmons W. *Burroughs Wellcome and AZT (A).* Boston: Harvard Business School; 1993 Feb 26. pp. 1–21. Available from http://harvardbusinessonline.hbsp.harvard.edu/b02/en/cases/cases_home.jhtml.

31. Ibid.

32. The Orphan Drug Act of 1983 (21 U.S.C. 360) provided pharmaceutical companies with three types of incentives to develop drugs for diseases that afflicted less

than two hundred thousand persons in the United States or in cases where there was no reasonable expectation that the costs of development and manufacturing could be recouped from U.S. sales. First, companies could receive a tax credit of 50 percent of clinical testing costs during the time the drug was under consideration for FDA approval. Also, the government would provide assistance during the clinical trials and approval processes. Finally, the company would obtain seven years of market exclusivity, regardless of whether the new orphan drug was patentable. During the early years of the AIDS crisis, several anti-AIDS drugs received orphan drug status that was not revoked as the AIDS epidemic grew, since the act also allowed orphan drug status to continue even if the patient population grew to greater than two hundred thousand during the seven-year exclusivity period. Burroughs Wellcome obtained orphan drug status for AZT to treat AIDS during the time that the disease affected less than two hundred thousand patients. But as the AIDS epidemic spread, the number of persons with the full-blown disease grew to more than 270,000 at the end of 1984, so that such drugs were no longer eligible for orphan drug status. In addition, AZT was denied orphan status in 1985 for the treatment of AIDS-related Complex or ARC, the name given to those patients who were infected with HIV but had not developed the full manifestations of AIDS. This orphan drug application was denied when Burroughs Wellcome failed to provide data to show that ARC affected fewer than two hundred thousand patients. However, FDA reversed its denial in 1987 when Burroughs Wellcome amended its application to apply to a smaller group of patients who had "advanced" ARC. This move by Burroughs Wellcome was viewed by company critics as having gamed the Orphan Drug Act by stacking the exclusive marketing periods for the two target patient populations and thereby blocking the competition for AZT, which would have introduced price competition. Peter Arno, associate professor in the Department of Epidemiology and Social Medicine at Albert Einstein College of Medicine, New York, believed that companies "stand to make a fortune" if they develop a successful AIDS drug and that seeking further economic assistance from the government was a "manipulation by the industry of the AIDS community."

33. President Hailger later told the *Wall Street Journal* that the company spent more than $80 million to test and develop AZT.

See also Note 30.

34. Centers for Disease Control. *HIV/AIDS surveillance*. Department of Health and Human Services. 1990 Feb.

35. See Note 30.

36. See Note 11.

37. The initial case study was prepared by Madhuri Mani Roy and Marko Curavic under the guidance of and with later revision by Margaret Eaton. The input and assistance of the members of the Crixivan Distribution Team, Bradley Sheares, Lisa Fettig, Carol Esch, and Mike Doodson, and especially of Kyra Lindemann at Merck & Co., are greatly appreciated. We also thank Steve Schalchlin who provided insight about people with AIDS and helped us teach this case study. The events described in this case study occurred up until spring 1996.

38. Merck 1996 annual report, Merck & Co. Inc.

39. Gilmartin RV. *Innovation, ethics and core values as keys to global success.* Text of a speech by Raymond V. Gilmartin, chairman, president, and chief executive officer of Merck & Co. Inc. New York; 1998 Oct 20; p. 15; Merck & Co. Inc. *The Merck story: Serving society.* 1994; p. 1; Merck 1996 annual report to security holders, Form 10-Q. Filing date: 1997 Mar.

40. Merck & Co. Inc. Overview and history of Merck's research activities. In *The Merck story: Serving society.* 1994; pp. 1–5.

41. Merck & Co. Inc. Corporate philanthropy report. 1998; p. 13.

42. Merck & Co. Inc. Corporate philanthropy report. 1998; p. 11.

43. See Note 39, Gilmartin.

44. Common infections and cancers seen in AIDS patients included pneumocystis carinii pneumonia, tuberculosis, Kaposi's sarcoma, cryptosporidiosis, yeast infections, such as from candida, cytomegolavirus, isosporiasis, toxoplasmosis, cryptococcosis, non-Hodgkin's lymphoma, varicella zoster, and herpes simplex. Most of these diseases were themselves severely disabling or lethal.

45. Centers for Disease Control and Prevention, National Center for HIV, STD and TB Prevention, Divisions of HIV/AIDS Prevention. *HIV/AIDS Surveillance Report* 1995; 7:1–38. Available from www.cdc.gov/hiv/stats/hivsur72.pdf.

46. Center for Disease Control and Prevention, National Center for HIV, STD and TB Prevention, Divisions of HIV/AIDS Prevention. *HIV/AIDS recommendations & guidelines.* Available from www.cdc.gov/nchstp/hiv_aids/.

47. Eventually it was learned that HIV could mutate so effectively that it could produce millions of different forms, even in one individual.

48. Centers for Disease Control and Prevention. *HIV/AIDS Surveillance Report* 1996; 8:1–40. Available from www.cdc.gov/hiv/stats/hivsur82.pdf.

49. Ho DD. Time to hit HIV, early and hard [editorial]. *New England Journal of Medicine* 1995; 333:450–51.

50. Centers for Disease Control and Prevention, National Center for HIV, STD and TB Prevention. *Milestones in the U.S. HIV epidemic.* Available from www.cdc.gov/nchstp/od/20years.htm.

51. Waldholz, M. Companies expect big costs, not huge profits. *Wall Street Journal* 1996 June 14; Sect. A:6.

52. Galambos L, Sewell JE. *Confronting AIDS: Science and business cross a unique frontier.* Business History Group and Johns Hopkins University, Merck & Co. Inc.; 1998.

53. Information for a large portion of this and subsequent sections of the case study was drawn from an extensive history of Merck's Crixivan development program: Galambos L, Sewell JE. *Confronting AIDS: Science and business cross a unique frontier.* Business History Group and Johns Hopkins University, Merck & Co. Inc.; 1998. Notes indicate when information was obtained from other sources.

54. Navia M, Fitzgerald P, McKeever BM, et al. Three-dimensional structure of aspartyl protease from human immunodeficiency virus HIV-1. *Nature* 1989; 337:615–20.

55. Fried S. Cocktail hour. *Washington Post* 1997 May 18; Sect. W:10.

56. Merck 1996 annual report, Merck & Co. Inc.

57. Waldholz M. Merck scientists find a chink in the armor of the AIDS virus. *Wall Street Journal* 1989 Feb 16; Sect. A:1.

58. Collins H, Vedantam S. 8 years and $700 million later, how a better drug was found; this breakthrough might save the lives of people once doomed by an HIV-positive diagnosis. *Philadelphia Inquirer* 1996 Mar 17; Sect. A:1.

59. Ibid.

60. Ibid.

61. Common side-effects from anti-AIDS drugs included abdominal pain, fatigue or weakness, dry mouth, flank pain, nausea, diarrhea, vomiting, acid regurgitation, loss of appetite, back pain, headache, trouble sleeping, dizziness, rashes, upper respiratory infections, dry skin, and sore throat. More dangerous side effects also occurred but were less common.

Attacking AIDS with a "cocktail" therapy. *FDA Consumer Magazine* 1999 July–Aug. Available from www.fda.gov/fdac/499_toc.html.

62. Spilker B. Production issues. In *Multinational pharmaceutical companies: Principles and practices*. 2nd ed. New York: Raven Press; 1994. pp. 596–611.

63. Waldholz M. Merck claims its AIDS drug is the best yet. *Wall Street Journal* 1995 Feb 23; Sect. B:1.

64. Tanouye E, Waldholz M. Merck's marketing of an AIDS drug draws fire. *Wall Street Journal* 1996 May 7; Sect. B:1.

65. See Note 63.

66. PR Newswire Association, Inc. FDA grants marketing clearance for Crixivan, new protease inhibitor for HIV: Merck's AIDS medication receives accelerated review. *Financial News* 1996 Mar 14. Available from http://aegis.com/news/pr/1996/pr960314.html.

67. Collins H, Vedantam S. A new drug in the race with death; researchers at Merck & Co. were closing in on a new medicine; but AIDS patients were dying daily. A group of activists felt they had no time to wait. So they stole the formula. *Philadelphia Inquirer* 1996 Mar 18; Sect. A:1; see also Note 55.

68. Personal interview with members of the U.S. Distribution Team for Crixivan. 1999 Nov 8; West Point, PA.

69. Taylor R. Allies against AIDS: Gay Men's Health Crisis and ACT UP. *Journal of NIH Research* 1993 July: 37–42.

70. See www.actupny.org.

71. See Note 55.

72. Ibid.

73. Emmons W, Nimgade A. *Burroughs Wellcome and AZT*. Harvard Business School, Case Study. 1993 Feb 26.

74. Personal communication, Kyra Lindemann, director of public affairs, U.S. Human Health, Merck & Co., Inc.; 1999 Nov 8; West Point, PA.

75. See Note 67, Collins, Vedantam.

Activists obtained the drug's formula and manufacturing information by culling the worldwide scientific literature, attending scientific meetings and lectures given by Merck scientists, and analyzing the contents of the capsules used in Merck's clinical trials. They eventually succeeded in working out the process but dropped the project when it appeared that FDA approval of Crixivan was imminent.

76. See Note 55.

77. *Expanded access and expedited approval of new therapies related to HIV/AIDS.* Office of Special Health Issues: Available from www.fda.gov/oashi/aids/expanded.html. See also, information on expanded access in the introduction to this chapter.

78. Personal interview with members of the U.S. Distribution Team for Crixivan, 1999 Nov 8; West Point, PA.

79. Hoffman-LaRoche's program was intended to supply 2,280 patients with the drug and in less than one month had received ten thousand calls from patients who wanted to register for the lottery. Associated Press Wire Service. Lottery for AIDS drug. *New York Times* 1995 July 18; Sect. C:3. Hoffmann-LaRoche was later criticized when the lottery was delayed until October 1995 and then shut down after the drug was approved in December 1995. Greene JB, Kramer L. On AIDS drug, profits over patients. [Letter to the editor] *New York Times* 1995 Dec 18; Sect. A:16.

80. See Note 67, Collins, Vedantam.

81. Lotteries set up for two experimental AIDS drugs. *American Journal of Health-System Pharmacy* 1995; 52:1848.

82. Associated Press Wire Service. Lottery for AIDS drug. *New York Times* 1995 July 18; Sect. C:3.

83. See Note 67, Collins, Vedantam.

84. FDA grants accelerated approval to third protease inhibitor to treat HIV. *FDA News* 1996 Mar 14. Available from www.fda.gov/bbs/topics/NEWS/NEW00528.html.

85. According to one newspaper article, "Because of the efforts of TAG (the Treatment Action Group), for the first time in pharmaceutical history, the development of a drug would be heavily influenced by the people who actually took it." The government reorganized its entire AIDS research program based on a TAG critique, and the group along with the Gay Men's Health Crisis and Project Inform, played a major role in getting FDA to set up an "accelerated approval" program that created a separate "fast track" for AIDS drugs. Galloro V. Abbott seeks FDA OK for stronger anti-AIDS drug. *Chicago Daily Herald* 2000 June 6; Sect. Business:1.

86. Accelerated development/review. *Federal Register* 1992 Apr 15. Available from www.fda.gov/cder/handbook/accel.htm.

87. Food and Drug Administration. *Expanded access and expedited approval of new therapies related to HIV/AIDS.* Office of Special Health Issues. Available from www.fda.gov/oashi/aids/expanded.html.

88. Public Law 102–571 as amended by Public Law 105–115. See www.fda.gov/cber/pdufa.htm.

89. See Note 55.

90. See Note 84.

91. In February 1999, based on clinical endpoint data submitted by Merck that demonstrated a medical benefit, the company received full FDA approval.

92. See Note 84.

93. Centers for Disease Control and Prevention. *HIV/AIDS Surveillance Report* 1996; 8:1–40. Available from www.cdc.gov/hiv/stats/hivsur82.pdf.

94. The scientist in charge of producing Crixivan was also a gourmet chef. He told one reporter that making Crixivan was "like cooking an intricate, multicourse meal— for 1000 people. If you wrote the 'recipe' for Crixivan, 14 steps in all, each step would cover 60 pages." See Note 58.

Merck & Co., Inc. Crixivan: A Test of MMD's Agility. *Merck World* 1996 Sept; pp. 2–3.

95. Merck & Co., Inc. Crixivan: A Test of MMD's Agility. *Merck World* 1996 Sept; pp. 2–3.

96. See Note 64.

97. The Merck Patient Assistance Program provided temporary access to Merck prescription medicines free of charge to qualified U.S. patients in need. To be eligible for participation in the program, the patient could not have pharmaceutical insurance coverage or afford to pay for medication, and a physician needed to determine that a Merck medicine was appropriate for treatment. There was a separate assistance program for Crixivan called SUPPORT, established in April 1996. Beyond providing medicine free of charge to those who qualified, SUPPORT also offered patient case management by a reimbursement counselor. These services, such as researching insurance policies and assistance with forms, were available to any patient or health-care provider, regardless of the patient's qualification for Merck medicine free of charge. Merck & Co., Inc. *Merck background information. SUPPORT: Accessing the reimbursement SUPPORT and Patient Assistance programs for Crixivan (indinavir sulfate).*

98. Personal communication, Kyra Lindemann, director of public affairs, U.S. Human Health, Merck & Co., Inc. 1999 Nov 8; West Point, PA.

99. See Note 64.

100. Ibid.

101. Waldholz M. Merck's newly approved AIDS drug is priced 30% below rival medicine. *Wall Street Journal* 1996 Mar 15; Sect. B:5.

102. See Note 64.

103. Jacobs A. neighborhood report: Greenwich Village: Agonizing delays for AIDS drug. *New York Times* 1996 Apr 7; Sect. 13:6.

104. ACT-UP/Philadelphia Press Release. *Activists win price break on new AIDS drug.* 1996 Apr 24. Available from www.actupny.org/reports/stadt.html.

105. Centers for Disease Control and Prevention, National Center for HIV, STD and TB Prevention. *Milestones in the U.S. HIV epidemic.* Available from www.cdc.gov/nchstp/od/20years.htm.

106. Merck 1996 annual report, Merck & Co. Inc.; see also Note 58.

107. These questions included: Should the protease inhibitors be taken early in the course of HIV infection or saved for later? What was the best drug to start with? What

were the best combinations? Would cross-resistance develop between the drugs? What were the comparative side effects of the compounds? Were the drugs any less powerful for those who had already been on AZT compared to those who had not? Would resistance ultimately develop to the cocktail therapies as it had with single drug therapy?

108. Sanford D. Back to a future: One man's AIDS tale shows how quickly epidemic has turned. Last year this editor wrote his own obituary; now, he writes of surviving. *Wall Street Journal* 1996 Nov 8; Sect. A:1.

109. Steve Schalchlin, *On line diary*. Available from www.bonusround.com.

12

Advertising Prescription Drugs Directly to Patients[1]

Until the early 1980s, prescription drug advertising was directed solely to physicians (either through sales staff or in medical journal advertisements or other medical venues) and was heavily regulated by the Food and Drug Administration.[2] FDA developed its Division of Drug Marketing, Advertising, and Communications (DDMAC) for this regulatory purpose. The regulations were to ensure that the advertising and other promotion was supported by scientific data and accurately reflected indications, contraindications, risks, benefits, use instructions, and warnings, and that it contained other information required by the FDA.[3] Drug advertising aimed at lay people, while not illegal, was considered ill-advised by manufacturers since the absence of formal FDA guidance or regulations created uncertainty about how FDA would treat any particular approach. It was also widely believed that consumer ads for prescription drugs were inappropriate because lay people lacked the education to understand the technical medical information that would be conveyed. However, during the late 1970s and early 1980s, with the advent of health consumerism in general, drug companies began to experiment with what subsequently became known as "direct-to-consumer" or DTC drug advertising. In 1982, FDA found many of these DTC ads to be objectionable (that is, not truthful or biased or misleading) and called for a voluntary moratorium while it set about determining the overall implications of this type of advertising to determine whether it should be allowed and, if so, with what oversight. The information collected convinced the agency that consumers legitimately wanted access to prescription drug information but that they easily could be misled by drug ads. In 1985, FDA announced in the *Federal Register* that DTC prescription drug advertising would be allowed and that current regulations governing prescription drug advertising to physicians provided sufficient safeguards to protect consumers.

In these drug promotion regulations, FDA focused on the accuracy of the advertised information, the *fair balance* between the benefits and risk information presented, and whether all *material* information was presented. To meet these requirements, the regulations specified that ads had to be accompanied by a *brief summary* of drug information, which included extensive details about side effects, contraindications, and effectiveness. Recognizing that it was not feasible to present the large amount of information required for print ads in a radio or television ad, the FDA regulations allowed broadcast advertisements to include a *major statement* of the drug's chief side effects and contraindications and either a brief summary—as was required for print advertisements—or an *adequate provision* for dissemination of the drug's full prescribing information.

Many manufacturers found that the regulations made it difficult to accomplish what they believed to be effective advertising. For instance, the brief summary required in print ads often took a full page of tiny print listing all of the indications, contraindications, and potential side effects of the drug. This requirement added to the cost and the complexity of the ad and, given the technical medical language used, led companies to question whether the information would be read or understood by consumers. With the extensive information required, it also was not possible to provide the brief summary in radio or television ads. But manufacturers were unclear about how to meet major statement or adequate provision requirements for DTC broadcast ads, and often were told by FDA to stop the ad or risk the imposition of sanctions. As a consequence, manufacturers attempted to produce ads that avoided these pitfalls. Since the regulations stated that the major statement of side effects and contraindications was required whenever the ad contained both the name of the drug and its purpose, some drug companies avoided the major statement obligation by omitting from the ad either the name or the purpose of the drug. Such ads, however, often left consumers guessing what the ad was all about.[4] For instance, an ad showing a wind surfer sailing through a wheat field with the name of a drug displayed at his feet prompted many viewers to wonder briefly about what it was promoting and then forget the ad altogether.[5] Such a reaction would be disappointing for the pharmaceutical company attempting (at high cost) to advertise this drug. In contrast, an ad that encouraged a consumer to see a physician about a particular disease did not accomplish the purpose of promoting the company's drug. Because of these problems, many manufacturers felt that the regulations made it virtually impossible to promote drugs on radio or television and began to lobby FDA to generate concrete and reasonable DTC broadcast rules.

DEVELOPMENT AND ENFORCEMENT OF FDA'S DTC BROADCAST AD GUIDELINES

Twelve years later, in 1997, FDA published proposed DTC broadcast ad guidelines.[6] These guidelines were not final nor were they mandatory at the time that Zeneca (the company featured in the following case study) was attempting to design its DTC ads in November 1998. But the guidelines did provide Zeneca and other companies with some boundaries within which to structure their broadcast ads. Two years after the publication of the proposed guidelines, in August 1999, FDA issued a final guidance on DTC broadcast advertising that was substantially similar to the draft guidance but with some distinct differences that again forced drug companies to alter their advertising strategies.[7]

The draft and final broadcast guidance reinforced the requirements that DTC ads be truthful and not misleading, clearly communicate the product's indication, and adequately communicate the most important risk information. To comply with the broadcast guidelines, pharmaceutical ads in broadcast media that named the drug and its indication were required to contain information about major side effects and contraindications in audio or audio plus visual format. In addition, the ad needed to contain the brief summary or make adequate provision for providing this part of the product labeling. The adequate provision requirement could be met with a multi-faceted approach to provide a diverse audience with the required product information, such as with (1) a toll-free number for information to be mailed, faxed, or read, (2) a reference to DTC print advertisements (which would contain the brief summary), (3) an Internet Web page address, and (4) a statement that directed consumers to physicians or pharmacists for additional information about the product. The choices were varied in order to address consumers' differing levels of use of or comfort with sophisticated technology, to accommodate active and passive information seekers, and to allow access for those who did not want to disclose personal information (such as their address) in order to obtain the product information.[8] FDA also requested, but did not require, that DTC ads be sent to the DDMAC for review prior to release.

As a consequence of the new FDA broadcast guidance, which, for the first time, effectively allowed brand name and drug purpose to be advertised together in a broadcast ad, drug companies began to move a large share of their DTC drug advertising from print to television. However, companies still did not see eye-to-eye with FDA about how to implement the drug advertising rules. In the first two years after the issuance of the proposed DTC broadcast guidelines (1997 and 1998), FDA objected to more than half of the DTC television ads produced (eighteen of thirty-five) and initiated enforcement actions against these companies, requiring that the ads be stopped or changed.[9] Using notices of violation, FDA had the authority to make companies change or stop ads, publish retractions, or send corrective letters to doctors. In egregious circumstances, FDA also could seize the advertised products or criminally prosecute the corporate executives responsible for issuing the ads.[10] However, these latter two remedies were rarely sought for drug advertising violations, and FDA had no authority to seek monetary penalties. When companies protested about the number of ads that had to be pulled, the agency responded that enforcement actions were the expected cost of adopting a new policy.[11] As time went by, pharmaceutical companies adapted to the new rules and the prevalence of enforcement actions decreased. However, they were never eliminated because innovative advertising strategies (including the advent of Internet advertising) would continue to challenge DDMAC's interpretations of what constituted appropriate consumer-directed drug advertising.[12]

According to FDA regulators who spoke frequently on this topic at industry meetings, common problems with DTC print ads were that the drug claims were too broad or incomplete, the ads contained incomplete explanations or were out of context, or there was a lack of fair balance between the risks and benefits of the drug. Lack of "fair balance" led the FDA to censure ads that had distracting or simultaneous presentation of risks and benefits, that minimized or omitted risk information, or in which risk information received too little prominence, was displayed too fast, or was less audible than the benefit information.

For example, FDA had required Wyeth-Ayerst Laboratories to withdraw a television commercial for one of its drugs, stating that "multiple distracting visual images and activity occur during the audio presentation of the risk information, but the drug's benefits are described clearly and cogently, against a visual background without any distractions."[13] Pfizer, Inc., and Pharmacia Corporation were told to cut a widely aired television ad for their arthritis drug Celebrex®; the FDA thought the ads overstated the drug's effectiveness, because supposedly arthritic seniors on the drug were seen using scooters and otherwise engaged in overly vigorous physical activity. Schering-Plough, manufacturer of the widely advertised allergy drug Claritin®, was told by FDA to change its telephone responses to consumers who called the advertised 800 number for drug side effect information. Callers were made to listen to a four-minute promotional message and then respond to a marketing survey before being given a second 800 number to call for what FDA considered only limited side effect information.[14] Other problems with some drug ads included the printing of side effect information in white letters on a white background, broadcasting an ad in Spanish with side effects presented in English, and broadcasting ads with a wide target audience that referred the consumer to a complete source of drug information in a publication with a more narrow target audience.[15] At the same time that FDA was publicizing information about the objectionable ads, its regulators also acknowledged the agency's limited resources to promulgate specific guidelines, review proposed ads in a timely fashion, conduct surveillance of published ads, and enforce existing guidelines.[16]

All of this activity within FDA and the prescription drug industry was accompanied by debates about whether DTC prescription drug advertising was good or bad for the medical profession and the public. These debates prompted the agency to publicize the message that it was interested in receiving empirical study data that could show whether the public health was being harmed, or was likely to be harmed, by FDA's actions in facilitating DTC prescription drug advertising. By 1999, no such data had been published, and the agency decided that it would conduct consumer surveys to evaluate whether DTC drug advertising had had any of the hypothesized ill effects.[17]

COST EFFECTIVENESS OF DTC PRESCRIPTION DRUG ADVERTISING

In the meantime, although there was insufficient research data available on the consumer impact or the cost effectiveness of DTC drug advertising, drug manufacturers pursued it initially on the general belief that such advertising would be as effective as it was for other products. Manufacturers soon learned that assessing the impact of consumer-directed pharmaceutical ads was a difficult task. Prescription records did not indicate whether a physician was encouraged by the patient to prescribe a particular drug. To learn more, companies began to hire consulting firms to conduct studies to provide conclusive evidence of the impact of these ads.

While this research was underway, anecdotes appeared showing how powerful DTC prescription drug advertising could be. For instance, in 1992, a nicotine patch that had been on the market relatively unnoticed for months was advertised during the Super Bowl. According to the American Association of Advertising Agencies, the public response to the ad was so great that within weeks demand for the patches exceeded supply. A DTC ad for a new osteoporosis drug was believed to have had a similar impact. In the year following the ad, patient visits to physicians for osteoporosis in the United States nearly doubled, from 409,000 visits in the fourth quarter of 1995 to 713,000 in the same period of 1996. Although there was no direct evidence to substantiate it, the firm conducting the research attributed a large portion of the increase to the new drug ads.[18] Likewise, when the male impotency drug Viagra® was first advertised to the public and reported on by the media, physician visits for impotency more than doubled from the same period of time the prior year. Health-care consulting firm research showed that nearly two-thirds of these visits involved a request for a prescription, with Viagra having been requested more than 80 percent of the time, and in 90 percent of these cases a prescription was written for the drug.[19]

As the use of DTC drug ads increased, the anecdotes were replaced by professional surveys and studies on the impact of the ads. Research and surveys showed, for instance, that 13 percent of patients requested a prescription drug from their physician after seeing an ad and that in as many as 50 percent of those times the physician wrote a prescription for that specific brand of drug.[20] Another health-care research agency study reported that, while overall visits to doctors increased 2 percent between January and September 1998, visits for heavily advertised conditions rose 11 percent. For particular drugs, such as the allergy drug Claritin and the anticholesterol drug Pravachol®, which were the most promoted drugs to consumers in 1997, physicians were honoring requests for these drugs 86 percent and 93 percent of the time, respectively.[21] At the same time, another consulting firm reported a study showing that 53 percent of two thousand physicians surveyed reported an increase in the number of patients requesting prescription drugs by name, and that two-thirds of physicians said that DTC ads were the source of brand awareness by their patients.[22]

Although the findings were not as dramatic, academic medical researchers too were confirming that DTC drug advertising was increasing patient requests for drugs. One such study involved telephone interviews with 329 randomly selected adults examining their awareness and understanding of, attitudes toward, and susceptibility to DTC drug advertising.[23] Among other things, the study showed that DTC advertisements had led one-third of respondents to ask their physicians for drug information and one-fifth to request a prescription.

The National Consumers League, an advocacy group, also conducted surveys, which showed that if a patient spoke to his or her doctor about a drug, the doctor would prescribe the drug 22 percent of the time.[24] A 1999 survey conducted by *Prevention* magazine of twelve hundred patients revealed that 31 percent of responders talked with their physician about a prescription drug they had seen in a DTC ad. Of these people, 28 percent asked for the drug, 84 percent of whom reported that their physician wrote them a prescription for that drug. This survey concluded that DTC drug ads had encouraged a projected 21.2 million consumers to talk to their doctors about a medical condition they had never discussed with the doctor before seeing the ad, and that as many as 12.1 million consumers received a prescribed drug as a direct result of seeing a DTC advertisement.[25] The results of these surveys led to the widespread belief that DTC prescription drug advertising did indeed increase physician visits by patients and lead to an increase in the number of drug prescriptions written. Data collected by marketing research firms also confirmed that DTC prescription drug advertising was a successful marketing technique and that it was cost effective for the companies to promote drugs in this manner.

One factor, however, that could detract from the positive financial aspects of DTC prescription drug advertising was an emerging legal climate that made such advertising potentially risky. It is widely established that drug manufacturers have a legal duty to warn about drug risks when marketing a drug. Traditionally, this duty to warn is fulfilled by including sufficient warnings in the product labeling made available to physicians and pharmacists, who use that information to make proper prescription drug choices for their patients. DTC advertising challenged the traditional legal notion that warning physicians and pharmacists was legally sufficient to protect patient interests. One court case in particular that tested this law was the long-standing New Jersey class action lawsuit by Norplant patients against Wyeth-Ayerst Laboratories, in which plaintiffs alleged that the company failed to adequately warn of side effects associated with the drug in the DTC advertising campaign the company ran in the early 1990s.[26] The trial court had initially dismissed the case by holding that the so-called learned intermediary doctrine could be used as a defense against patients who claimed that the company did not properly warn of drug side effects in DTC ads. The learned intermediary doctrine in pharmaceutical product liability law allows a drug company to fulfill its duty to warn patients of prescription drug and device risks by supplying doctors and pharmacists with this information.[27] The basis for the doctrine stems from the fact that all prescription medical products are ordered by physicians, who have an obligation to select the proper drugs for patients aided by the information provided by the manufacturer. Relying on the learned intermediary doctrine, Wyeth had argued to the trial court that the doctors who prescribed Norplant had the sole duty to inform their patients of the device's side effects and that the manufacturer's legal duty to the patient was fulfilled if it properly warned the physician. The trial court accepted this long-standing legal precedent and dismissed the case against Wyeth. However, the plaintiffs had appealed to the New Jersey Supreme Court, arguing that the doctrine had not contemplated that drug manufacturers would advertise their drugs directly to consumers and that the law had to change to hold manufacturers accountable for information disseminated in this way.

In 1999, the Supreme Court of New Jersey ultimately ruled in favor of the patients, holding that the learned intermediary doctrine could not be relied upon to discharge the company's duty to warn when the prescription drug was marketed directly to consumers. The court accepted the argument that DTC advertising encouraged patients to seek specific drugs and pressure their doctors to prescribe them, thus altering the traditional doctor-patient relationship on which the learned intermediary doctrine was originally based. Now that drug manufacturers were legally responsible to patients for their DTC ads, the case raised the ugly prospect that drug companies and the doctors who prescribed their drugs would be pointing fingers in lawsuits over who failed to adequately warn the patient of dangerous side effects. Even though the court stated that compliance with FDA advertising regulations and guidance should constitute a rebuttable presumption that an ad was legally adequate, this ruling and a growing number of others in the lower courts gave drug companies reason to worry about the negative consequences of engaging in DTC advertising.[28]

DTC PRESCRIPTION DRUG ADVERTISING EXPENDITURES

Drug companies deciding how much of their advertising budgets to devote to DTC ads had to contend with the high costs for such promotion compared with promotion directed to physicians.[29] In 1998, for example, Hoechst spent $580,000 on one sixty-second ad for its prescription antihistamine Allegra®

during the popular television show *The X-Files*. By comparison, a full-page ad in a leading medical journal cost less than $11,000.[30] An executive from the biotechnology company Genentech told one reporter that in 1997 a one-month television campaign during which ads ran four or five times a day in major cities cost anywhere from $5 million to $15 million and needed a patient customer base in excess of 250,000 to be economically feasible.[31]

But analysts following the "DTC spend" and comparing it with drug sales were noting that there was often a positive correlation between the two. One study showed that between 1998 and 1999 twenty-five drugs, most of which were heavily advertised to consumers, accounted for 43 percent of the growth in prescription drug sales. By contrast, all other prescription drugs produced sales growth of only 13.3 percent. Some classes of drugs seemed to have benefited more than others from DTC advertising. For instance, the prescription allergy drugs with the most money devoted to DTC advertising in 1998, Claritin, Allegra, and Zyrtec®, experienced sales increases over the prior year of 32 percent, 50 percent, and 56 percent, respectively, making the advertising well worth the costs. Top-selling drugs to lower cholesterol and treat arthritis and gastrointestinal ulcers were also heavily advertised and produced above average sales growth.[32]

Statistics such as this caused pharmaceutical advertising to become one of the fastest-growing categories of the advertising industry.[33] The total amount of money spent on DTC prescription drug advertising in 1987 was $35 million. By 1994, this amount had grown to $308 million. In 1999, total pharmaceutical company promotional spending directed to U.S. physicians and consumers reached $13.9 billion, 13 percent ($1.8 billion) of which was DTC prescription drug advertising and most of that ($1.1 billion) devoted to televisions ads. The most active DTC marketers were spending between 3 percent and 20 percent of annual prescription drug sales on DTC advertising. The number of drugs advertised directly to consumers also grew from ten in 1990 to over one hundred by 1999. In addition, companies were shifting their spending so that DTC advertising budgets for some drugs began to exceed physician-directed promotion (that is, medical journal advertising, sales representatives). Ex-FDA commissioner David Kessler noted that, with the advent of DTC advertising, some pharmaceutical companies had marketing and promotion budgets almost as big as their R&D budgets.[34] Advertising in popular magazines became widespread. In one 1997 issue of *Time* magazine, for example, eight of the first twenty-six pages were ads for Pravachol (which lowers cholesterol), Lamisil® (for nail fungus), and Accolate® (for asthma), plus an ad in the back of the magazine for

Valtrex® (a treatment for genital herpes).[35] From that point on (after the FDA broadcast guidelines were available), companies began to shift large amounts of advertising dollars from print to the more expensive but presumably more effective broadcast media.[36]

As the advertising boom expanded, strategies to reach consumers became more sophisticated. Some companies were hiring advertising agencies such as Foote, Cone & Belding, which had affiliated with an academic behavioral scientist to develop theories about how best to promote prescription drugs to consumers. According to one of these theories, consumers were either "information-actives" (who sought health information and would call 800 numbers or order brochures to learn about treatments), "indifferents" (who were indifferent about health), and "passives" (who needed to be pushed to participate in their health care). To make use of these insights into consumer behavior, pharmaceutical advertising executives sought to learn whether the targeted patient market fit one of these categories and then adjusted their advertising strategy accordingly.[37]

MEDICAL COMMUNITY REACTIONS TO DTC PRESCRIPTION DRUG ADVERTISING

Physician Concerns

Physicians and others in the medical community had a difficult time dealing with DTC prescription drug advertising.[38] Polls taken in the 1990s showed that the majority of physicians were opposed to these ads. In one survey of five thousand physicians, more than 60 percent wanted pharmaceutical companies to cut back on or eliminate television advertising of prescription drugs.[39] The American Medical Association was initially opposed to DTC prescription drug advertising but after it saw that FDA would allow it, changed its view to one that stressed more stringent control, tighter policing, and greater punishment for irresponsible advertising.

Reasons for physician opposition were many.[40] A prevalent view was that the ads would confuse and mislead consumers, artificially stoke demand, and inflate expectations more than they would educate patients. This was especially true for newly marketed anticancer and other life-saving drugs and for the so-called life-style drugs, such as weight loss, hair loss, impotency, and anti-aging products, some of which could produce significant side effects.[41] Physicians also objected that the featured ad material would promote the use of one drug only, so that patients had no information about the use of the drug in the context of other treatment choices (for example, no information about other treatments or the consequences of no treatment would be given), and consumers would not read or understand the fine print (or the fast-paced recitation) about the drug's side effects or contraindications. It was expected that these problems would be most prevalent in the elderly, the highest users of prescription drugs. In one survey, 55 percent of physicians did not believe that patients had the ability to fully understand DTC drug ads.[42] Other surveys confirmed this view, such as one that showed that 43 percent of consumers thought that only "completely safe" drugs could be advertised and 22 percent thought that advertising of drugs with serious side effects was banned.[43] In another consumer survey, 43 percent of consumers (skewed to the older respondents) said they read none or very little of the small print, technical language (that is, the brief summary) on drug adverse effects. This survey was inconclusive about whether consumers felt that their knowledge of medicines was increased after reading an ad—53 percent of those interviewed said this "sometimes" happened, while the rest were evenly split between "always" and "rarely/never."[44]

The view that drug ads could be misleading was also bolstered by reports of problems with drug ads in medical journals. In some studies of these ads, which assessed both scientific accuracy and compliance with FDA standards, researchers reported statistics such as that 35 percent of the ads lacked fair balance between drug efficacy and risks, or that in 40 percent of the ads studied the physician would be led to prescribe the drug improperly. The fact that these ads had been published led the researchers to conclude that FDA did not have sufficient resources to police its drug advertising regulations.[45]

Others were troubled by the manner in which some advertisers promoted their drugs. Behavioral science research had shown that the manner in which a product ad message was conveyed was crucial to its success. However, critics believed that DTC ads should not use motivational tools commonly used in other consumer product advertising. Some DTC drug ads were believed to be too coercive, such as the one that offered to enroll consumers in a contest to win a trip to Hawaii if they tried the allergy drug Claritin, or another that offered money-back guarantees for the patients dissatisfied with their first six months of the cholesterol-lowering drug Zocor®.[46]

The extent to which fear was a motivational tool in DTC ads was also a subject of comment.[47] Drug ads that dealt with serious diseases could evoke emotional responses in consumers about mortality and disability, and, because of this, questions were raised about whether such ads contributed to or detracted from rational decision making on the part of the patient. Also, fear could work for or against the advertiser by either evoking consumer interest and motivation to seek out the advertised treatment or triggering denial and avoidance, especially in consumers who lacked the belief that something could be done to prevent illness, disability, or death. Consequently, according to one agency that specialized in DTC advertising:

> The use of fear in promoting prescription drugs should be based on a careful assessment of target consumers' level of confidence that they can take the advocated action (contact the physician, acquire the prescription, and comply with the regimen), and their belief that the product is effective. Therefore, for each individual product and condition, precise research into the target audience's existing knowledge and attitudes must be undertaken to determine whether fear appeals will lead to adaptive or maladaptive responses.[48]

Other physicians argued that consumer drug ads led to a loss of professional control, undermined their authority, and harmed their ability to maintain a therapeutic relationship with patients. Patients who requested advertised drugs would put pressure on doctors to prescribe, which sometimes led to patient dissatisfaction when the drug was deemed inappropriate and not prescribed or led the physician to acquiesce and prescribe a less-than-optimal or inappropriate drug.[49] Some doctors feared that refusing requests for a glowingly described drug could undermine the patient's trust in the doctor and lead the patient to seek the drug from a less scrupulous physician. Indeed, one survey showed that when asked what they would do if a physician refused to prescribe a requested drug, 46 percent of consumers said they would be disappointed, 25 percent said they would try to persuade the physician, 24 percent would try to obtain the prescription from a different physician, and 15 percent said they might switch physicians.[50]

Even for some physicians who believed that their patients should be active decision makers in accepting or rejecting treatment options after hearing the physician explain the merits and risks of various alternatives, there was a worry that powerful DTC ads could lead the patient to select treatment based on which was better advertised rather than on medical merit. Another anticipated problem was that the prevalence of drug ads would increase the number of what physicians called the "worried well"—people with a too-ready tendency to believe they were sick, who self-diagnosed, and who consumed too much physician time for reassuring medical visits. Taking the time to discuss (and sometimes debate) the various attributes of advertised drugs with both well and sick patients would strain physicians' overcommitted schedules and was not a reimbursable activity under most health plans. Still other physicians worried that expansion in advertising would add to the already high cost of prescription drugs. Many physicians worked in medical organizations with built-in cost controls, such as a drug formulary that would not allow them to prescribe every advertised brand name drug, and felt that ads for drugs they could not prescribe made the practice of medicine more difficult.[51]

Some physicians and others thought that the FDA guidelines and enforcement practices were too lenient to prevent abuses. Companies that violated the guidelines were usually told only to modify the ad or stop it. FDA notices could lag ad publication or broadcast by days or weeks and, since companies were not obliged to send advance copies to FDA, it was sometimes a matter of chance that FDA noticed and took action against an improper ad. Given the large number of television viewers or magazine readers who saw the initial offending ads, some physicians believed that the damage was allowed to occur and that companies were given little incentive to stop offensive ad practices. Indeed, some companies did seem to be repeat offenders. In less than a four-year period, FDA had cited Schering-Plough Corporation eleven times and Glaxo Wellcome PLC fourteen times for improprieties in their DTC ads for three widely advertised prescription allergy and asthma medications.[52] Companies responded that it was not their intention to test the agency's willingness to enforce the regulations. Rather, they claimed that they were feeling their way in an environment in which the FDA response to DTC ads was unpredictable and where the time and cost constraints of broadcast ads made it difficult to decide what drug information to include or cut. However, critics thought that instead of preventing the release of inappropriate ads, FDA enforcement practices encouraged companies to continue to push the envelope of acceptability.

Physicians and industry representatives who supported DTC prescription drug advertising thought that the objectors were being overly paternalistic and had not learned to adapt to the modern environment in which patients were active participants in their medical care. Under this "patient empowerment" view of medical care, patients were encouraged to become as knowledgeable as possible about their medical care and, after seeking physician and other advice about various treatment options, select the treatment deemed most personally suitable. DTC drug ads fit into this construct because they had the potential to lead patients to visit their physicians and to receive treatments for ailments they might otherwise have ignored or chosen not to pursue because they were unaware of the availability of treatments. The FDA survey confirmed this belief when it revealed that about 25 percent of people who had seen a prescription drug ad asked their doctor (for the first time) about a medical condition.

Also, about 85 percent reported that these ads helped them become more aware of new drugs.[53]

Statistics showed, for example, that among U.S. adults, there were an estimated eight million undiagnosed cases of diabetes, a disease that can be treated with prescription drugs. Ads that alerted people to the symptoms of diabetes and encouraged physician treatment could save people from the devastating effects and costs of the disease, and extend lives. The Air Force/Texas Coronary Atherosclerosis Prevention Study concluded that use of a cholesterol-lowering drug could lower the risk of heart attacks, chest pain, and cardiac arrest by 37 percent, even in people with no symptoms of heart disease. The authors of the study estimated that six million Americans currently not recommended for this treatment could benefit. Studies such as this led some physicians to welcome the fact that drug ads could bring patients to their offices with requests for treatments and that ads could prompt patients to seek health information or become more responsible for their health. Others felt that anything to reduce the stigma of such diseases as herpes, impotency, or mental illness with encouragement to seek treatment was bound to have an overall positive public health effect. Worries about undue pressure leading to inappropriate prescribing practices were dismissed as exaggerated, since most physicians were believed to be professional enough to resist irrational requests for drugs and to continue to exercise their professional judgment to select the most appropriate treatment for a given patient.[54]

Eventually, as experience with DTC prescription drug advertising grew, physician opposition lessened but did not abate. Thirteen years after the advent of DTC prescription drug advertising, the American Medical Association's Council on Ethical and Judicial Affairs wrote:

> While there is legitimate opposition to this form of information delivery, there also is reason to believe that patients' health and medical care may benefit. In this report, the Council on Ethical and Judicial Affairs (CEJA) of the American Medical Association (AMA) considers the potential strengths and pitfalls of DTC advertising to provide guidance for physicians when such activities affect their practices. This is the summary advice given by the AMA—Ultimately, physicians are expected to remain vigilant to ensure that DTC advertising does not promote false expectations. When confronted with the influences of advertising, physicians should maintain professional standards of informed consent by denying requests for inappropriate prescriptions, educating patients as to why certain advertised drugs may not be suitable treatment options, and including, when appropriate, information on the cost

effectiveness of prescription drug options. Upholding professional standards may entail reporting to pharmaceutical companies or FDA, advertisements that raise concerns about the promotion of patients' health and safety. It also may entail promoting, participating in, or conducting studies regarding DTC advertising's effects on patients health and medical care.[55]

Managed Care Organization and Health Insurers

Along with physicians, public and private payers of health care such as the Health Care Financing Administration, managed care organizations, and health insurance companies were worried that increased drug advertising would increase prescription drug costs.[56] Estimated retail spending on prescription drugs had risen from $78.9 billion in 1997 to $111.1 billion in 1999, with estimates that future yearly spending would increase by 12 to 18 percent, making prescription drugs the fastest growing health-care expense. Primarily, these increases were attributed to an increase in the number of prescriptions being written and in the shift to newer, more expensive drugs. Commentators were wondering about the extent to which DTC advertising contributed to these increases and whether the increased costs were worthwhile. A June 1998 survey of 2,015 people conducted by Louis Harris & Associates for the Harvard School of Public Health, Andersen Consulting, and London & Associates showed that nearly three in ten patients who had taken any prescription drug said they had talked with their doctors about a drug they saw advertised. But only 40 percent said the doctor had prescribed the drug they had discussed. About this finding, one pharmaceutical management and economics professor said, "The Harvard study means half the effort caused by the advertising is probably wasting the doctor's time and wasting expense within the H.M.O., which drives up the cost for everybody."[57] At a time when spending on prescription drugs was growing twice as fast as total health-care spending, these were disconcerting conclusions. But, despite the concerns, there was no consensus or comprehensive data on how DTC ads influenced overall health-care costs. Some postulated that if patients were motivated by ads to seek treatments for certain conditions and hospitalization was therefore averted, an overall health-care cost savings could be achieved. One contrary view, expressed in a presentation at the American Chemical Society, postulated that even the positive health effects from DTC advertising could be unacceptably costly:

> Creating more demand for a (drug) product can put a company in conflict with HMOs, which must keep costs down while delivering adequate care. Indeed, the growth in expenditures for hospitals and physician-related

expenses has gone down over the past decade. Growth in spending on pharmaceuticals, however, has gone up. Over this period, the consumer price index for drugs has fallen while the sales volume for drugs has risen indicating that growing demand, not increases in the prices, is driving cost growth.

DTC advertisements increase demand, sales, and profits. Some of these profits are at the expense of the HMOs' bottom line. Moreover, if DTC advertisements can increase compliance and the rate of diagnosis for certain diseases, they will create yet more demand for particular drugs. From the point of view of HMOs, then, the more DTC advertisements succeed, the harder it will be for them to make a profit.[58]

CONCLUSION

Fifteen years after the advent of DTC prescription drug advertising in the United States, it was clear that this activity was on the rise with both positive and negative consequences, the magnitude of which remain unquantified. What is certain is that DTC advertising had become an established practice for those pharmaceutical companies that could afford it, and that these companies were still grappling with FDA and medical professionals over the acceptable boundaries for ads. Perhaps because the ads increased the visibility of pharmaceutical companies, DTC prescription drug advertising had become a subject of public focus. Press and medical journal reports on the subject continued to be numerous. Also, consumer groups and watchdog organizations, like RxHealth Value, a group composed of consumers, physicians, and health-care organizations, and EthicAd, a nonprofit organization started by a pharmaceutical industry consultant and some university physicians, were devoted to monitoring DTC prescription drug advertising activity and proposing improved standards for ads.[59] These developments, along with changes in the medical and legal climates, would make corporate management of DTC prescription drug advertising in the next decade a continued challenge. Pharmaceutical companies were obviously interested in using DTC advertising to increase the sales of their drug products. FDA and patient consumer groups were more interested in having the impact of this advertising further public health by educating consumers about prescription drugs and empowering them to become more involved in rational health-care decision making. The extent to which DTC prescription drug advertising could meet both of these goals remains the subject of lively debate.

Case Study

Zeneca's Direct-to-Consumer
Advertising of Nolvadex®[60]

In May 1999, a cross-functional team named "Moon Shot" at Zeneca Inc., a pharmaceutical, agrochemical, and specialty products company, gathered to review the results of a $54.4 million direct-to-consumer ad campaign. This campaign was to promote the use of the drug Nolvadex (Zeneca's brand name for tamoxifen citrate) for use in reducing the risk of breast cancer in women at high risk—an estimated nine million women in the United States. Tamoxifen had been used since 1977 as a cancer chemotherapy agent and since 1990 to prevent the recurrence of tumors in women with early-stage breast cancer. The new campaign for Nolvadex resulted from the approval of a new indication for its use granted by the Food and Drug Administration in November 1998. The Moon Shot team members had known from the outset that DTC prescription drug advertising was one of the most complex aspects of product marketing. They were eager to assess the results of the print and television ad campaigns for the product. Since July 1998, when campaign development began, the team had worked hard to comply with FDA regulatory requirements and those of the Division of Drug Marketing, Advertising, and Communications, the FDA arm responsible for enforcing all prescription drug promotion activity regulations and guidelines. In addition, during the development of the ads, the team had responded to comments from advocacy groups, such as the Susan B. Komen Foundation and the American Cancer Society. First on the team's agenda were comments from the activist community and concerns voiced in the lay press about the propriety of the Nolvadex ads. With the clarity afforded by hindsight, the team began to assess the ambiguities and uncertainties associated with market opportunities and costs, patient needs and tendencies, clinical study data, regulatory requirements, physician prescribing practices, the efficacy of advertising, and activist responses. Their goal was to use this assessment to inform future DTC advertising.

ZENECA INC.

Zeneca Inc. was the U.S. unit of a large pharmaceutical and agricultural/industrial chemical company, Zeneca Group PLC of the United Kingdom.[61] In 1997–98, pharmaceutics represented 51 percent of the overall company business and generated 73 percent of the company's operating profit (see corporate financial information in Table 12.1). This division was considered a top-tier pharmaceutical company with a diversified business that included oncology, cardiovascular, and critical care drugs. In 1998, the company employed more than thirty-two thousand people and generated over $9 billion in sales, up 6 percent from the prior year with operating profit up 1 percent and net profit down 2 percent.[62] Over 91 percent of Zeneca's 1998 sales were obtained in foreign currencies, and the weakness in sterling had driven sales down 4 percent and profits down 12 percent.

To maximize the potential of its established products, Zeneca pursued developing them for other uses.[63] Nolvadex was a case in point. Zeneca had been selling Nolvadex since 1977 as a treatment for women suffering from breast cancer and had leveraged knowledge gained through the development of Nolvadex to expand its oncology drug portfolio. Oncology drugs produced one-third of Zeneca's total pharmaceutical sales, which in 1998 were about $4.6 billion, up almost 10 percent from 1997 with pharmaceutical operating profits up 4 percent. Sales in oncology drugs had grown 15 percent in 1998.[64] Yet by the late 1990s, sales of Nolvadex had flattened, and competing drugs had emerged (see Table 12.2). Despite this, Nolvadex contributed significantly to Zeneca's profits, since research expenses were virtually nil in the late 1990s and manufacturing and marketing costs were also quite low. Zeneca's U.S. patent on Nolvadex, however, would expire in 2002 and had already expired in most other major markets.

EVOLUTION OF ATTITUDES ABOUT DISEASE
AND TREATMENT

In the late twentieth century, patients were beginning to seek more information about their diseases and treatments and were becoming more involved in their health-care choices. Gone were the days when the U.S. medical establishment advised that drug labeling was to be written "only in such medical terms as are not likely to be understood by the ordinary individual" (United States *Federal Register*, 1938), and gone forever were the days when physicians could be fined for disseminating information to their patients about their medicines:[65]

> "Let no physician teach the people about medicines or even tell them the names of the medicines, particularly the more potent ones . . . For the people may be harmed by their improper use. Violations: 40 shillings."
>
> Royal College of Physicians Ethical Statutes (circa 1555)

More open ways of thinking about the dissemination of medical information began to replace paternalistic and patronizing attitudes about the public's need for and ability to understand medical information. During the late 1990s, FDA restrictions on patient drug advertising were lifting, and drug manufacturers were eager to educate patients about new drugs and treatments. Some were even developing information-intensive Web sites to communicate to patients the benefits and drawbacks of medication (as an example, see Appendix 12.1).

Many types of patients benefited from this medical information trend. Specifically, and pertinent to Zeneca, women at risk of breast cancer had access to more information about diagnosis and treatment. In addition, political action on the part of women and their families—aimed at both the National Institutes of Health (which funds cancer and other medical research) and pharmaceutical companies—resulted in substantial increases in funding for breast cancer research. These two developments directly impacted Zeneca's Nolvadex marketing.

BREAST CANCER EPIDEMIOLOGY, POLITICAL ACTION,
AND RESEARCH

In 1999, breast cancer was the most frequently diagnosed cancer in women (aside from skin cancers), and the cumulative lifetime risk for developing breast cancer for American women was one in eight.[66] Over 175,000 cases would be diagnosed in 1999 alone, and more than 43,500 of these women would die from the disease. Except for lung cancer, no other cancer killed as many women in the United States.[67] Although the incidence of breast cancer had remained steady since 1988, it was likely that the actual number of cases would rise in the future, as the population of American women became older.[68] The economic and emotional costs of breast cancer were staggering, and advancing research in breast cancer treatments, causes, and prevention were prominent goals of NIH, the American Cancer Society, and many private foundations.

Breast cancer was almost exclusively a disease of women, and historically financial support for research into women's health issues had trailed that of men's. Because it affected so many women, the disease had become the call to arms for many groups interested in increasing general funding for women's health research and education. These groups spanned a wide range of political viewpoints and goals but collectively represented a huge number of women and their families. Breast cancer advocacy organizations had been so successful that other patient advocacy groups emulated them when trying to increase research funding for their own diseases.

The growth in funding for breast cancer research had led to a wealth of new treatment and early detection campaigns and the introduction of genetic tests, all of which aimed to better diagnose and treat the disease, educate patients, and calm the fears of millions of women who saw breast cancer as a highly unpredictable and uncontrollable killer.[69]

FDA APPROVAL FOR TAMOXIFEN CITRATE: 1977

Zeneca initially received FDA approval in 1977 for the use of tamoxifen citrate (Nolvadex) as a chemotherapy drug in women with advanced-stage breast cancer. Nolvadex was the first hormonal therapy to be approved for treatment of the disease. Tamoxifen had a chemical structure similar to that of the natural hormone estrogen, but the drug acted as an anti-estrogen in breast tissue. Normal breast cells, and many cancerous breast cells, depend on estrogen for growth. By binding to the estrogen receptor on breast cancer cells and blocking estrogen's progrowth effects, Nolvadex halts tumor progression and prolongs survival in women with breast cancer.

Compared to many other cancer drugs, most of the systemic side effects of Nolvadex were relatively mild. Nolvadex had a similar side effect profile to other estrogen-containing drugs, such as the hormone replacement therapies (HRT) used by many women in their menopausal years. These side effects included blood clots in the legs and lungs, hot flashes, flushing, irregular menstrual cycles, and other menopausal symptoms. In addition, use of Nolvadex increased the risk of endometrial (uterine lining) cancer. This side effect was quite rare; endometrial cancer was expected to occur in less than 1 percent of Nolvadex users.[70] However, the "traditional" side effects of cancer chemotherapy—such as uncontrollable nausea, hair loss, and life-threatening bone marrow toxicity—were noticeably absent with this drug.[71] Because of its efficacy and overall favorable side effect profile, the drug had been widely prescribed as a breast cancer treatment in conjunction with more traditional chemotherapeutic drugs. As use of Nolvadex increased, it was also discovered that it reduced recurrence of the original cancer and prevented the development of new cancers in the opposite breast.

FDA APPROVAL FOR A NEW INDICATION FOR
TAMOXIFEN CITRATE: 1990

In 1990, following further research, Nolvadex was also approved for use as an adjuvant treatment to prevent the recurrence of tumors in women with early-stage breast cancer.[72] Encouraged by these later studies, scientists and clinicians wondered whether tamoxifen might also prevent breast cancers in healthy women, and thus the $68-million Breast Cancer Prevention Trial (BCPT) was launched in 1992.[73] The trial was overseen by the National Surgical Adjuvant Breast and Bowel Project, a cooperative group of over three hundred medical centers coordinating U.S. cancer research and clinical trials. Funding was largely provided by the federal government's National Cancer Institute, a division of NIH. The BCPT was a large, double-blind, placebo-controlled clinical trial, the gold standard for evaluating the efficacy and safety of a pharmaceutical product. In the study, half of the women received tamoxifen daily for five years and half received a placebo. Neither the women nor the investigators knew which women were in which group until the study was "unblinded."

The trial enrolled 13,388 high-risk women, defined as women with a substantially higher than average risk of breast cancer, specifically, a 1.7 percent or greater chance of developing breast cancer within five years as predicted by a statistical model. This statistical prediction analysis, the Gail Model, took into account the major risk factors for breast cancer.[74] Previous epidemiological studies identified the risk factors as: current age, age at menarche (onset of menstruation), age at first live birth, number of previous breast biopsies, presence of atypical hyperplasia (an abnormal microscopic finding on a breast tissue biopsy), and number of first-degree relatives (mothers or sisters) with breast cancer.[75] Although this model was not a perfect risk predictor, it was widely felt to be the best statistical risk assessment tool available at the time of the study.

The results of the BCPT were so dramatic that investigators stopped the study in March 1998, fourteen months earlier than expected. A 45 percent reduction in the incidence of breast cancer was noted in the treated group of women who had taken Nolvadex as compared to the women on placebo medication.[76] The 45 percent relative risk reduction figure was derived from data that showed that tamoxifen lowered the breast cancer risk in women age thirty-five years or more from 2.6 percent to 1.3 percent.[77] Given these new data about tamoxifen, the investigators felt it was unethical to allow the control group to continue taking a placebo pill when the tamoxifen-treated group experienced such a decrease in the number of breast cancer cases. Thus, the study was stopped, the patient groups unblinded, and Nolvadex was offered to the women in the control group.

The announcement of the study results was met with much fanfare among physicians, patients, and the popular press. For the first time, investigators had demonstrated that a drug could reduce the number of breast cancer cases in healthy, high-risk women. Using Nolvadex to decrease cancer risk presented an opportunity to address an unmet need. Many women with a family history of breast cancer who were worried about their own future had two mostly unacceptable options—get frequent cancer check-ups and mammograms, which would hopefully detect cancer early, or undergo prophylactic mastectomy (surgical removal of both breasts). Nolvadex now offered a more palatable option for many of these women. In April 1998, using the results of the BCPT trial, Zeneca applied to FDA to approve the new indication, which would allow Zeneca to market Nolvadex for breast cancer prevention.[78] The FDA review was extensive, requiring Zeneca to submit an additional thirty-three supplements and amendments to the initial application. In September 1998, FDA's Oncologic Drugs advisory group recommended that the agency approve Nolvadex for the new indication. The advisory group, a committee of expert physicians, felt that although the use of Nolvadex carried certain risks (the major ones being blood clots, embolisms, and endometrial cancer), these risks were considered to be outweighed by the drug's potential for reducing the number of breast cancer cases.[79]

As is typical with FDA submissions, there was some "back and forth" about the exact language that would be contained in the new labeling for the drug.[80]

For instance, Zeneca favored the use of the word "prevention" to describe the Nolvadex effect on breast cancer, something FDA was not inclined to allow since there were no data available on what happened to the women in the study after five years of treatment. Breast cancer activist groups following the FDA approval process for Nolvadex opposed such wording and presented testimony to the agency in an attempt to limit what they believed to be Zeneca's intended overpromotion of the drug.[81] In November 1998, following its outside advisory group's recommendation, FDA formally approved Zeneca's application. The approved labeling would state that Nolvadex was indicated to "reduce the incidence of breast cancer in women at high risk for breast cancer" and that there was no impact of the drug on overall or breast cancer-related mortality. Physicians who prescribed Nolvadex for this indication were instructed in the labeling to identify high-risk women using the Gail Model Risk Assessment Tool (the same mathematical model used in the BCPT) that Zeneca would provide. In approving the new use and labeling, FDA also required that Zeneca submit advance copies of any initial promotional material for Nolvadex.[82]

TEMPERED OPTIMISM: QUESTIONING THE BREAST CANCER PREVENTION TRIAL

At the same time, there was ambivalence about and even criticism of BCPT and the resultant FDA approval.[83] Studies of the use of tamoxifen in the treatment of early-stage, estrogen-responsive breast cancer had validated the BCPT data.[84] However, British and Italian studies similar to BCPT had failed to show that tamoxifen was associated with a cancer risk reduction benefit.[85] Other physician researchers downplayed the discrepancies, claiming that the European trials were statistically underpowered, studied fewer women, and (in the Italian study) had high numbers of women who dropped out of the study. Others noted that, compared to BCPT, the European studies included generally younger, higher-risk women, all with strong family histories of breast cancer. In such populations, tamoxifen might not have an effect or such an effect could take longer to demonstrate.[86] Nonetheless, the lack of uniformity of the trial results led some to question whether stopping the American trial early had been wise. According to one clinical scientist, "The failure of these [European] trials to confirm the results of the U.S. study, however, casts doubt on the wisdom of the rush, at least in some places, to prescribe tamoxifen widely for prevention. Longer follow-up of completed and current trials is clearly required to clarify the relative preventive benefits and risks in different populations and to confirm the BCPT findings. Most importantly, none of these trials provides reliable data on mortality, which should be the ultimate endpoint."[87]

The lack of mortality data was an issue among clinical researchers and epidemiologists in this field. Although a reduced number of breast cancer cases was seen in the BCPT tamoxifen-treated group, it was unclear if tamoxifen prevented breast cancer in these patients or merely delayed its onset. Therefore, the study did not address what some believed was the more important question—could five years of tamoxifen administration delay or reduce the overall death rate from breast cancer in high-risk women? Continuing the trial would have helped address this question.[88] The lack of mortality data was the reason that FDA did not approve Nolvadex for use as a breast cancer prevention agent per se, but approved instead its use "to reduce the incidence of breast cancer in women at high risk for breast cancer."[89]

Others were concerned that the drug's indication for "high risk" women (according to the Gail Model, women older than thirty-five years with a 1.7 percent risk of developing breast cancer in five years) was too inclusive, since about twenty-nine million American women would fall into this category. According to the Gail Model, every woman over the age of sixty (regardless of any other risk factors) was at sufficiently high risk for breast cancer that she was eligible to take tamoxifen.[90] Given the endometrial cancer potential of the drug, some felt that the breast cancer risk level should be higher to justify prescribing the drug to so many women for five years.[91]

The financial aspect of Nolvadex use was also in question since it was too early to know if the drug could delay the onset of cancer and thereby add years to life or prevent breast cancer altogether. If cancer was delayed by just five years of treatment, significant health-care savings could be achieved. Insurers would much rather spend the $6,000 it would cost for five years of Nolvadex treatment rather than the much high cost for breast cancer treatment, the last year of which (that is, the most expensive year) could cost as much as $20,000. However, if only half the number of women in the BCPT (6,500 women) took Nolvadex for five years, that would cost almost $40 million compared to spending $5.6 million for the last year of cancer care for the estimated 280 cases of breast cancer Nolvadex treatment would prevent.[92]

Some cancer support groups were pleased that Nolvadex offered a new option to reduce breast cancer risk. Others were not. Some groups would have preferred that the government research money had been spent on discovering causes of cancer. According to Breast Cancer Action, "Tamoxifen is a known carcinogen. Why is it that when we demand prevention the government responds by testing a pill and a known carcinogen at that instead of focusing on what is causing the increased incidence of breast cancer?"[93] Other complaints focused on the expanded recommendations for use of tamoxifen beyond women similar to those in the BCPT study group. It was known that the incidence of breast cancer was not the same in all ethnic and racial groups. The BCPT patients primarily were Caucasian (97 percent), and thus it was unclear if Nolvadex would have the same effects in the non-Caucasian population.

Some activists and women's health advocates also were worried about the small but significant risk of endometrial cancer in women taking the drug. They felt that, although the risk could be downplayed in women who already had breast cancer and who might die without the drug, it would be unacceptable to give healthy women a drug that could more than double the risk for endometrial cancer. Since the BCPT was stopped early and the incidence of endometrial cancer increased with extended exposure to the drug, they said, the real risk for this cancer was not known for women who would be taking Nolvadex for the full five years. To compound the problem, there was no medical consensus about the most accurate and effective means of screening women for endometrial cancer, which meant that early diagnosis of this side effect might not occur.[94] The activists eventually vented these complaints beyond their newsletters and Web sites to the lay and science press.[95] As Jacqueline Miranda of the Berkeley Women's Cancer Resource Center stated, it was "completely unethical to use a classified carcinogen on healthy women." The National Women's Health Network, an advocacy group based in Washington, D.C., had long argued against the BCPT, feeling that "tamoxifen should only be studied in ultra high risk women, as it is likely to merely substitute one disease for another in women at average or moderately high risk."[96] Breast Cancer Action put it this way: "We have every reason to be concerned about how doctors in the field will respond to women who, terrified of developing breast cancer, demand immediate access to tamoxifen believing that, if they take the drug, they will not develop breast cancer."[97]

Uncertainty about the newly indicated use of tamoxifen prompted more studies, which would add to existing knowledge about the advisability of using the drug to lower the risk of breast cancer. European oncologists were continuing the process of attempting to reconcile the different tamoxifen study results.[98] Also, under the direction of the American Society of Clinical Oncology, a U.S. group of oncologists was reviewing all of the studies published between 1990 and 1998 that collected data on the cancer-risk-cutting potential of tamoxifen and another related drug, raloxifene (Evista® by competitor Eli

Lilly).[99] About one month after Nolvadex had received FDA approval to market the drug to reduce breast cancer risk, Eli Lilly announced preliminary research data that showed that Evista could also reduce the risk for breast cancer (in their case, by 55 percent or more) but without producing an increased risk for endometrial cancer.[100] Eli Lilly was seeking FDA approval to add a breast cancer risk reduction indication to its Evista labeling and clearly intended to compete with Zeneca for this market. Eli Lilly also announced that in spring 1999, a five-year study of twenty-two thousand women would start comparing both the efficacy and side effects of Nolvadex with Evista. Depending on the results of this study, the market for Nolvadex could rise or fall.

NEW LIFE FOR NOLVADEX[101]

With the new information obtained through BCPT and the FDA approval in hand, Zeneca deployed the cross-functional team Moon Shot to examine all of these issues and develop an appropriate marketing campaign. At the time in 1998, Nolvadex generated about $526 million per year as a cancer treatment.[102] If Nolvadex was to be sold for reducing the risk of breast cancer, it would need to be taken twice daily and would cost the patient about $100 per month. Clearly, selling Nolvadex to reduce the risk of breast cancer opened the doors to an expanded market while also providing help to millions of high-risk women. However, questions remained about the BCPT findings, and the side effect profile of the drug was not insignificant. The company quickly had to decide how to market Nolvadex for the new indication.

One question that came up early was whether, in addition to traditional marketing efforts, the company should market the cancer preventive drug directly to women. At the time, FDA was still evaluating the draft DTC guidelines and studying the impact of DTC drug ads in general. The company knew that some policy makers considered consumer ads to be harmful for patients since they could easily be misunderstood and the extra advertising costs would add to the overall price of the drug.[103] At the same time, pharmaceutical companies were attempting to adjust to the FDA guidelines for broadcast ads and were pressuring FDA to develop still more concrete DTC regulations, which were slow in coming. As a consequence, the Zeneca advertising team was very much operating in a shifting regulatory environment. Guessing wrong was not without hazard, since FDA had the authority to sanction a company for producing objectionable ads. The sanctions ranged from the issuance of warning letters requesting that manufacturers change the ads, notices of violations to stop the ads, and other remedial measures, such as issuing retractions or sending corrective letters to doctors likely to have seen the ad. In egregious situations, the agency could seize the advertised products, or criminally prosecute the corporate people responsible for issuing the ads.[104] However, these latter two remedies were rarely sought for drug advertising violations, and FDA had no authority to seek monetary penalties. It was clear nonetheless that FDA was increasing its surveillance of promotional activity and was issuing more warning letters and notices of violation than in the past.[105]

THE NOLVADEX DTC CAMPAIGN[106]

While the Zeneca Moon Shot team's decision to market Nolvadex as a cancer risk reducer was not an easy one, the company ultimately committed wholeheartedly to market Nolvadex to physicians and consumers for the newly approved indication. Although some American physicians were still debating the question at the time, Zeneca team members were convinced that Nolvadex was a valuable product for high-risk women and therefore held promising commercial potential beyond its original market of breast cancer patients. Their position was supported by many leading U.S. cancer specialists. However, realizing the commercial potential of Nolvadex for this new use would not be easy. In addition to the opposition from some of the smaller breast cancer activist groups, Zeneca quickly learned that a number of physicians were not anxious to prescribe the drug for use in healthy women. For some doctors, this reluctance was due to previous bad experiences with hormone replacement therapy. For others, the side effect profile of the drug was simply too serious to prescribe for women who did not have breast cancer and might never get it, despite being classified as higher risk by the statistical model. These physicians wanted to wait for more data about the drug and for the results of the new trial comparing Nolvadex with Eli Lilly's Evista, which some believed to be as effective but safer than Nolvadex. However, the Nolvadex versus Evista trial was planned to begin in mid-1999 and would not conclude until long after the Nolvadex patents had expired. To protect its market in the meantime, Zeneca sued Eli Lilly, alleging that it was illegally promoting Evista for breast cancer risk reduction before there was FDA approval to do so.

In order to be most effective in its Nolvadex ad campaign, Zeneca decided that it would market the new indication to physicians and women directly and do so with broadcast and print ads. This strategy was founded on the belief that the choice to use Nolvadex was one that women would make themselves.

The Zeneca team decided that physicians on their own were not likely to offer the drug to women as much as the company would like. But prompted by patients, physicians could inform them of the benefits and risks of Nolvadex, and ultimately each woman would make her own decision. This conclusion made it abundantly clear to the company that Nolvadex needed a DTC campaign. Other market dynamics also boded well for DTC ads. For example, it was expected that high-risk women (as compared to women already suffering from cancer) would most likely discuss breast cancer risks with their primary care physician or gynecologist. These physicians were typically not familiar with Nolvadex because it had been marketed primarily to cancer specialists in the past. Additionally, the estimated market size for Nolvadex was large enough to justify the expense of a DTC campaign. Zeneca estimated that there were twenty-nine million women in the high-risk category under the Gail Model, nine million of whom were eligible for Nolvadex treatment. The nine million patient target was a reasonably large market in the pharmaceutical industry. With these factors under consideration, Zeneca decided to start developing a Nolvadex DTC campaign.

Zeneca hired Linda Pfeiffer from D'Arcy, Masius, Benton, & Bowles (DMBB), a leading advertising agency, to develop the Nolvadex ad campaign. DMBB was recognized for its successful brand development work for clients, including Proctor & Gamble, General Motors, Mars Inc., and Coca-Cola, and the agency had recently entered the burgeoning market for pharmaceutical advertising. Of particular importance to Zeneca was the fact that DMBB had developed the first branded television campaign for a drug as part of its work on the Allegra[107] DTC campaign. Zeneca felt that the agency's experience with Allegra would be valuable as it worked with FDA to develop acceptable ads for Nolvadex.

DMBB began the campaign development process in July 1998 by conducting preliminary research through a series of focus groups. The purpose of the initial focus groups was to understand how women felt about breast cancer. The studies primarily included women who had some experience with breast cancer—those with a family member or close friend who had contracted the disease. Women who were aware of the high risk of breast cancer were also included. The focus groups included over one hundred women in seven cities throughout the United States. After asking participants about their general attitudes toward breast cancer, the studies presented more specific ideas about the disease, its detection, and treatments. The results of the focus groups showed that denial was an overwhelming theme. Despite knowledge of the disease and, in many cases, firsthand experience with it, most women did not see themselves as high-risk individuals. They consistently talked about breast cancer in an abstract manner rather than as something that could happen to them.

From the focus group research, Pfeiffer and her team developed several television ad concepts. These concepts, which each adhered to one of two major themes, were retested on additional groups of women. The first theme was that of empowerment: commercials focused on the idea that "there is something you can do" and that "it is your decision." The second theme had a more emotional appeal about a woman's role in her family. Its commercials employed messages such as "you owe it to your loved ones" or "people depend on you." While preferences were split between the two themes, Pfeiffer felt that women who preferred the empowerment theme were more likely to take action. Women who responded to the empowerment theme were characterized as being between the ages of forty and fifty-nine years, of higher income (at least $30,000 annually), and more educated (education beyond high school). This group became a primary target market for the DTC campaign.

With the target demographic and basic theme of the campaign clearly identified, the DMBB team began developing the actual television and print advertisements, some of which would be sent for prescreening to FDA's DDMAC.[108] Zeneca started with a print ad that was a "coming soon" placeholder ad, to be used only once or twice while the main Nolvadex campaign was under development. The ad ran with a handful of pictures of women and the statement, "There is something you can do: Nolvadex®" Since the ad did not discuss breast cancer or any of the uses for Nolvadex, Zeneca felt it would not require a brief summary statement of the benefits and risks of the drug.[109] To Zeneca the ad was similar to branding ads used by Pfizer for the impotency drug Viagra, which featured a couple dancing, the name Viagra, and no indications for the drug nor any brief summary information. FDA disagreed and sent Zeneca a notice that its ads were unacceptable, should have included risk and other information, and must be withdrawn.[110] The warning letter from the FDA to stop the print ad (this letter also includes a notice about the deficiencies of a Nolvadex brochure accompanying a medical journal reprint) is in Appendix 12.2.

To Zeneca, this turn of events was an example of how difficult it was to determine what drug promotion activity was acceptable to FDA. Not only were the FDA DTC ad regulations and guidelines changing during the development of the Nolvadex campaign, but also the existing rules could be interpreted in different ways.[111] The initial Nolvadex print ad had not been precleared with DDMAC because Zeneca thought it to be rather innocuous, not the type of ad that required prescreening, and seemingly in compliance with the existing regulations and guidelines.

When it came time to develop the initial television DTC Nolvadex ads, the team decided to use an unbranded ad. If a branded ad was used, Zeneca would be required to disclose the full side effect profile in the advertisement, and it was agreed that citing endometrial cancer as a side effect would immediately limit the commercials' effectiveness. In fact, it was believed that mentioning this side effect would be so damaging that women would probably not even go through the risk assessment process to determine if they were a candidate for the drug. Independent marketing research supported this conclusion with a finding that the percentage of patients willing to visit a doctor after viewing DTC ads increased from 18 percent following ads with product warnings to 33 percent without product warnings.[112] Hence, the team felt that an unbranded broadcast ad was the only feasible option. This decision, combined with DMBB's previous experience with Allegra, made the FDA screening process relatively painless. Since the ad was unbranded, FDA was less concerned about its content.

The television ad showed a variety of healthy women who held stereotypical but incorrect assumptions about breast cancer (for example, that you can only get breast cancer if you have a family history or that the risk of breast cancer decreases with age). These assumptions were corrected for the viewing audience with a series of graphics and text. Viewers were then told there was a way to find out their personal risk, and that "now there was something you could do" by seeing a physician. The commercial provided a toll-free number to call for more information. Since the ad was unbranded, the drug Nolvadex was not mentioned. Only one round of FDA review was required for this television commercial. During this review, FDA's comments were minor, focusing mainly on simplifying the description of the risk assessment test so that it was understandable to all.

The final step for the television ad was to develop the response package—the set of materials that consumers would receive after calling the toll-free number included in the commercials. The primary component of the Nolvadex response package was a videotape that provided detailed information about breast cancer risk and Nolvadex. Gaining DDMAC's approval for the video proved more difficult. Since the video was heavily branded, FDA was concerned about fair balance in the benefit and risk information presented. For example, Zeneca was required to include a four-part disclaimer (including side effects) whenever the name Nolvadex was mentioned. Zeneca felt that

DDMAC's requirements were harsh because DTC advertisements for many other drugs had only to disclose "major" side effects that occurred in greater than 3 percent of users. Endometrial cancer occurred in less than 1 percent of Nolvadex users, but Zeneca was forced to display this side effect prominently and repeatedly. This DDMAC requirement was an example of another regulatory difficulty—in practice, the agency's DTC ad requirements were different for different types of drugs and diseases, making FDA reactions difficult to predict. For example, DDMAC had allowed DTC campaigns for the "statin" class of cholesterol-lowering drugs to be broadcast with only brief mention of the fact that many such drugs could cause serious liver damage. DDMAC treated Zeneca's Nolvadex ads quite differently. One of the biggest disappointments for Zeneca, however, came when DDMAC refused to allow Nolvadex to be described as a breast cancer preventative. Instead, Zeneca could refer to it only as risk reduction therapy. The Nolvadex video was finally approved by DDMAC after five rounds of editing and reviews, and the television DTC campaign was finally launched in February 1999.

Zeneca followed the Nolvadex television ads with branded print ads. These ads contained advertising material and the required brief summary containing descriptions of the indications, risks, and contraindications for the drug. The print ads ran in mainstream and specialty women's magazines.

CRITICAL RESPONSE TO NOLVADEX DTC ADS

Having been in the oncology drug business for many years, Zeneca had developed good, long-term working relationships with consumer and patient groups, such as the Susan B. Komen Foundation and the American Cancer Society. Aware of the key role that activist groups could have in the public success of marketing efforts, such as the one for Nolvadex, Zeneca gave these groups the opportunity to comment during the development of the Nolvadex marketing campaign and made modifications to the ads based on the groups' insights.

Despite careful planning, the multiple FDA reviews and approvals, and the input of the cancer patient groups, some concerns were voiced in the activist community and in the lay press about the propriety of the Nolvadex ads.[113] Some activists believed that pharmaceutical companies were not a legitimate source of drug information for their own products. Others were not so global in their views but still had problems with the Nolvadex ads, namely, that they were going to frighten and mislead women into thinking that their cancer risk was high, causing them to seek therapy that they did not need and that could cause irreparable harm in the form of false hopes or serious side effects. Most of the activist outcry over the ads was from five main groups: Public Citizen (founded by Ralph Nader), National Women's Health Network, Boston Women's Health Book Collective, Massachusetts Breast Cancer and DES Action, and Breast Cancer Action (a San Francisco–based organization).[114]

The print ad was also criticized because of the use of a provocative photo and the suggestion that women were more interested in their body shape than their health. This ad showed the back of a slim young white woman sitting on a bed and dressed only in a black lacy bra and black panties. Another version of the "black bra" ad showed this woman only from the waist up. The copy of the ad headline read: "If you care about breast cancer, care more about being a 1.7 than a 36B." The ad text explained that the 1.7 referred to the results of a test assessing a woman's risk of getting breast cancer. The print ads were also criticized for highlighting the risk of breast cancer without presenting the actual risk statistics. Even though it did not mention the name of the drug or its use, the broadcast ad was also disparaged. Ironically to the Zeneca team, the breast cancer activists' main criticism of the Nolvadex broadcast ad was that it was

> so benign that our organizations have received calls from women who saw them and wanted to get the toll free number from us because they thought they would get information about diet and exercise. The ads are misleading and dangerous for several reasons . . . they do not tell viewers what they are talking about, or that the drug that is the unstated subject of the ad is a dangerous drug with serious potential side effects.[115]

In addition to their own press releases detailing criticisms of the ads, two breast cancer activist groups (Public Citizen and the National Women's Health Network) petitioned FDA to require stronger warnings to physicians and consumers about the risks of Nolvadex.[116] According to one activist, "Women need to know that although they might have a slightly smaller chance of getting breast cancer by using tamoxifen, that benefit might be completely offset by the risk of contracting another deadly disease."[117] Despite what was felt to have been a thorough evaluation of the drug's benefits and risks, FDA reported that it would review the need to alter the drug's labeling requirements. This was a potentially troublesome development for Zeneca since ad copy about Nolvadex was governed by the language of the drug's FDA-required labeling.

The concern over the DTC ads was the latest in a long-term battle with some activist groups. For example, Breast Cancer Action, a perennial critic of

Zeneca, had the following to say about Zeneca's long-standing corporate sponsorship of Breast Cancer Awareness Month (BCAM):

> It's a smooth move for an outfit like Zeneca. These folks are the fourth largest producer of pesticides in the U.S., the manufacturer of the most widely prescribed drug for breast cancer (tamoxifen, also listed under Proposition 65 as a carcinogen), and now sole owner of Salick, Inc., a management company which runs a chain of cancer care centers. With BCAM it's got breast cancer all wrapped up in the pretty little pink ribbon.[118]

Zeneca felt that much of the ad criticism came from an outspoken, vocal minority of women who would be difficult if not impossible to satisfy, especially since these critics did not seem interested in establishing a dialogue with Zeneca about the issues. Public Citizen and National Women's Health Network did not approach Zeneca directly with their concerns over Nolvadex advertising; rather, the groups went directly to the press and FDA. Even if dialogue had been established, the company felt that satisfying every constituency in this difficult arena would not have been possible.

20/20 HINDSIGHT?

In 1999, Zeneca spent $54.4 million on Nolvadex DTC ads, ranking the product ninth in the top ten DTC drug products advertised that year.[119] Mary Lynn Carver (Zeneca's public relations staff member assigned to the Nolvadex campaign), Pfeiffer, and the Zeneca Moon Shot team strongly believed they had done the best possible job in developing their marketing campaign to meet the difficult and sometimes conflicting regulations, guidelines, and concerns of FDA, physicians, and the major breast cancer advocacy groups.

Although it was clear that patients were seeking more information about their diseases and treatments and were becoming more involved in directing their health care choices, it was unclear whether Zeneca's investment in the Nolvadex DTC campaign would produce the desired results. Zeneca executives who worked on the Nolvadex campaign believed that more corporate and regulatory experience and better data were needed in order to make DTC advertising a less risky proposition for drug manufacturers. In spite of the risks involved, however, the Moon Shot team believed that it would be facing these issues again soon. DTC drug advertising was likely to accelerate in the years ahead as a result of corporate pressures and the sea change in patient requirements for information about diseases and treatments.

Questions

1. What uncertainties (medical and regulatory) did Zeneca face when they decided to advertise Nolvadex direct to consumers? Did the company decisions appropriately take these into consideration when designing the ad campaign?

2. What ethical and social ramifications were relevant in developing the ad campaign? Were these issues adequately addressed?

3. Were the Nolvadex ads irresponsible as the breast cancer activists claimed?

4. How should Zeneca have managed the protests of the breast cancer activists?

Discussion

Three groups had a major stake in the manner in which Zeneca advertised Nolvadex—women who were the targets of the ads, prescribing physicians, and Zeneca itself. An interesting way to approach the question of whether Zeneca appropriately balanced the interests and the issues is to divide discussants into the three groups and, from the points of view of each group, have them propose an optimal marketing approach. Each group would need to discuss the certainty of the scientific data, the potential benefits and risks of the drug, and to what extent they should take the needs and capabilities of the other groups into consideration. After comparing and contrasting the recommendations, a combined approach may result in the optimal utilitarian solution of the greatest good for the greatest number of relevant individuals. Again, as with other case studies in this book, the issue arises here about the right of patients to be treated as ends, whose ability to choose should be developed. As with consent for research, patients have a right to make fully informed medical choices, and this right can only be exercised if women are provided high-quality information in ways that do not undermine their ability to assess that information. Considering Zeneca's role as an advertiser and a provider of health information compared to the role of physicians places consumer advertising in the entire health-care context and can broaden the discussion about Zeneca's advertising obligations to both physicians and patients. Finally, this case can also be used to discuss the extent to which companies have an obligation to interact with activists who protest company activity, even when the activists' points of view seem irrational.

TABLE 12.1

Zeneca Group PLC Financial Data,
Sales and Financials 1997 and 1998

	Sales of Key Products			
	1997 Sales (£m)	*Growth % over 1996*	*1998 Sales (£m)*	*Growth % over 1997*
Phamaceuticals				
Oncology				
Zoladex	348	17	377	14
Casodex	122	94	147	14
Arimidex	51	180	73	47
Nolvadex	306	1	316	6
Others	8	n/a	13	63
Primary Care				
Zestril	632	14	677	10
Tenormin	337	-5	302	(6)
Accolate	53	n/a	92	78
Zomig	12	n/a	61	408
Others	83	16	86	8
Specialists/ Hospital Care				
Seroquel	31	n/a	39	29
Diprivan	347	9	393	17
Merrem	60	119	77	40
Others	175	-6	158	(5)
Total	2,565	16	2,811	10
Salick Health Care	121	16	126	4
Agrochemicals	1,631	6	1,738	7
Specialties	885	(6)	840	(5)
Miscellaneous	(8)	n/a	(14)	n/a
Total Sales[a]	5,194	7	5,510	6

NOTE: Based on constant currency; £m means millions of pounds sterling.
[a] After interbusiness eliminations.

(continued)

TABLE 12.1 *(continued)*

Operating Profit

	1997 Profit (£m)	Growth % over 1996	1998 Profit (£m)	Growth % over 1997
Pharmaceuticals	786	17	815	4
Salick Health Care	3	(33)	(9)	(400)
Agrochemicals	223	24	216	(3)
Specialties	85	51	88	4
Miscellaneous	(14)	n/a	(13)	n/a
Total Sales	1,083	21	1,097	1

NOTE: Based on constant currency; £m means millions of pounds sterling.

Profit and Loss Account for the Year Ended December 31

	1996 (£m)	1997 (£m)	1998 (£m)
Turnover	5,363	5,194	5,510
Operating costs	(4,421)	(4,190)	(4,528)
Other operating income	101	79	115
Operating Profit	1,043	1,083	1,097
Share of profits less losses of associated holdings	(19)	8	2
Profits less losses on sale or closure of operations	(36)	—	(28)
Profit on sale of fixed assets	—	—	10
Profit on ordinary activities before interest	988	1,091	1,081
Net interest payable	(13)	(10)	(36)
Profit on ordinary activities before taxation	975	1,081	1,045
Profit before exceptional items	1,011	1,081	1,063
Exceptional items	(36)	—	(18)
Taxation	(320)	(345)	(330)
Profit on ordinary activities after taxation	655	736	715
Attributable to minorities	(12)	(6)	(1)
Net profit for financial year	643	730	714
Dividends to shareholders	(332)	(365)	(399)
Profit retained for the year	311	365	315
Earnings per 25p Ordinary Share before exceptional items	70.6p	77.0p	76.3p
Earnings per 25p Ordinary Share	67.8p	77.0p	75.2p
Weighted average number of Ordinary Shares in issue (millions)	947	948	950

NOTE: £m means millions of pounds sterling; p means pence.

TABLE 12.1 *(continued)*

Statement of Total Recognized Gains and Losses
for the Year Ended December 31

	1996 (£m)	1997 (£m)	1998 (£m)
Net profit for the financial year	643	730	714
Net unrealized holding gains on short-term investments	1	1	1
Exchange adjustments on net assets	(128)	(63)	36
Translation differences on foreign currency borrowings	46	(3)	(4)
Tax on translation differences on foreign currency borrowings	(15)	1	1
Total recognized gains and losses relating to the year	547	666	748

NOTE: £m means millions of pounds sterling.

General Financial Information
(in U.S. dollars)

	1993	1994	1995	1996	1997	1998
Sales ($ million)	6,569	7,010	7,597	9,184	8,579	9,144
Net income ($ million)	651	539	521	1,101	1,204	1,185
Income as % of sales	9.9%	7.7%	6.9%	12.0%	14.0%	13.0%
Earnings per share	0.76	0.61	0.55	1.16	3.82	1.25
Stock price—FY high	12.45	14.03	20.69	28.64	38.34	49.95
Stock price—FY low	8.95	10.07	13.40	18.36	26.72	31.00
Stock price—FY close	12.40	13.69	19.44	27.97	35.96	44.88
P/E—high	16	19	38	25	10	40
P/E—low	12	14	24	16	7	25
Dividends per share ($)	0.17	0.44	0.49	0.56	0.00	0.28
Book value per share ($)	0.93	0.93	1.02	1.22	1.21	4.38
(Employees	32,300	30,800	30,800	31,100	31,400	34,000)

1998 Year end:
  Debt ratio
  Return on equity   28.0%
  Cash ($ million)   342.0
  Current ratio   1.28
  Long-term debt
    ($ million)   764.0

SOURCE: Zeneca Group PLC and AstraZeneca PLC financial reports

TABLE 12.2

Nolvadex Sales History
(in U.S. dollars)

	1995	*1996*	*1997*	*1998*	*1999*[a]
Nolvadex sales ($ million)	567	515	502	526	566
Sales growth rate	—	-9%	-2.5%	5%	8%
Nolvadex sales as percentage of total AZN oncology sales	57.0%	43.8%	36.7%	34.2%	33.5%
Nolvadex sales as percentage of total AZN pharmaceutical sales	7.3%	5.9%	5.6%	4.8%	3.9%

[a] 1999 sales are estimated using first three quarters of actual sales
plus average fourth-quarter sales in 1997 and 1998.
SOURCE: Zeneca Group PLC and AstraZeneca PLC financial reports

Communicating Risks and Benefits of Medications via the Web

The following statement is from a 1999 press release from Immunex Corporation.

> In an effort to better educate patients and health care providers about ENBREL
> a breakthrough treatment for rheumatoid arthritis (RA), Immunex Corporation
> and Wyeth-Ayerst Pharmaceuticals have launched the ENBREL Web Site.
> ENBREL is used to treat moderately to severely active rheumatoid arthritis. . . .
> The comprehensive internet site explains how ENBREL works in the body, offers
> a question and answer section, provides an interactive quiz to help RA sufferers
> and their doctors determine if ENBREL may be right for them, and highlights
> several patients' personal experiences with ENBREL. Color photography and
> animation add to the graphic interest of the site. Enbrel.com also offers two toll-
> free numbers to provide support to patients who are considering or are currently
> taking ENBREL. For questions about insurance coverage, patients can call the
> Reimbursement Support Line (1-800-282-7704) where they will be connected
> with an insurance specialist. To answer any non-insurance questions about
> ENBREL and RA in general, trained telephone counselors are available at
> 1-888-4ENBREL. A link to the Arthritis Foundation Web Site is also
> provided.[120]

Warning Letter from the FDA to Zeneca Pharmaceuticals

From the Department of Health & Human Resources, Food and Drug Administration, Rockville, MD, posted 2/17/99 at www.fda.gov/cder/warn/warn1999.htm

William J. Kennedy, Ph.D.
Vice President, Drug Regulatory Affairs
Zeneca Pharmaceuticals
1800 Concord Pike, Wilmington, DE 19850-5437

RE: NDA 17-97-/S-040 Nolvadex (tamoxifen citrate) MACMIS ID# 7432

Dear Dr. Kennedy,

As part of its routine monitoring project, the Division of Drug Marketing, Advertising, and Communications (DDMAC) has become aware of promotional labeling and advertising materials for Nolvadex (tamoxifen citrate) disseminated by Zeneca Pharmaceuticals (Zeneca) that violate the Federal Food, Drug, and Cosmetic Act (ACT) and its implementing regulations. Reference is made to a direct-to-consumer (DTC) Journal Advertisement (NL1203) that appeared in the December/January 1999 issue of *Mamm* magazine. Reference is also made to a Fisher reprint carrier (NL1210), submitted under cover of Form FDA 2253 on December 24, 1998. DDMAC has reviewed these materials and has determined that they contain promotional claims that are false or misleading and lacking fair balance. DDMAC requests that the use of the above referenced materials and those containing similar promotional claims cease immediately.

JOURNAL ADVERTISEMENT

The advertisement in its entirety makes a representation about the product and its intended population (making it a product ad rather than a reminder ad). The pictorial representation only of women makes a representation concerning the intended patient population of Nolvadex. Therefore, DDMAC considers this advertisement to be a full product ad and in violation of the Act for the following reasons:

- it fails to provide adequate information regarding Nolvadex's approved indication and usage;
- it fails to include *any* risk information; and
- it fails to present a brief summary of information related to side effects, contraindications and effectiveness.

FAILURE TO COMPLY WITH 314.81 (b) (3)(i)

Since the journal advertisement was not submitted on form FDA 2253 at the time of initial dissemination, Zeneca has violated the postmarketing reporting requirements of the Act (21 CFR 314.81 (b) (3) (1)). Moreover, reference is made to Zeneca's letters dated December 9, 1998, and January 7, 1999, wherein Zeneca did not reference the aforementioned journal advertisement as being continued or discontinued.

FISHER "REPRINT CARRIER" (BROCHURE)

The Fisher brochure containing the reprint Fisher, B. MD et al., "Tamoxifen for prevention of breast cancer: Report of the National Surgical Adjuvant Breast and Bowel Project P-1 study," *J NCI*, 1998; 90: 1371-88, is in fact a promotional detail aid or brochure. This brochure contains promotional claims that are false or misleading and lacking in fair balance. DDMAC objects to the use of this material for the following reasons:

Zeneca's failure to discuss the *Gail Model Risk Assessment Tool* in the brochure undermines the importance of an accurate risk assessment. This material omission is dangerously misleading because Zeneca fails to adequately define women at high risk;

Promotional materials are lacking in fair balance, or otherwise misleading if they fail to present information relating to the contraindications, warnings, precautions, and side effects associated with the use of the drug in a manner reasonably comparable to the presentation of efficacy information. The risk information contained in the reprint carrier lacks the prominence, readability, scope, and depth that Zeneca dedicated to the presentation of efficacy information;

Zeneca's use of the word "uncommon" to modify endometrial cancer is misleading because it minimizes the significance of this serious risk. This description does not adequately communicate the fact that healthy women had a 2 1/2 times increased risk of getting endometrial cancer on Nolvadex as compared to placebo;

The brochure fails to provide sufficient emphasis for the information relating to side effects or contraindications, when such information is distorted because of repetition or other emphasis on claims for effectiveness. The presentation of safety information was selectively intertwined with the benefits so as to minimize the risks associated with therapy. For example, the perceived benefits of Nolvadex therapy (fewer fracture events and no effect on ischemic heart disease) were presented with proximity to risk information so as to minimize the adverse events associated with therapy;

Zeneca's use of the chart listing "criteria for evaluating high risk" is misleading because it promotes the use of Nolvadex in an unapproved patient population. Although one of the BCPT criteria for participation in the study was women over 60 years old, such women are not included in the indicated population *unless* they also have a 5-year predicted risk of breast cancer >1.67%, as calculated by the Gail Model.

Misleading efficacy data contained in the brochure that is inconsistent with the approval product labeling (PI) include:

49% reduction in the incidence of breast cancer vs. 44% (PI);

4.6 years median follow-up time vs. 4.2 (PI);

36.8% of women had follow-up >5 years vs. 25% (PI).

Material information that is missing from the reprint carrier but contained in the approved product labeling includes:

Nolvadex does not normalize the risk of breast cancer in high risk women;

In the BCPT study, Nolvadex had no impact on survival;

Nolvadex may not be appropriate for all women at high risk.

The claims relative to fewer fracture events are misleading because they are not supported by statistically significant evidence.

While prevention of breast cancer in women at high risk may have been the hypothesis tested in the trial (and thus influenced the name of the study), the results, in fact, did not demonstrate that Nolvadex prevents breast cancer. Rather, the data showed that Nolvadex may reduce the incidence of breast cancer in women at high risk. Hence, Zeneca was informed, in previous discussions with the Agency, that use of the term "prevention" would be false and/or misleading. DDMAC has no objection to the cover of the brochure that accurately presents the title of the study. However, page 2 of the brochure repeatedly refers to the "Breast Cancer Prevention Trial." This presentation promotes Nolvadex for "prevention."

Zeneca should immediately cease using the journal advertisement, Fisher reprint carrier, and all other promotional materials for Nolvadex that contain the same or similar claims or presentations. Zeneca should submit a written response to DDMAC, on or before February 5, 1999, describing its intent and plans to comply with the above. In its letter to DDMAC, Zeneca should include a list of all promotional materials that were discontinued, and the discontinuation date.

Zeneca should direct its response to the undersigned by facsimile at (301) 594-6771, or by written communication at the Division of Drug Marketing, Advertising, and Communications, HFD-40; Room 17B-20; 5600 Fishers Lane; Rockville, MD 20857. DDMAC reminds Zeneca that only written communications are considered official.

In all future correspondence regarding this matter, please refer to MACMIS#7432 and NDA 17-970/S-040.

Sincerely,
Michael A. Misocky, R.Ph., J.D.
Regulatory Review Officer
Division of Drug Marketing, Advertising, and Communications

Notes

1. Unless otherwise specified, information in this chapter came from Findlay S. *Prescription drugs and mass media advertising*. National Institute for Health Care Management Research and Education Foundation, 2000 Sept.

2. There were also voluntary marketing practice codes such as the one developed by the International Federation of Pharmaceutical Manufacturers Associations, available from www.ifpma.org. However, this code was voluntary and had not been adopted by U.S. companies.

3. The FDA regulates all prescription drug advertising in accordance with section 502(n) of the Federal Food, Drug, and Cosmetic Act (21 *United States Code* 352(n)) and the implementing regulations (21 *Code of Federal Regulations* Part 202).

Pines WL. A history and perspective on direct-to-consumer promotion. *Food and Drug Law Journal* 1999; 54:489.

4. *Direct-to-consumer advertising*. Pharmaceutical Research and Manufacturers of America. Available from www.phrma.org/facts/bkgrndr/advert.html.

5. The ad was for a nasal allergy drug.

6. Food and Drug Administration. Draft guidance for industry: Consumer-directed broadcast advertisements. 62 *Federal Register* 1997:43,171.

7. Food and Drug Administration. *Guidance for industry: Consumer-directed broadcast advertisement*. Washington, DC: Food and Drug Administration; 1999. Available from www.fda.gov/cder/guidance/index.htm.

8. Ibid.

9. Hayes TA. The Food and Drug Administration's regulation of drug labeling, advertising and promotion: Looking back and looking ahead. *Clinical Pharmacology & Therapeutics* 1998; 63:607–16.

10. Food and Drug Administration. Direct-to-consumer promotion. 61 *Federal Register* 1997:24,314–24,315.

11. See Note 3, Pines.

12. See Note 6.

13. Pear R. Drug companies getting FDA reprimands for false or misleading advertising. *New York Times* 1999 Mar 28; Sect. 1:28.

14. Adams C. FDA scrambles to police truthfulness of drug ads. *Wall Street Journal* 2001 Jan 2; Sect. A:1.

15. Stifano TM. *Direct-to-consumer promotion of prescription drugs and biologics*. BIO West Conference, 1999 May.

16. Ostrow NM. *Update on DTC promotion.* Washington, DC: Food and Drug Administration, Division of Drug Marketing, Advertising and Communications; 2000. Available from http://fda.gov/cder/ostrFDL1900/tsld001.htm.

17. Food and Drug Administration/Center for Drug Evaluation and Research. *Guidance for industry; consumer-directed broadcast advertisements; questions and answers.* 1999 Aug. Available from www.fda.gov/cder/guidance/1804q&a.htm.

18. Holmer AF. Direct-to-consumer prescription drug advertising builds bridges between patients and physicians. *Journal of the American Medical Association* 1999; 281:380–82.

19. *Physician drug and diagnosis audit: Patient visits up for DTC conditions.* Scott-Levin Agency; 1998. Available from www.scottlevin.com/news/rel_archive.cfm?rel_id= 10&prsearch=dtc.

20. Aikin K. Attitudes and behaviors associated with direct-to-consumer (DTC) promotion of prescription drugs. Washington, DC: Food and Drug Administration, Division of Drug Marketing, Advertising, and Communications, Office of Medical Policy; 1999. Accessed at www.fda.gov/cder/ddmac/DTCtitle.htm.

21. *Physician drug and diagnosis audit: Direct-to-consumer pharmaceutical ads "raising consumer awareness."* Scott-Levin Agency; 1998. Available from www.scottlevin.com/ news/rel_archive.cfm?rel_id=10&prsearch=dtc; see also Note 19.

22. *IMS Health reports direct to consumer advertising increases prescription pharmaceutical brand requests and awareness.* 1998 Sept 15. Available from www.imshealth.com/ html/pr_arc/09_15_1998_104.htm.

23. Bell R, Kravitz R, Wilkes M. Direct-to-consumer prescription drug advertising and the public. *Journal of General Internal Medicine* 1999; 14:651–57.

24. Consumers want details about prescription drugs: Many use "alternative" medicines. *American Journal of Health System Pharmacy* 1999; 56:307.

25. See Note 18.

26. Norplant is a female contraceptive contained in four silastic rods that are implanted under the skin of the upper arm of the patient.

Perez v. Wyeth Laboratories, Inc. 734 A.2d 1245, 161 N.J. 1 (1999 Aug 9). Although many of the pharmaceutical companies that produce DTC drug ads are multinational, this case deals only with DTC drug ads in the United States, since such ads were not allowed in Europe. At the time, one other court had reached an opposite conclusion in a similar case involving Norplant. In re Norplant Contraceptive Prod. Liability Litigation v. American Home Products Corp., 165 F.3d 374 (1999). It was unclear which legal opinion would be followed in other jurisdictions.

27. The rationale behind the learned intermediary doctrine is based upon a number of factors including that physicians have superior training and experience and are better able to determine what is medically appropriate prescribing for individual patients. This legal doctrine assumes that the physician is also better situated than the manufacturer to convey the appropriate and applicable warnings to the patient. In addition, courts believed that warnings given to consumers might interfere with the traditional physician-patient relationship. See Allen MC. Medicine goes Madison Av-

enue: An evaluation of the effect of direct-to-consumer pharmaceutical advertising on the learned intermediary doctrine. 20 *Campbell Law Review* 1997; 113:Winter.

28. McMenamin JP, Tarry SL, Whelan DJ. Corporate strategy: How Perez v. Wyeth Laboratories will affect direct-to-consumer drug advertising. *Product Liability Law & Strategy* 1999; 18:7.

29. In 1999, a total of $13.9 billion was spent on promoting prescription drugs, divided as follows: 52 percent retail value of drug samples, 26 percent doctor's office sales calls, 13 percent DTC ads, 5 percent hospital sales calls, and 4 percent journal advertising.

30. Ono Y. Drug makers learn to craft a slicker path. *Wall Street Journal* 1998 Feb 10; Sect. B:1.

31. Hamilton J, Bogan T. The promise and peril for biotech in direct-to-consumer drug advertising. *Signals Magazine* 1997 Aug 18. Available from www.signalsmag.com.

32. Freudenheim M. Influencing doctor's orders. *New York Times* 1998 Nov 17; Sect. C:1.

33. Wilkes MS, Bell RA, Kravtiz RL. Direct-to-consumer prescription drug advertising: Trends, impact, and implications. *Health Affairs* 2000; 19:110–28.

34. Sampey K. Former FDA chief raises alarm over drug ads. *AdWeek* 1999 June 18. Available from http://members.adweek.com/archive/adweek/daily/june/aw/wo61999-52.asp.

35. DTC ads: Just what the doctor ordered. *MediaWeek* 1997 Oct 20. Available from http://members.adweek.com/archive/adweek/mediaweek/1997/w102097/w_80.asp.

36. According to one pharmaceutical industry market research firm, U.S. and Canadian pharmaceutical sales in 1998 and 1999 were rising about 11–12 percent per year with annual sales of $72 billion to $80 billion. IMS Health, Global Services, 5/22/98 and 4/21/99, accessed at www.imshealth.com/html/tw_arc/05_22_1998_3.html and at www.imshealth.com/html/news_arc/04_21_1999_191.html.

Suydam LA. *Advertising and promotion in the new millennium.* Food and Drug Law Institute Conference, Food and Drug Administration; 1999 Sept 13. Available from www. fda.gov/oc/speeches/offlabel.html.

Fox JL. Industry-linked groups, geneticists, hoard data. *Nature Biotechnology* 1997; 15:504–5.

Morgan C, Levy D. Direct marketing: To their health. *BrandWeek* 1998 Jan 19. Available from members.adweek.com/cgi-bin/query.asp.

IMS Health reports U.S. pharmaceutical promotional spending reached a record $13.9 billion in 1999. 2000 Apr 20. Available from www. imshealth.com/html/news_arc/04_20_2000_352htm.

See also Note 3, Pines; Note 4.

37. See Note 30.

38. Rosner F, Kark P, Packer S, et al. Direct-to-consumer drug advertising: Education or anathema? *Journal of the American Medical Association* 1999; 282:1226–28.

39. Loden DJ, Schooler C. How to make DTC advertising work harder. *Medical Marketing & Media* 1998 Apr. Available from www. cpsnet.com/reprints/1998/04/DTCAdvertis.pdf.

40. See Note 3, Pines.

41. For instance, in the mid-1990s, many physicians began prescribing two weight-loss drugs, dexfenfluramine and fenfluramine, the combination of which was nicknamed "fen-phen." Physicians reported that this was such an effective weight-loss regimen that patients were demanding it even after they were told that the treatment could be seriously toxic. In September 1997, FDA recalled dexfenfluramine after it had been associated with potentially fatal heart valve abnormalities in a substantial percentage of women who took the drug. Ault A. Anti-obesity drugs recalled from global market. *Lancet* 1997; 350:867.

42. See Note 22.

43. See Note 23.

44. See Note 24.

45. Wilkes M, Doblin B, Shapiro M. Pharmaceutical advertisements in leading medical journals: Experts' assessments. *Annals of Internal Medicine* 1992; 116:912–19; Stryer D, Bero L. Characteristics of materials distributed by drug companies: An evaluation of appropriateness. *Journal of General Internal Medicine* 1996; 11:575–83.

46. See Note 32.

47. See Note 39.

48. Ibid.

49. Pirisi A. Patient-directed drug advertising puts pressure on US doctors. *Lancet* 1999; 354:1887; Hollon MF. Direct-to-consumer marketing of prescription drugs: Creating consumer demand. *Journal of the American Medical Association* 1999; 281:382–84.

50. See Note 33.

51. A drug formulary is a list of approved drugs carried by a hospital pharmacy. The list is intended to limit physician choices for prescribing to necessary drugs with reasonable benefit versus risk profiles. Committees of doctors and pharmacists in the institution decide which drugs to include or delete and process requests from doctors who want to prescribe their favorite drugs. Formularies are a hospital's attempt to prevent unneeded drug duplication (e.g., stocking only one antihistamine among several on the market) and to keep drug costs down (e.g., stocking equivalent generics instead of brand name drugs or refusing to list a new expensive drug when there is doubt about its incremental benefits over existing drugs). Drug companies and insurers often lobby the chief pharmacist to either include or exclude certain drugs from the hospital formulary. See Note 33.

52. See Note 14.

53. See Note 20.

54. *Half of Rx drug consumer ad spending goes to TV, Scott Levin reports.* Scott-Levin Agency; 1998 June 2. Available from www.scottlevin.com/news/rel_archive.cfm?rel_id=17&prsearch=dtc; see also Note 18.

55. Council on Ethical and Judicial Affairs, AMA. Direct-to-consumer advertisements of prescription drugs. *Food and Drug Law Journal* 2000; 55:119–24.

56. See Note 49, Hollon.

57. See Note 32.

58. See Note 3, Pines.

59. Kranhold K. New groups seek remedy to drug ads. *Wall Street Journal* 2000 June 22; Sect. B:16.

60. The initial case study was prepared by Jason Ehrlich and Naveen Chopra under the guidance of and later revision by Margaret Eaton. The input and assistance of Mary Lynn Carver, oncology communications leader at AstraZeneca, is greatly appreciated. We also thank Steven Bateman of FCB Healthcare for his insights into the DTC prescription drug advertising process. The events described in this case study occurred up until spring 1999.

61. Zeneca Group PLC was formed in 1993 as a spin-off of the large British company, Imperial Chemical Industries. Zeneca's four main businesses were (1) Zeneca Pharmaceuticals, which produced nearly half of sales, developed drugs for cancer, cardiovascular, central nervous system, metabolic, infectious, and respiratory diseases, (2) Zeneca Agrochemicals, which developed herbicides, insecticides, and fungicides for horticulture and crop protection, (3) Zeneca Specialties, which developed industrial chemicals, resins, and life science molecules, and (4) Salick Health Care, which operated cancer treatment and dialysis centers in the United States. Zeneca Inc. was the U.S. unit of Zeneca Group PLC. In April 1999, Zeneca Group PLC merged with another large pharmaceutical company, Astra AB of Sweden, to become AstraZeneca PLC. Given that the major events described in this case study occurred prior to the merger, the company will be referred to as Zeneca Group and the U.S. unit as Zeneca.

62. Zeneca Group, 1998 annual report and account.

63. Zeneca 1997 annual report and account, p. 10.

64. Zeneca Group, 1998 annual report and account.

65. From a presentation given by Toni Stiffano, Office of Compliance and Biologic Quality, Center for Biologics Evaluation and Research, BIO West Conference; 1999 May.

66. CancerNet, National Cancer Institute. Available from www.cancernet.nci.nih. gov/.

67. *Breast cancer facts and figures, 1999–2000: Who gets breast cancer?* American Cancer Society. Available from www.cancer.org/statistics/99bcff/who.html.

68. *Breast cancer facts and figures, 1999–2000: How has the occurrence of breast cancer changed over time?* American Cancer Society. Available from www.cancer.org/statistics/99bcff/occurrence.html.

69. Kinsinger L, Harris R, Karnitschnig J. Worry about breast cancer in younger women: A major problem. *Journal of General Internal Medicine* 1998 Apr; 13:99.

70. According to the Zeneca Press Release of 9/2/98: "An increased risk of changes in the endometrium (lining of the uterus), including endometrial cancer, has been associated with NOLVADEX treatment. Healthy women in the general population have reported endometrial cancer of 0.7 cases per 1,000 women. Women with breast cancer, regardless of any treatment they may receive, have an increased risk of endometrial cancer: about 1 case per 1,000 women. Among breast cancer patients treated with NOLVADEX, between 2 and 3 cases per 1,000 women per year may be diagnosed."

71. From the Nolvadex U.S. prescribing information for physicians. Available from www.tamoxifen.com.

72. Adjuvant treatment refers to medical treatments given along with the primary treatment of surgical removal of the tumor.

73. The research study was initiated in April 1992 and closed enrollment in September 1997 after 13,388 women had been enrolled.

74. This model was developed by Dr. Mitchell Gail, a National Cancer Institute (NCI) scientist. According to Zeneca, "The Gail model was derived using 4,496 matched pairs of breast cancer cases and controls from the Breast Cancer Detection and Demonstration Project, a mammography screening project carried out between 1973 and 1980, which involved more than 280,000 women. Using logistic regression techniques, Gail and colleagues examined a number of possible risk factors for breast cancer, among them, hormones, cigarette smoking, alcohol consumption, height, gynecological history (including first period and first childbirth), history of breast biopsy, and family history. The risk factors were adjusted simultaneously for the presence of the other risk factors, and only five factors emerged as significant predictors of the lifetime risk: current age, age at first period, number of breast biopsies, age at first birth, family history of breast cancer in first degree relatives." See www.tamoxifen.com/assessing.asp. The Gail Model Risk Assessment Tool was used by the NCI to identify which women were "high risk" and therefore qualified to enroll in the Breast Cancer Prevention Trial.

75. CancerNet, National Cancer Institute. Available from http://cancernet.nci.nih.gov/clinpdq/cancer_genetics/Genetics_of_breast_and_ovarian_cancer.html and http://rex.nci.nih.gov/massmedia/pressreleases/riskasses.html.

76. Fisher B, Costantino JP, Wickerham DL, et al. Tamoxifen for prevention of breast cancer: Report of the National Surgical Adjuvant Breast and Bowel Project P-1 Study. *Journal of the National Cancer Institute* 1998; 90:1371–88.

77. There were 85 cases of invasive breast cancer in the tamoxifen group (of 6,694 subjects) compared with 154 in the same-sized placebo group. Women who received tamoxifen also had fewer noninvasive breast cancers.

78. See 11/3/98 letter from Robert Temple, M.D., director of drug evaluation, Center for Drug Evaluation and Research, FDA, to Zeneca Pharmaceuticals. Available from www.fda.gov.

79. According to the FDA-approved Nolvadex labeling (called the package insert), in the BCPT trial, there were thirty-three cases of endometrial cancer in the Nolvadex group, compared to only fourteen in the placebo group; there were thirty cases of deep vein thrombosis (blood clots in major veins) in the tamoxifen group, compared to nineteen in the placebo group; and there were eighteen cases of pulmonary embolism (blood clot that has traveled to the lung and is potentially lethal) in the tamoxifen group, compared with six in the placebo group. There were thirty-four strokes in the Nolvadex group and twenty-four in the placebo group. There were three deaths from breast cancer in the tamoxifen group, compared with five in the placebo group. Two women on tamoxifen who developed pulmonary emboli also died. There-

fore, there were five drug-related deaths in both the tamoxifen and the placebo groups. There was a small increased incidence of cataracts. There were also cases of minor side effects in the tamoxifen group, the most common of which were hot flashes and vaginal discharge, with fewer women experiencing irregular menstrual periods, dizziness, headaches, fatigue, loss of appetite, nausea and/or vomiting, vaginal dryness or bleeding, irritation of the skin around the vagina, and liver toxicities. See also, National Cancer Institute. Breast cancer prevention trial shows major benefit, some risk. Press release. 1999 Apr 6. Available from http://rex.nci.nih.gov/massmedia/pressreleases/prevtrial.htm.

80. FDA considered all manufacturer information that accompanied a drug and all promotional material to constitute a drug's "labeling."

81. Ault A. Tamoxifen prevention claim will not be allowed in USA. *Lancet* 1998; 352:883. See also www.bcaction.org/news/9812-06.html.

82. See 11/3/98 letter from Robert Temple, M.D., director of drug evaluation, Center for Drug Evaluation and Research, FDA, to Zeneca Pharmaceuticals. Available from www.fda.gov.

83. Bruzzi P. Tamoxifen for the prevention of breast cancer; important questions remain unanswered, and existing trials should continue. *British Medical Journal* 1998; 316: 1181–82; Ault A, Bradbury J. Experts argue about results of tamoxifen trial. *Lancet* 1998; 351:1107.

84. Early Breast Cancer Collaborative Group. Tamoxifen for early breast cancer: An overview of the randomized trials. *Lancet* 1998; 351:1451–67.

85. Powles T, Eeles R, Ashley S, et al. Interim analysis of the incidence of breast cancer in the Royal Marsden Hospital tamoxifen randomised chemo prevention trial. *Lancet* 1998; 352:98–101; Veronesi U, Maisonneuve P, Costa A, et al. Prevention of breast cancer with tamoxifen: Preliminary findings from the Italian randomised trial among hysterectomised women. *Lancet* 1998; 352:93–97.

86. Kmietowicz Z. Latest studies fail to show that tamoxifen prevents breast cancer. *British Medical Journal* 1998; 317:162.

87. Pritchard KI. Is tamoxifen effective in prevention of breast cancer? *Lancet* 1998: 352:80–81.

88. Ibid.

89. Letter from Robert Temple, M.D., Center for Drug Evaluation and Research, FDA, to W.J. Kennedy, Ph.D., vice president, Drug Regulatory Affairs, Zeneca Pharmaceuticals. Available from www.fda.gov/cder/foi/appletter/1998/17970s040.pdf.

90. Cancer statistics showed that the risk of breast cancer increases throughout a woman's lifetime and the annual incidence of breast cancer in U.S. women eighty to eighty-five years old was fifteen times higher than for women thirty to thirty-four years old. See Notes 66–68, supra.

91. Norton A. Cancer researchers still not sure who should take Tamoxifen. *Medical Tribune News Service* 1999 May 19. Available from www.personalmd.com/cancercenter_update1.shtml.

92. Ross, PE. Drugs to cure cancer have little success: We need new ones to pre-

vent it. *Forbes Magazine* 1999 May 13. Available from www.forbes.com/forbes/1999/0531/6311238a.html.

93. Less than meets the eye: The Breast Cancer Prevention Trial. *Breast Cancer Action* 1998 Apr 8. Available from www.bcaction.org/news/9804-01a.html.

94. Suh-Burgmann E, Goodman A. Surveillance for endometrial cancer in women receiving tamoxifen. *Annals of Internal Medicine* 1999; 131:127-35.

95. Ibid.

Ginsburg M. Breast cancer recommendation faces criticism. *San Francisco Examiner* 1999 May 20. Available from www.personalmd.com/cancercenter_update1.shtml.

96. Tamoxifen for healthy women. National Women's Health Network. Available from www.womenshealthnetwork.org/clearinghouse/tamox.htm.

97. See Note 93.

98. At the European Cancer Conference in September 1999, the lead researcher of the British tamoxifen trial questioned "whether exposing tens of thousands of healthy women to tamoxifen was preferable to the treatment of the hundreds of breast cancers that would otherwise arise." European studies were continuing so that definitive data could be collected. Other researchers, however, defended the use of tamoxifen. According to one American physician at the same meeting, "The toxicities from tamoxifen have been highly over-rated for many reasons, including politics, economics, and pure bias. The side-effects were not unexpected or fatal, and so-called 'effective' treatment for breast cancer still fails to cure many women." So, he said, "we cannot deny tamoxifen to those at increased risk." McNamee D. Debate on whether to use tamoxifen for cancer prevention continues. *Lancet* 1999; 354:1007.

99. See Note 91, Norton. In May 1999, these researchers presented their unpublished findings that most research confirmed the tamoxifen benefit and recommended that doctors at least discuss the drug with higher-risk women. The researchers were of the opinion that a similar recommendation for raloxifene was not justified at the time. See First independent assessment of breast cancer risk reduction drugs supports a role for tamoxifen therapy. ASCO press release; 1999 May 18. Available from www.asco.org/people/nr/html/tue_techassess.htm. See also, Chlebowski RT, Collyar DE, Somerfield MR, et al. American Society of Clinical Oncology technology assessment on breast cancer risk reduction strategies: Tamoxifen and raloxifene. *Journal of Clinical Oncology* 1999; 17:1939-55.

100. Burton T. Lilly's Evista shows promise in cancer test. *Wall Street Journal* 1998 Dec 11; p. A:3.

The study showing that that Evista could lower the risk of breast cancer without the endometrial cancer side effect was eventually published: Cummings S, Eckert S, Krueger K, et al. The effect of raloxifene on risk of breast cancer in postmenopausal women: Results from the MORE randomized trial. *Journal of the American Medical Association* 1999; 281:2189-97.

101. Information on Nolvadex marketing and advertising was provided by various Zeneca managers.

102. Zeneca Group, 1998 annual report and account.

103. See Note 34.

104. See Note 10.

105. The FDA's Division of Drug Marketing, Advertising, and Communications (DDMAC) issued sixty-one Notices of Violation in 1997, distributed as follows: false and/or misleading claims (38 percent), unsubstantiated comparative claims (23 percent), unapproved uses (23 percent), promotion of lack of fair balance (18 percent), and unsubstantiated cost-effectiveness claims (10 percent). Source: see Note 9.

106. Information on Nolvadex marketing and advertising was provided by various Zeneca managers.

107. Allegra is Aventis Pharmaceutical's antiallergy drug. Some of the biggest DTC drug ad campaigns to date had been for this class of drug.

108. Although it was not required for companies to have their DTC ads pre-screened by DDMAC, FDA had required Zeneca to do so for ads stating Nolvadex's new indication.

109. See introductory information in this chapter on DTC prescription drug promotion regulations.

110. Grady D. Drug marketing starts legal battle. *New York Times* 1999 Mar 28; p. 28.

111. FDA general regulations for DTC ads had been promulgated in 1985. However, these regulations had made it extremely difficult to develop understandable DTC broadcast ads. In August 1997, FDA issued a nonmandatory Draft Guidance for Industry on DTC broadcast advertisements. These guidelines were made final with some changes in August 1999. The Nolvadex DTC ads were developed in the interim between the draft and final guidelines. For a full description of the regulations, see the introductory information at the beginning of this chapter.

112. Direct-to-consumer marketing 1999: A long term strategic perspective. Abstract. *DataMonitor* 1999 Apr. Available from www.datamonitor.com.

113. Salter S. Risqué hype sends wrong message about cancer drug. *San Francisco Examiner* 1999 May 23; p. D:5.

114. Available from www.inmotionmagazine.com/zeneca.html, www.citizen.org, www.womenshealthnetwork.org, and www.bcaction.org.

115. Zeneca's Tamoxifen (Nolvadex®) ads. Breast Cancer Action. Press release. DES Action, Boston Women's Health Book Collective, National Women's Health Network, Massachusetts Breast Cancer Coalition. 1999 May 5. Available from www.inmotion-magazine.com/zeneca.html.

116. Public Citizen, National Women's Health Network urge FDA to require warnings about risks associated with Tamoxifen. Public Citizen news release. 1999 May 4. Available from www.citizen.org/hrg.

117. Richwine L. Groups urge more warnings about cancer drug risks. *New York Times* 1999 May 4.

118. Brady J. Public relations and cancer. *Breast Cancer Action Newsletter* 1998 Oct/Nov; No. 50. Available from www.bcaction.org/Pages/SearchablePages/1998Newsletters/Newsletter050F.html.

The mention of a pink ribbon was a reference to the widespread use of a small pink ribbon used as a symbol of breast cancer awareness and support for research. Since this statement was made, Zeneca's merger and spin-off activity resulted in its no longer selling pesticides.

119. By comparison, the spending leader Schering Plough spent $137.4 million on DTC ads for its Claritin antiallergy products. IMS Health reports U.S. pharmaceutical promotional spending reached record $13.9 billion in 1999. IMS Health. 2000 Apr 20. Available from www.imshealth.com/html/news_arc/04_20_2000_352.htm.

120. Immunex Corporation press release. 1999 Apr 6.

Using Corporate Ethics Advice

What motivates a company to develop a corporate ethics program? Many times, this motivation comes from a recognition that the company cannot afford the cost and other ramifications of misconduct or needs to reform to prevent future misconduct. Avoiding trouble prompted many companies to develop ethics programs after the Federal Sentencing Guidelines held organizations responsible for the illegal conduct of individual employees and offered lenient treatment for convicted organizations with an effective ethics program.[1] Other companies develop ethics programs because company leadership believe in the compatibility of business and ethics. Regardless of the motivation, companies that became serious about developing a corporate ethics program set up internal departments that developed a code of ethics, provided ethics training for employees, set up communication and reporting mechanisms to discuss ethical questions or report misconduct, conducted ethics audits, and developed remedial solutions when misconduct was discovered. Hundreds of large and small U.S. companies have such programs and hire an ethics officer to run them. The goals of such programs range from ensuring legal compliance to fostering company integrity and encouraging employees to act ethically.[2]

Most bioscience companies do not have such advanced programs and gained an appreciation for the ethical aspects of their business when public debates began about the propriety of biotechnology advances. As biotechnology and pharmaceutical companies work on the frontiers of new medical and genomics technologies, more are seeking the assistance of ethics advisors to review the social, moral, and religious implications of their activities. In the 1990s, the new medical technologies, especially in the field of genetics and genomics, were generating a host of tricky ethical and social questions. By the late 1990s, several companies were realizing that managing these issues required more than simply referring them to the public relations department. Geron Bio-Med chief executive officer Simon Best (originally from the company that sponsored the Dolly cloning research) recognized the need for ethics advice when he said, "We in the industry are not experts in ethics. Forming an ethics advisory board to deal with both scientific discoveries and the conduct of business is therefore a strategic and moral necessity."[3] Statements such as this prompted one science reporter to write, "The industry has come to understand that it can not afford to alienate the public—which includes investors and consumers—with its science, for it is with the public that its fate ultimately lies."[4]

In part, this recognition had been prompted by the public relations disaster brought on by the manner in which bioengineered foods had been introduced in Europe. Monsanto Company, a leader in the commercialization of agricultural biotechnology, triggered widespread protests when it made two decisions —not to segregate transgenic from naturally grown products, and refusal to label products as containing transgenic food. The consumer protests were based on fears that these products were unnatural, unsafe, and environmentally destructive, and these fears led to boycotts, picketing, sabotage of Monsanto croplands, lawsuits, moratoria on the further production of transgenic plants, and other regulatory reversals.[5] See Chapter 3 for the difficulties Monsanto faced with its Posilac labeling. Monsanto's problems were attributed to a failure to appreciate and address Europe's relative lack of trust in science and technology, consumers' need to know what is in their food, and the continent's strong proenvironment political movement. Not long afterward, American companies were beginning to see this antibiotechnology backlash cross the Atlantic. Indeed, by the mid-1990s, some biotechnology companies were already the target of protests, and consumer, patient, antiglobalization, and environmental activists were picketing the Biotechnology Industry Organization each year at its annual meeting.

Another catalyzing event was the 1997 announcement of the cloning of the sheep Dolly, an activity that was partially funded by private money and that quickly led to widespread alarm about the potential for human cloning and calls to ban the use of the technology.[6] Commenting on the impact of this scientific feat, Steven Holtzman, the chief business officer of Millennium Pharmaceuticals, said, "Many companies have become savvy enough to understand that the single greatest obstacle to utilizing new technologies is the potential for a public backlash. In 1995, it was more difficult to get companies involved in these issues, because they didn't see the relevance to them. That changed for the most part when Dolly came along." Holtzman added that since then, a growing number of companies have recognized that larger issues in biotechnology beyond the business and scientific aspects of their work could have an impact on their future prospects.[7]

These events led some biotechnology companies to decide that it was time to deal proactively with the ethical and social impact of their corporate work. Since there was no established precedent for the optimal manner in which to obtain ethics advice, companies took different approaches, which produced different results. Early examples of these different approaches and results include those described below.

MILLENNIUM PHARMACEUTICALS, INC., CAMBRIDGE, MASSACHUSETTS

When the founders of genomics company Millennium Pharmaceuticals started their company, they incorporated an ethical aspect into the company mission. The Millennium founders knew, for instance, that their R&D in genetic testing would raise issues related to privacy of genetic information and genetic discrimination. The founders also knew that they would have to deal initially with questions about corporate ownership of human tissue and gene patenting, both of which had been a source of social and ethical conflict and public debate. With these issues in mind, CEO Mark Levin wrote a preliminary ethics vision for the company that included a set of core values and commitments to integrity and corporate and social responsibility. He then hired Holtzman to be Millennium's chief business officer. Holtzman, a biotechnology business executive who also held advanced degrees in philosophy, was asked to spend part of his work time initiating an ethics program for the company. "Written into my job description—literally—was a mandate to bring an awareness of sensitive ethical issues to the staff that our work would raise," Holtzman said. "Millennium's founders and board of directors believed that in order to realize the full potential of its technologies and to guarantee their socially responsible use, it was necessary to have a strong, informed public discourse within the company about issues the science was raising."[8] Holtzman started with the premise that the ethical perspective of the business should not be brought to the company by an outside expert but rather that the company should develop it from within.

To accomplish this, Holtzman worked to extend the strong leadership focus on ethics into the workforce. He hired Dr. Philip Reilly, a University of Massachusetts Medical School clinical geneticist with a law background, to set up a bioethics, law, and social policy course and related seminars for employees. Employees were released from other work responsibilities to attend classes that included such topics as the history of the eugenics movement in the United States, genetic privacy issues, population screening for genetic defects, genetic counseling, genetic discrimination, DNA banking, new reproductive technologies, legal issues raised by behavioral genetics, and ethical responsibilities to human research subjects. For the human research aspect of the course, three facets of the work were emphasized: (1) what are the goals of the research and are they ethical? (2) is the manner in which the research will be performed ethical? and (3) will the fruits of the research be made available in an ethical manner? The company Web site also included resources for employees on ethics and social responsibility, and employees were encouraged to submit bioethical articles to the company newsletter. With all of these initiatives, Holtzman intended to incorporate moral discourse into the overall corporate dialogue. The core values of the company are incorporated in various ways, including in the hiring and employee evaluation process (does the person display the requisite integrity?), in assessing business relationships (do the values and culture of the other group or company fit with ours?), and in research decisions (is the goal of the research ethical?). In one instance, the company decided that integrity required that Millennium consent forms for human research contain a statement that the research the company was conducting would likely result in profit for the company, in which research participants would not share. The decision was made not because it was required but because potential subjects might want to know this information.[9] Holtzman extended his ethics work when he started an ethics task force for BIO, the Biotechnology Industry Organization, and was named as the only corporate member of President Clinton's National Bioethics Advisory Commission, which provided advice about the preeminent biomedical ethical issues of the day. Because of these internal and external efforts, the company has developed a reputation as an ethical and socially responsible company.

AFFYMETRIX, INC., SANTA CLARA, CALIFORNIA

Affymetrix produces "gene chips" to detect the presence or absence of thousands of different genes or their variations. These chips are valuable research tools that can also be used in clinical practice to predict human disease risk or responsiveness to medications. Soon after the company went public in 1996, it formed a multidisciplinary advisory committee consisting of biomedical ethicists, health lawyers, scientists, and others to advise on the ethical and social implications of the company work. The names of these advisors were not made public, according to Dr. Thane Kreiner, vice president of business operations, because the company wanted advice, not public endorsement of its work. Affymetrix initially paid the advisors a consulting fee of $125 an hour for up to four meetings a year. Many of the advisors declined or directed their fees to a charity in their name. The advisory committee work was confidential, but Kreiner disclosed that, based on committee advice, Affymetrix contracts contain a clause requiring its customers and collaborators to use "the highest standards of informed consent" for those who donate samples for genetic analysis.[10] Input from the company ethics advisory committee also helped the company decide to turn away potentially profitable business from a company that wanted to put a disease gene mutation test on an Affymetrix chip. The reason for the refusal was that no prevention or treatment was currently available for patients who tested positive for the mutation. The ethics committee meetings are often attended by senior management, who rely on the committee for its objective outsider input into corporate activity.[11]

THE INSTITUTE FOR GENOMIC RESEARCH, ROCKVILLE, MARYLAND

TIGR, a private, nonprofit genomics research organization, gave a $75,000 grant to the bioethics center at the University of Pennsylvania, led by bioethicist Arthur Caplan, to study some of the institute's work. One such project was the creation of the minimal genome—to answer the question of how few genes it would take to create a living organism. This work was halted to allow Dr. Caplan's group to study the ethical ramifications involved and to create ethically acceptable guidelines for future similar research. "We knew the work had profound ethical public policy implications, and we decided to set a new precedent and have an ethical review before we went ahead," said board president Dr. J. Craig Venter. "It's important when you're creating life in the lab or even thinking about it." With this in mind, questions such as safety and the possibility that such an organism could be used as a bio-terror weapon were addressed. For his part, Caplan was interested in consulting for this institute and for other companies because "we're going to have this genetics explosion complete with patents and lawyers and stocks and investments and no oversight. The secrets of life will be in private hands. Can we trust industry to act responsibly?" Whether or not the outside ethicists would play the role of corporate overseers, the fact that scientists were analyzing the implications of their research in advance was viewed as having allayed some of the fears associated with this project.[12]

DNA SCIENCES, MOUNTAIN VIEW, CALIFORNIA

The genomics company DNA Sciences set up an Internet Web site asking for volunteers to provide blood samples for DNA testing along with detailed health histories. With this tissue and information, the company planned to develop a large data base of human genetic information to discover which genetic variations were responsible for disease susceptibility or differing responses to drugs. Gene tests and drug therapies could be developed with such knowledge.[13] Knowing that this work would raise questions about corporate ownership and commercialization of human DNA and medical information, company executives were committed to incorporating an ethical perspective into their business and hired a group of prominent academic bioethicists to advise them. When DNA Sciences posted its Internet solicitation, all of the names and credentials of the outside ethics advisors were also posted on the same site, which implied that the request for volunteers had been endorsed by the advisors. However, this turned out to be a premature move since none of the advisors had been asked to approve the solicitation and, in fact, had not even had a first meeting to advise the company about any of its activities. Responding to press inquiries about the company solicitation, one of the advisors, Nancy Neveloff Dubler, a professor of bioethics at the Albert Einstein College of Medicine in New York City, said, "We were startled to find our names on the Web site. My guess is that every one of us was prepared to resign, but none of us did so."[14] Although well intentioned, this glitch almost caused a wholesale defection of the advisors and led to some early negative publicity for the company.

ADVANCED CELL TECHNOLOGIES,
WORCESTER, MASSACHUSETTS

In November 1998, Advanced Cell Technologies publicly announced that scientists paid by the company had performed the ethically controversial feat of using cloning techniques to fuse the nucleus of a human cell with the cytoplasm from a cow's egg to create a hybrid human embryo.[15] The company made the public announcement not "to be sensational, but we felt it was unethical to do such work behind closed doors," said president and chief executive officer Dr. Michael West.[16] According to the company, the announcement was to test the public acceptance of trans-species research. The reaction was immediate. By the next day, reporters and scientists were asking if the research violated a ban on the use of federal funds for embryo research, if FDA research rules had been violated, and if the company had properly described its research plan to the institutional review board at the federally supported University of Massachusetts, where the research was performed. Others criticized the company for using the lay press to make the announcement rather than publishing the research in a scientific peer-reviewed journal so that scientists could assess, for instance, whether the embryo created could be viable.[17] In response to the furor, Congress and the FDA began investigations and President Clinton asked the National Bioethics Advisory Commission to advise him on the appropriateness of the work. Soon after, the company set up an ethics advisory board as an alternative to using public announcements to obtain feedback and guidance on ethical and social issues raised by its work.[18]

CONCLUSIONS

This range of experience indicates that there are both benefits and risks to using corporate ethics advisors. Among the benefits are that ethics advisors can assist with difficult internal decisions, such as what products to develop and whether it is premature to market them. They can also provide enlightenment about the ethical implications of company work and can inform companies about the history of different ethical challenges, the prevailing views of different groups, and the public reactions to expect. With this knowledge, business decisions can be made with a better appreciation for the impact of various options. In addition, a company that heeds ethical advice could avoid potential stumbling blocks in the process of research and product development. There are also strategic advantages for companies that foster ethical conduct and that gain a reputation for integrity.

Some companies that have used outside ethics advice, however, have also discovered the associated risks. Problems such as those experienced by DNA Sciences can easily lead to public skepticism about the intentions of companies that employ ethics advisors. For instance, one science reporter who interviewed several corporate executives from companies using ethics advisors asked whether ethicists were "engaging in rigorous analyses of these issues, or just providing window dressing?"[19] In part, such a reaction comes from a widespread notion that "business" and "ethics" make strange bedfellows, implying that business is solely concerned with profit making. Also, the use of ethics advice after a problem has developed can seem like image burnishing, although it may be the result of a belated recognition of the ethical consequences of corporate activity. According to BIO president Carl Feldbaum, the concern about ethicists window-dressing is reasonable, "but sometimes research leads you into areas that you don't expect. You may not realize you need [ethics advice] until you're halfway through."[20]

Other problems can develop when a company disregards the advice of its ethicists. "They could choose to take our advice or not," said one of the DNA Sciences advisors. "If we find out later on that they are not really serious about it, we will leave. And if we are really unhappy about it, we will make public why we leave."[21] This power can be limited, since corporate ethicists usually sign confidentiality agreements about the matters they review—a practice that can lead to another set of unique concerns. The fact that ethical concerns are kept confidential led one reporter to comment:

> The ethicists have become proxies for all of us, precisely because so much of this technology, for political reasons, is unfolding in the private sector. . . . It's very hard to have a national debate on issues as socially and ethically important as cloning and the creation of embryonic stem cells when every conversation may ultimately bump up against corporate confidentiality. The problem of openness is compounded by the editorial policy at a number of leading scientific journals, which refuse to publish research if the results have previously been disclosed in public. That almost guarantees that breakthroughs in a controversial and competitive field of research like stem cells will land in the public's lap as scientific faits accomplis, just as Dolly did.[22]

There were others who wondered what qualified a person to provide biomedical ethics advice. Current professionals had myriad backgrounds and degrees from philosophy, medicine, genetics, law, nursing, anthropology and other social sciences, and religion. Few academic programs existed to train biomedical ethicists, and, as Alta Charo, professor of law and medical ethics at the University of Wisconsin, said, "Anybody can stand up and claim to be an ethicist—there is no licensing, there is no accreditation."[23] Obviously, individuals with disparate backgrounds would bring different skills and approaches to ethics, but there was no consensus on what qualified someone as an expert who can analyze the conflicting values at stake and provide competent advice. What makes an ethicist authoritative? There was no agreement on this question. And there was suspicion that, with so many different individuals holding themselves out as ethicists qualified to advise bioscience companies, opinion shopping could occur. "This is a semi-scandalous situation for my field," said Dr. Daniel Callahan, of the Hastings Center, a medical ethics center in Garrison, New York. "These companies are smart enough to know that there are a variety of views on these subjects, and with a little bit of asking or shopping around you can find a group that will be congenial to what you are doing."[24]

Consistent with the difference in backgrounds, bioethicists were also consulting with bioscience companies for different reasons. Some viewed it as a public service. Others viewed it as a job. Some were interested in the ability of the consult work to enhance and broaden their academic work. Others wanted to hold companies accountable or to have a hand in controlling what happened to the technologies as they were turned into products. According to Barbara Handelin, a geneticist with a background in diagnostics who consults on ethics for biotech companies, "I knew if I wanted to be part of the solution, I had to be on the inside. Squawking from the outside would be of limited use. And, once a product or procedure is developed, it's too late to start asking questions, for at that point, there's no going back," she said.[25] Again there was no consensus about whether the motivation of the consultant should matter to the company. The question raised issues such as whether the consultant would be prone to provide opinions that pleased the company or was likely to keep company information confidential.

Still others wondered if corporate ethics advice, no matter how competent, could ever be effective in changing corporate behavior. Companies were free to keep information from their ethics consultants; one consultant, Glenn McGee, a philosopher and assistant professor of bioethics at the University of Pennsylvania, had publicly resigned from the board of a private biotech company because the company had kept too much information from the consultants. McGee reported that he heard only through the media that the company had cloned an endangered animal that died soon after birth, something that the ethicist thought was akin to "playing God" and should have undergone an ethical review.[26] Whether ethics consultants could alter company action was another question. According to George Annas, a lawyer and biomedical ethicist at Boston University, "It's totally unlikely that ethical consultants are going to have an impact on corporate technology if it's going to cost them money. . . . The companies are trying to deflect criticism, nothing more. It's a matter of good corporate strategy."[27]

Comments and views such as these suggest that companies operating in ethically complex areas need to be cautious not only about their R&D strategy but also about the manner in which they seek, obtain, and consider ethics advice. Adjustments in this uneasy and relatively recent alliance between business and bioethics will be needed as the public and private expectations of such arrangements are worked out.

Case Study

Geron Corporation and the Role of Ethics Advice [28]

"Is it ever permissible to use one human life—or, if you will, potential life—in service of the lives of others?"

—A Stem Of Hope, By Marjorie Williams, *Washington Post*, Friday, August 25, 2000; Page A31

"Imagine being paralyzed by a spinal cord injury in your teens, watching for decades as medical treatment progresses but not quite fast enough, and knowing that it could have been faster."

—Reason, Faith and Stem Cells, By Michael Kinsley, *Washington Post*, Tuesday, August 29, 2000; Page A17

In the spring of 1999, scientists, biotechnology companies, ethicists, religious leaders, patient advocates, abortion opponents, the National Institutes of Health, and members of Congress were all engaged in a protracted debate about human embryo research. In the middle of and fueling this debate was Geron Corporation, a publicly traded biotechnology company in Menlo Park, California, founded in 1990. Thomas Okarma, M.D., Ph.D., vice president of research and development, was largely responsible for how Geron would respond to the debate. Okarma had joined Geron as vice president of cell therapies in December 1997, when Geron had been financing research at three U.S. universities to isolate human embryonic stem (hES) cells, the primordial or master cells from which all human tissues evolve. Geron executives had known from the outset that this research was likely to stir public debate on the ethics of the science, and as early as 1996, senior managers suggested that the company might benefit from a board that could provide an external evaluation of the ethics of the research methods and goals. Okarma implemented the concept in March 1998, and the Geron Ethics Advisory Board (EAB), a novelty among biotechnology companies when the idea was conceived, was born. The EAB's first pronouncement, the Statement on Human Embryonic Stem Cells, on the ethics of Geron's decision to pursue the isolation of hES cells, was published in the spring 1999 issue of the *Hastings Center Report*, a prominent ethics journal. The statement was published alongside articles by other medical ethicists. Although many of the commentators lauded Geron for its actions, others questioned whether a company-based EAB could exercise effective oversight. Because Geron's future research work was likely to be as ground-breaking and controversial as its work on hES cells, Okarma needed to assess the role and efficacy of the EAB. Had the board served its purpose? Would the board play an effective role in helping Geron direct its future technology development in an ethically and socially responsible manner? Okarma reflected on both the research and the ethical discourse surrounding the current debate to focus his thoughts on the role the EAB should play in assessing future research at Geron.

TECHNOLOGY BEHIND THE ETHICAL ISSUES

Embryonic stem (ES) cells—cells present in the developing embryo that are the starting point for the creation of the adult organism—have long held the fascination of biologists. These rare cells multiply within the embryo, exist for a short period of time, and then, dividing further, begin to develop into all of the more than two hundred specialized cells of the adult organism, including the cells that make up muscle, bone, the nervous system, and the immune system. Researchers had been successful in isolating ES cells from animals but, until Geron's research, no one had done the same for humans.[29] For a scientist to prove that he or she has isolated and could maintain ES cells in culture, the cells must possess several characteristics. They must be pluripotent, that is, capable of maturing and differentiating into virtually any cell or tissue in the body. They also must be able to self-renew and replicate an indefinite number of times, approaching immortality as much as possible. This special characteristic is unlike most tissue cells, which can replicate only a limited number of times before dying. Geron scientists had previously discovered that ES cell immortality was conferred in part by their expression of telomerase, an enzyme that enables cells to defy the aging processes undergone by adult cells.[30] Last, the ES cells must be unaffected by the process of isolation, meaning that the resulting cells must have normal chromosomal structures.[31]

The various characteristics of ES cells contribute to their high value as scientific and medicinal tools. Once isolated, hES cells could have a major impact in three areas of biomedicine: human developmental biology, pharmaceutical research and development, and transplantation medicine.[32] These cells might be studied to unravel the key molecular events responsible for their transformation from primordial cells into functional cell types, thus providing invaluable insight into how organs and tissues form at the very earliest stages of human development. Such knowledge could contribute to the treatment of fertility disorders (which affects one out of every six U.S. couples) and to the successful diagnosis and prevention of birth defects. These cells could also be developed for use in identifying, screening, and testing new drugs, thus extending the capability of current assays. Streamlining the drug development process with the use of such assays has been a dream of pharmaceutical and biotechnology companies faced with the daunting costs and uncertainties of product development. But perhaps the most exciting potential application of all lay in coaxing hES cells to differentiate into specialized cells for replacement of damaged or diseased tissue. Neurons derived from hES cells could, for instance, be used for treating the more than one million people in the United States suffering from Parkinson disease, or the over five million Americans diagnosed with Alzheimer disease, or the seventy-eight hundred individuals who experience spinal cord injuries each year. Similarly, hES cell-derived cardiac cells could be used for therapy in congestive heart failure, and immune cells originating from hES cells could be used for transplantation into AIDS patients. Although far in the future, hES cells could theoretically be grown outside of the body into whole organs that could then be used for replacing damaged or diseased hearts, livers, or kidneys.[33] Dr. Harold Varmus, director of the National Institutes of Health, commented that "there is almost no realm of medicine that might not be touched by this innovation."[34]

LONG PATHWAY TO THE SUCCESSFUL
ISOLATION OF HUMAN STEM CELLS

The search for ES cells began in earnest in 1981, when several researchers succeeded in isolating the cells from mice and growing them in the artificial conditions of a laboratory dish (such lab work is called *in vitro*, as opposed to *in vivo* research, which is conducted in a living organism). Over the past decade, scientists learned how to add and delete genes from mouse ES cells to create genetically altered adult mice, and these new mice have served as powerful tools in biological research. In recent years, the technology developed to successfully isolate and grow ES cells from other animals, such as rabbits, cows, sheep, rhesus monkeys, and marmosets. While these advances were valuable, scientists knew that animal models are often imprecise substitutes for learning about human biology. Prior to 1997, however, no group of researchers had reported success in isolating primordial cells from humans. The search for human ES cells had been a Holy Grail for some scientists.[35] Geron, interested in leveraging its telomerase technology into the field of cell therapy, played a key role in the scientific hunt for hES cells. The company provided research funds to support hES cell development work to Dr. John Gearhart, a professor of gynecology and obstetrics at Johns Hopkins University School of Medicine, Dr. James Thomson, an associate research veterinarian at the University of Wisconsin's Regional Primate Research Center, and Dr. Roger Pedersen, the director of the In Vitro Fertilization Laboratory at the University of California, San Francisco.[36] In exchange, Geron obtained exclusive licensing rights to the technology developed at Johns Hopkins and Wisconsin.[37]

Human ES cell development work had been progressing slowly. From a scientific standpoint, hES cells had been difficult to isolate and grow, because the correct conditions for keeping the cells alive outside of the body were difficult to create. Special ingredients (including macerated mouse embryonic tissue) were needed to keep cells growing in laboratory dishes and to prevent them from spontaneously differentiating into more specialized cells. These problems had stymied scientists for years. Then came the exciting news that a breakthrough had occurred. In July 1997, Dr. Gearhart of Johns Hopkins University announced at a scientific meeting that he and his group had for seven months been successfully culturing human embryonic germ cells (hEG), which originate from the primordial reproductive cells of the developing fetus and have characteristics that are close but not identical to those of hES cells.[38] Scientists attending the meeting were immediately impressed with the scientific and medical possibilities this advancement represented. "I attended his talk, and I was blown away by the possibilities," recalled Leon Browder, a professor of biology.[39] At the time, however, there was little commentary in the scientific or lay press about this work or its ethical and social implications. Because the hEG cells were derived from aborted fetuses, the research was acceptable according to U.S law and regulation, although the source of the material, aborted fetuses, remained controversial.

In the meantime, Thomson's work was also coming to fruition. In November 1998, the results of the research conducted by the scientists at Johns Hopkins and Wisconsin universities were officially published.[40] Both groups of researchers demonstrated that they had for the first time successfully isolated and grown human pluripotent embryonic germ and stem cells (collectively called human stem cells or hES cells from now on, with the understanding that the cells are pluripotent). David Gottlieb, a stem cell expert at Washington University in St. Louis, described this breakthrough at the time as "a great big advance that will really open up a large number of applications. The implications for basic science and biotechnology are huge."[41]

ETHICAL CONTROVERSIES SURROUNDING THE ISOLATION OF HUMAN STEM CELLS

As soon as these two advances were published, commentary began to appear about their ethical, legal, and social consequences.[42] Scientists hailed the breakthrough. Just as quickly, however, the research was heavily criticized as having violated moral principles related to the sanctity of life. Thomson, Gearhart, and Okarma, along with the director of the NIH and several biomedical ethicists and religious leaders, were called to the U.S. Senate to explain the impact of the technology.[43] President Clinton immediately asked his National Bioethics Advisory Commission to study the ethical issues raised by the discoveries.[44]

The stem cells grown by the scientists from Johns Hopkins and Wisconsin were derived from two sources, and the initial issue generated by this research was related to these sources. At Johns Hopkins, Gearhart's group had taken cells destined to become eggs and sperm (primordial germ cells) from human fetuses aborted at five to seven weeks after conception. The fetuses used for this research resulted from therapeutic (as opposed to spontaneous) abortions.[45] Consistent with federal law related to research involving human fetuses, the mothers' decisions to abort were made independent of and prior to consent being given to use the fetus for research purposes.[46] Despite these protections, which were intended to eliminate any coercion or undue influence on the decision to abort, the fact that abortions occurred and that research was conducted on fetal tissue was linked to the prolonged and unresolved debate surrounding abortion and the rights of the fetus. The abortion debate had caused the federal government to ban research using fetal tissue from 1988 to 1993. Because the funding ban had significantly slowed medical research progress on important diseases (such as the use of fetal tissue to treat Parkinson disease), the ban was lifted by presidential decree the day after Bill Clinton was inaugurated. But the controversies remained. Three leading U.S. biomedical ethicists deplored the intractability of the debate and the fact that it was very difficult to reach any consensus on medical issues linked to abortion. In their view, "Crucial issues such as human-embryo research, prenatal genetic screening, and the manipulation of embryos before their implantation must be disengaged from the abortion issue to receive the public debate they require."[47]

Thomson's group at Wisconsin used blastocysts for their research.[48] The blastocysts were early preimplantation human embryos (some call them preembryos) created in *in vitro* fertilization clinics and intended for implantation into the uterus of a woman attempting pregnancy.[49] It is common practice to create a number of embryos during the process of *in vitro* fertilization, since the fertility physicians never know how many it will take to achieve a successful pregnancy. In most cases, multiple implantations and several pregnancies are needed to produce one child. Excess embryos are frozen and stored until the man and woman who produced the sperm and eggs decide they no longer need or want them. Typically, the couple is then given a choice to store, discard, or donate the leftover embryos to another couple or, in Thomson's case, donate them to research. Thomson and his colleagues retrieved the embryos when they were one week old, then isolated cells taken from the inner surface of the hollow center and coaxed them to grow in laboratory dishes. The process of isolating the stem cells necessarily destroyed the embryo. The debates about Thomson's work centered around three issues: (1) the manner in which the stem cells were produced, that is, by destroying a potential human life (similar objections were raised to Gearhart's work), (2) the moral status of hES cells themselves, and (3) concerns about potential harmful uses of these cells.

Research on spare embryos has been a controversial subject for many years, since some believe that all embryos—no matter how early and regardless of whether they are implanted into a woman's womb—have moral status as potential human lives, and thus should not be casually discarded, or utilized or destroyed for research purposes.[50] Because the embryos have rights and interests, according to this view, it is unethical to destroy them to obtain stem cells, even to save other lives. As Judie Brown of the American Life League put it, "It doesn't matter if it's done in the womb or a petri dish, it's still killing."[51] The opposite position held that these embryos were too rudimentary in structure and development to have moral status or interests in their own right since they could not, without incubation in a uterus and other major interventions, become a fetus. Others took a somewhat middle ground, which did not accord these embryos' rights and interests, but accorded them symbolic meaning as a potent representation of human life that should be used only for important and essential research. Ethicists and others who held this view believed that the donation of spare embryos for important medical research that could not be conducted by other means was ethically superior to either destroying the embryos or keeping them perpetually frozen.[52]

Neither Thomson nor Gearhart had major reservations about the means used to derive the stem cells, nor did they believe that the cells had a special moral status, since they could not grow into a fetus. However, Okarma stated that he believed that the blastocysts used by Thomson deserved to be treated seriously due to their "moral authority," but that use of the cells was justified because they were something less than a living embryo, and life-saving treatments might be derived from them. He went on to explain that "we are not saying the ends justify the means, but that given that the moral authority of these cells is subordinate to that of the embryo, the work we contemplate with them is appropriate."[53]

Others disagreed with this distinction since they were not convinced that a human being could not be derived from the stem cells. The disagreement was based on practical aspects of the stem cell use (the cells would not be implanted into a uterus) and a debate about whether the stem cells were pluripotent or totipotent, that is, capable of forming most body tissues or all of them. Thomson and Gearhart knew that their cells were pluripotent since they had done the laboratory tests to prove it. But the tests for human totipotency would involve injecting stem cells into another human blastocyst to see if the growth of all human cells would result. Such an experiment was considered uncontrovertibly unethical, so totipotency of the human stem cells could not be proven. Those who based their opinion of the moral status of the stem cells on whether they were capable of forming a fetus were stumped. "Assuming the cells are not totipotent, reservations go only to the source [of the stem cells]," said Kevin T. FitzGerald, a geneticist and Jesuit priest at Loyola University Medical School. If they are totipotent, he said, he would conclude that their use could not be justified. But he noted the complexity of the issue, saying, "We are getting closer and closer to the lines of demarcation of the beginning of human life."[54]

There were also scientists to whom the difference between pluripotency and totipotency did not matter. One was geneticist Lee Silver at Princeton University, who believed that the stem cells derived by Thomson and Gearhart were capable (with further laboratory intervention) of developing into a fetus, that they therefore were the moral equivalent of an embryo, and that research using these stem cells should be allowed regardless.[55]

Others had further concerns about the use of the human stem cells that had been produced. What if these human stem cells were genetically modified and genetically altered humans were the result? What if the technology led to cloning embryos or even entire humans?[56] While it was not technically feasible at the time and other methods of gene therapy were easier, the belief and fear that humans could now be modified "will be the knee-jerk reaction of the academic community," Thomson told one reporter.[57]

Others combined their distaste for the research with the fact that commercial use would be made of it. Following a *Wall Street Journal* article about Geron's funding of the stem cell derivation research entitled "Labs Make a Major Advance in Biotechnology," one reader criticized Geron's involvement and suggested that the article should have been entitled "Wall Street Mines Profit from Abortions."[58] An editorial in the scientific journal *Nature Biotechnology* also lamented that the press seemed to have been primed to hype these and other similar discoveries so that the companies involved could enjoy a stock price run-up and attract more funding.[59]

POLITICAL AND POLICY DEBATES

The U.S. Congress played a major role in the politics and ethics of embryo research since the early 1990s. The federal government position on the research use of human embryos had flip-flopped over the years, and in some cases, the position differed between the executive and legislative branches. Consistent with the public debates on abortion and the moral status of the embryo and fetus, the federal views were divided. In 1994, recognizing that scientific advances on embryo development (including stem cells) would generate ethical and legal concerns, the National Institutes of Health, which funds the majority of university-based biomedical research, created the Human Embryo Research Panel to recommend guidelines for the funding of research involving human embryos. Included in an extensive set of guidelines developed by the panel was a recommendation that federal funding be allowed under strict conditions for research involving preimplantation embryos, and that in very limited cases, it might be ethically acceptable to create an embryo *in vitro* for research purposes only.[60] These guidelines, developed over a period of nine months by eleven researchers and eight nonresearchers (ten men and nine women), were never adopted because of a series of events that occurred immediately after their completion. On the very day that the panel delivered its report to then NIH director Harold Varmus, President Clinton issued a statement requesting that the NIH ban funding for research using embryos created solely for research purposes. However, research using "spare" embryos (those created for procreation but no longer needed) from *in vitro* fertilization clinics was presumably allowed to proceed. However, no funding for this research would occur because in 1995 the House Appropriations Committee (which authorizes the NIH budget) voted 30 to 23 to bar all federal funding for any research involving human embryos. Despite attempts at a compromise that would allow federal funding for the research use of spare embryos but not for embryos created expressly for research, the newly elected Republican Congress implemented the total ban in 1996. The ban, commonly called the Dickey-Wicker Amendment after the two Congressmen who authored it, stated that "grant, cooperative agreement, and contract funds may not be used for (1) the creation of a human embryo for research purposes; or (2) research in which a human embryo or embryos are destroyed, discarded, or knowingly subjected to risk of injury or death greater than that allowed for research on fetuses *in utero*."[61] This ban was attached to subsequent NIH authorization bills and remained in effect at the time Geron was grappling with this issue.

There were many critics who deplored the NIH funding ban. The effect (and some thought, the goal) of federal government bans on certain types of research was to stop the research completely, even if no federal funds were used. Indeed, the federal ban seemed to have a chilling effect. Many of the best scientists were dissuaded from conducting research considered illegal by the government, and consequently, many feared that the science would not advance. Thomson agreed. "I am convinced that in my lifetime there will be therapeutic applications [for hES cells], but exactly when that happens depends on whether there is federal funding," he said. "Without public involvement it will take much longer."[62] Also, banning federal funding changed the nature of the research that did take place with private funds. Private company research tended to be product-driven, whereas university scientists were more prone to engage in research on basic scientific questions. Others thought that by driving controversial research into the private sector, important public oversight and accountability was eliminated. According to Ronald Green, professor of religion and director of the Ethics Institute at Dartmouth College and former member of the NIH's Human Embryo Research Panel, "The best way of fostering responsible research in human reproduction is to federally fund it by supporting the best and most responsible researchers and by making sure there's continual dialogue on the moral guidelines affecting it."[63] Others warned that confining research to the private sector could lead to a corporate stranglehold and restrict access to the technology. "Not only will progress be slow, it will be hidden," said Arthur Caplan, a University of Pennsylvania bioethicist.[64]

Patient advocates also voiced strong opinions about the federal research ban. These support groups and advocates recognized that the ban had slowed the research, and they lobbied Congress to lift it. "We're definitely going to do everything we possibly can . . . to push Congress to reverse itself," said Joann Tompkins of the National Spinal Cord Injury Association, which represents the four hundred thousand Americans who suffer from such injuries.[65] One group, the Patients' Coalition for Urgent Research, was created to support stem cell research and to lobby Congress to lift the funding ban. The coalition believed that the potential medical benefits for desperately ill children and adults outweighed the ethical reservations about embryo cell research. According to the coalition's spokesperson, "What the patient groups have been saying all along is, 'Get on with it. We want this for our loved ones.'"[66]

Thomson's stem cell derivation work was not illegal since he was funded by Geron's private money, and he was very careful to segregate the stem cell work from his NIH-sponsored research. Thomson's successful isolation of hES cells raised immediate questions about whether the NIH funding ban would apply to future research using these stem cells. This question was important to Geron, since Geron's business plan in part depended on benefiting from research discoveries made by federally funded university scientists using stem cells derived by Thomson and others. Initially, things did not look promising. "I feel just as strongly as I ever did that an embryo is still a life," said Representative Jay Dickey, the cosponsor of the original funding ban. He predicted that the ban would remain in place. "It's not a spare life, one that you can just throw away. It's still killing."[67]

However, NIH director Harold Varmus was anxious to fund research on these new cells, and lawyers in the Department of Health and Human Services were asked to determine if the federal ban precluded federally funded researchers from conducting experiments on the already isolated stem cells. Using a strict legal definition of "embryo," HHS general counsel Harriet Rabb responded in the negative. In a memorandum to Varmus dated January 15,

1999, Rabb concluded that the statutory prohibition on the use of HHS funds for human embryo research would not apply to research utilizing existing human pluripotent stem cells because such cells are not a human embryo within the statutory definition since they cannot develop into an embryo even if implanted into a women's uterus.[68] Based on this interpretation, the NIH decided that, although it could not fund the development of cell lines from embryos, it could fund research on hES cells; the decision was met with much enthusiasm by the scientific community. The American Society for Reproductive Medicine commented that the HHS opinion was "an accurate interpretation of bad law."[69] In a public letter published on March 19, 1999, in the journal *Science*, seventy-three prominent scientists, including sixty-seven Nobel Prize winners, lauded the NIH's decision as "forward-thinking" and stated that the NIH plan "succeeds in protecting the sanctity of human life without impeding biomedical research that could be profoundly important to the understanding and treatment of human disease."[70]

Following this announcement, the President's National Bioethics Advisory Commission went further when it published its report concluding that federal funds could be used not only for research using human stem cells but also for the isolation of these cells, stating that "there is no compelling ethical justification for distinguishing between the derivation and use of human stem cells."[71] The commission also recommended that a higher degree of oversight be put into place over such research, including the establishment of a new body to oversee hES cell research at the national level.

These decisions and recommendations caused an uproar. "Today's announcement . . . is the latest step by the Clinton administration to treat human beings as property to be manipulated and destroyed," said Representative Christopher Smith of New Jersey. NIH money would allow researchers to "experiment with cells obtained from human beings ruthlessly killed in the first weeks of life," he said.[72] Smith responded to the scientists' published letter by saying that "some scientists resent any moral limits on their use of taxpayer funds for harmful experiments." He rejected "the claim that a degree in science—even a Nobel Prize in science—makes scientists our supreme arbiters of morality and human dignity."[73] Smith led a group of seventy pro-life Congress members (some of them Democrats) who wrote letters to the NIH opposing Varmus's plans to fund research using stem cells.[74] One letter stated that this "area of law has provided a bulwark against government's misuse and exploitation of human beings in the name of medical progress. It would be a travesty for this Administration to attempt to unravel this accepted ethical standard." According to Richard Doerflinger of the National Conference of Catholic Bishops, the NIH decision meant that the federal government would "not fund the act of destruction itself, but will reward those who destroy embryos by paying them to develop the cells and tissues they have obtained by destructive means."[75]

The NIH was committed to developing draft guidelines to help ensure that NIH-funded research using hES cells was conducted in an ethical and legal manner, and decided that it would not fund research using human pluripotent stem cells until final guidelines were published in the *Federal Register* and an oversight process was in place.[76] In 1998, when Geron's EAB was reviewing the issue, the NIH's recommendations on this question were not developed. Nor was it known whether Thomson's stem cells specifically would qualify for federal funding under the future guidelines. Some thought that the goal of the NIH to fund this research would be thwarted if the guidelines were finalized under a new Republican and more conservative administration, which would begin in January 2001. There were also plans in Congress to schedule further hearings and to introduce legislation both permitting and banning research using human stem cells.[77] Because of these uncertainties, the fate of this research remained an open question.

GERON CORPORATION'S STEM CELL HOPES

Geron was founded in 1990 to commercialize the application of molecular information and technology in the processes that control aging.[78] Founder Dr. Michael D. West, a cell biologist who started the company while still in medical school, had been researching telomerase's effect on cellular longevity, and, although the science was quite new, he realized the market potential of using this information to develop therapies for many degenerative diseases and cancers.[79] In 1992, West convinced the venture capital firm Kleiner Perkins Caufield & Byers to invest $7.6 million, and work on investigating cellular life extension began in earnest.

Geron went public in mid-1996 and obtained a major patent in 1997 for cloning the human gene for telomerase. In addition to pursuing product development based on anti-aging, West was interested in combining telomerase technology with a renewable source of cells and tissues, and as early as 1992 explored the possibility of deriving the first hES cells. Initially, scientists were not willing to work with Geron on such a sensitive project, preferring public funding. However, after the NIH funding ban, Geron signed up the three university scientists who had developed animal stem cell lines—Thomson, Gearhart, and Roger Pedersen—and funded them to derive human embryonic and germ stem cells. In exchange, Geron obtained the intellectual property rights to the technology developed by the researchers. In 1997, Thomas Okarma was hired to run Geron's stem cell research program. Okarma, who obtained his graduate and medical education from Stanford University, was a Stanford faculty member and the scientific founder of Applied Immune Sciences prior to joining Geron. West left Geron about the same time, citing differences in strategic goals, and joined a new company, Advanced Cell Technologies, in 1998 to continue his own stem cell work. In May 1998, Okarma became vice president of research and development at Geron. By the spring of 1999, Geron employed approximately one hundred people, eighty-five of whom worked in the laboratory. Geron's major asset was ownership of a vast array of technologies that could be applied to the commercialization of telomerase and stem cell technologies, including twenty-nine issued U.S. patents, thirteen allowed U.S. patent applications, and three granted/accepted foreign patents.[80] Combined with the rights to the Wisconsin and Johns Hopkins stem cells, the company was in an excellent product development position.

Geron sought strategic partners in industry and academia to complement the company's R&D work both for telomerase and stem cells. Several large pharmaceutical companies (such as Kyowa Hakko Kogyo Co., Ltd., Pharmacia & Upjohn S.p.A., and Roche Diagnostics GmbH) were collaborating with Geron to expand research and develop therapies and diagnostics. These companies provided Geron with large infusions of cash. Other relationships with smaller companies typically provided specific services, such as clinical development and marketing support for Geron. These relationships (along with many collaborations with university researchers) had expanded to the point where management estimated that for every four full-time employees at Geron, there were three people employed at partner companies.

In anticipation that the stem cell technology would have such vast possible applications that no one company could fully exploit the technology, Geron initially planned to sell stem cell technology to other pharmaceutical companies for research use.[81] Thereafter, Geron intended to identify the genes that either started or maintained the generation of specific tissue cell types and use those genes to design new therapies and develop drug screening tests for pharmaceutical R&D. But the real commercial payoff would come from the use of stem cells to generate specific tissue cell therapies for diseases such as heart attack, diabetes, stroke, Parkinson and Alzheimer diseases, and spinal cord injuries, and for bone marrow transplantation, all of which have tremendous market potential.[82] Robert Alonso, CEO of Layton BioScience (Atherton, California), a competing company, commented on the potential market for just the neuron stem cells: "Conceivably, any [central nervous system] problem can be fixed by neural stem cells. That puts their commercial possibilities way beyond mind boggling."[83] Estimates placed the number of Americans with neurodegenerative (spine and brain) diseases at more than ten million, accounting for over $150 billion in annual health-care costs. As the population ages, these numbers are expected to grow dramatically. Among these diseases, stroke is the third leading cause of death and the most common cause of adult disability in the United States. And because no effective treatments existed for many of these diseases, Geron's therapies had the potential to expand the market rather than force the company to compete for market share against existing companies' products. Some industry insiders expected that promising therapies would be available in five to seven years, sooner than any genomics-based treatments.

That timeline may have been overly optimistic, given the scientific and regulatory hurdles Geron had to jump to get to market. For instance, for cell therapies, scientists had to figure out how to stimulate stem cells to develop into particular cell types (for example, cardiac, neuronal) to make therapeutic cell products for heart and nerve diseases. Up until then, hES cells had proven to be unpredictable differentiators. "You smile at them and they become heart, you frown and they become brain," complained Okarma to one reporter, adding that "the challenges ahead are formidable."[84] Another significant hurdle lay in making grafted cells compatible with the patient's immune system. Following that, the stem cells would be immortalized with the telomerase gene so that cells would divide indefinitely instead of growing old and dying after a set number of divisions. No one could predict how long it would take to perfect these techniques to make stem cells grow into the right tissue at the right time in the right place.[85] And, even after acquiring this knowledge, Geron would face the traditionally expensive, difficult, and uncertain path through clinical trial product testing, regulatory approvals, and subsequent market acceptance. Uncertainty was great, since the FDA had never been faced with questions about what data were necessary to ensure the safety and efficacy of medical products based on stem cells. In this respect, the path ahead was indeterminate and investors in the company needed to recognize that Geron could be years away from profitability. (See Table 13.1 for company financial information.)

In spite of these hurdles, Geron had difficulty encouraging Wall Street to keep expectations realistic and may even have fueled expectations with its frequent press releases of astonishing scientific breakthroughs. Geron's stem cell announcement was the fourth major "uptick" in share price since the company went public in 1996. With each new announcement of a technological breakthrough, Geron's stock would soar so high that analysts called it "crazy"; then investor optimism in the company would fade, profit taking would occur by institutional investors, and the stock price would fall quickly and steadily back down.[86] After a tripling of the share price following the telomerase gene cloning announcement in August 1997, Kenneth Kam, a fund manager at the San Jose–based Technology Value Fund, worried that investors were being unreasonably optimistic about the company's prospects. "I don't think that many of the investors that are so excited about this company right now realize how far away Geron is from getting clinical approval for its most important products and bringing them to market," he told the *Wall Street Journal*.[87] Sure enough, the share price began to fall steadily soon thereafter. The same thing happened in January 1998 following the announcement that Geron had been able to extend the life span of cells with its telomerase technology. When it was reported in November 1998 that Geron owned the commercial rights to Thomson's and Gearhart's stem cells, Geron's stock rose by 148 percent, with trading volume more than 180 times the average daily volume. This rise was followed again by a downfall, and the stock had lost about half of that gain by year's end.[88]

Despite Geron's early remarkable scientific innovations, competitors existed both for telomerase and stem cell products.[89] At least three companies were developing products derived from neural stem cells: Layton BioScience, CytoTherapeutics (a public company), and NeuralStem Biopharmaceuticals. Some of these companies had their own patented methodologies and were attempting to exploit the same market that Geron was trying to reach.[90] However, Okarma emphasized that the point was not so much that other companies would pursue stem cell work but that other types of stem cells could become commercially competitive. For example, work was being done by Osiris Therapeutics to derive bone and cartilage stem cells from fully differentiated adult human cells. The process, which was about to be tested in Phase I clinical trials, involved extracting stem cells from a patient's bone marrow, growing them in culture, and transplanting them back into that same person where the cells were needed. The process took weeks in animals. If that company succeeded, products could be developed to replace tissue lost to bone cancer, osteoporosis, injury, or dental disease.[91] Similarly, Nexell Therapeutics and Aastrom Biosciences were attempting to isolate adult human immune stem cells to restore cancer patients' immune systems after intense radiation or chemotherapy.[92] If adult cells could be converted to stem cells, the fetal and embryo cell derivation could become a much less attractive technology. The benefits of using already differentiated adult stem cells were that there was no need to go through a differentiation process; stem cells taken from adults and then transplanted back avoided rejection problems; and scientists avoided the ethically difficult issues surrounding use of fetuses and embryos as source tissue. Geron's detractors, specifically Richard Doerflinger, associate director of the Secretariat for Pro-life Activities at the National Conference of Catholic Bishops, used the promise of the "morally acceptable" adult stem cells as another reason that fetal and embryo cell work should cease.[93] Many scientists, however, believed that the work with adult stem cells was too premature to abandon explorations using fetal- and embryo-derived stem cells.

GERON'S ETHICS ADVISORY BOARD

The initial concept for Geron's EAB was raised as early as 1996, when Geron's management was first considering funding hES cell research at Johns Hopkins and Wisconsin. The idea arose out of concern for how ethically sensitive technology would be handled once it left the oversight of a university's institutional review board and entered the hands of the corporate sector. The advisory board concept remained on the shelf until Okarma took on the responsibility of searching for appropriate individuals to serve on the company's EAB.

In early 1998, Okarma approached various bioethicists at local institutions, such as the Graduate Theological Union in Berkeley, California, and Stanford University's Center for Biomedical Ethics, to ask if they would serve as members of Geron's EAB. No bioethical advisory board had ever been created for the purpose that Geron intended, so there was no known procedure or pool of people to draw from to form the board. Nonetheless, the company had several criteria in mind. Geron wanted leaders in bioethics who were also geographically convenient to the company. They also wanted diverse theological backgrounds to provide alternative viewpoints, but at the same time needed ethicists with a common interest in technology. Finally, the company searched for a group of people who were comfortable working with limited data, had good decision-making abilities, and felt comfortable treading into unmarked territory. The board that was finally impaneled in March 1998 was made up of five academics, all with religious backgrounds, all well known and widely published in the field of ethics, and some of whom had served on national ethics committees and commissions. Two were faculty members at the Pacific School of Religion in Berkeley, California (one an ordained minister and one a Catholic lay person), one taught theology at the Graduate Theological Union in Berkeley, one was an ordained Methodist minister and Codirector of the Stanford University Center for Biomedical Ethics, and the last was a professor of Jewish studies at San Francisco State University.

The newly formed board, working under Okarma's guidance, quickly decided on operating procedures. The board arranged to meet every two months to discuss issues raised by the company—usually company developments that were nearing a need for public disclosure. The meetings were entirely private and confidential and were to be attended by a Geron representative, almost always Okarma, to provide any technical or other information that might be required during the discussion. Consultation with anyone inside the company, or with outside researchers who were being funded by Geron, was encouraged. The results of the discussions were kept confidential and required the approval of the company prior to any release of information. As a final administrative matter, a stipend of $500 was offered to each board member for each meeting; not all members accepted the stipend. Geron considered this payment to be a token gesture, since the company expected that EAB members might spend considerable time preparing for any given meeting.

Decisions rendered by the EAB were not intended to be binding on Geron, and there was no explicit contract between the parties regarding how the company would respond to EAB findings. There was, however, an understanding among the board members that Geron would be responsive to their concerns. The members of the EAB all agreed that they were free to take any stand on the issues that they thought was justified and were free to disagree with one another. However, some feared that the fast-paced scientific advances would drive the bioethics agenda, leaving little time for ethical reflection and debate. This potential problem would be exacerbated by the fact that the EAB members' confidentiality promises would prevent them from testing their ideas and opinions on colleagues, a common practice among bioethicists.

The pressing issue facing the newly formed board in 1998 and early 1999 was whether Geron's decision to pursue isolation of hES cells was ethical. Lengthy meetings with lively debate among the board members and with Okarma's active participation led to the first major conclusions of the EAB. These conclusions were incorporated into a Statement on Human Embryonic

Stem Cells that was drafted in September 1998, revised, and then finalized on October 20, 1998. The EAB did not offer carte blanche approval of stem cell research but "unanimously affirmed that such research can be undertaken ethically, contingent upon meeting a range of qualifying conditions."[94] Geron then submitted its EAB report for publication in a leading ethics journal.

In the spring of 1999, the statement, which explained the qualifying conditions for the research and the qualifying conditions of the EAB, was published in the *Hastings Center Report*. Geron believed that the released decision of the EAB and the supporting reasoning provided company management with solid support for its decision to pursue stem cell research. Okarma also believed that this helped Geron in its public relations and in the internal management of its research. Okarma reasoned that having the decision and the published results out of the hands of the company helped the company to anticipate and respond to the ethical issues in a more objective and professional manner. An ethical framework had been effectively put in place that allowed the company to comfortably deal with concerns about the direction of the work and focus primarily on the work itself. In addition, from a public relations standpoint, the creation of the EAB appeared to be a fundamentally sound business strategy.

Geron's EAB report had been given to other medical ethicists for commentary, and their articles were published alongside the statement in the same issue of the *Hastings Center Report*. Geron's efforts were praised as "laudable," the EAB was described as composed of "independent thinkers," and Geron was "commended for establishing the EAB, and even more for allowing its work to be published, discussed, and critiqued at this time."[95] Some ethicists liked the EAB report as far as it went but were disappointed that it did not do more. One author wanted the EAB to say whether they believed the frozen embryos were legally property or persons, and who should be allowed to profit from the use of this human tissue.[96] The challenge was posed in the following way: "If it is wrong to commercialize embryos because of their nature, then it is wrong for everyone. It is simply inconsistent to argue that couples should act altruistically [by donating embryos] because commercializing [selling] embryos is wrong, while permitting corporations . . . to profit financially from cells derived by destroying these embryos." This same author went on to decry Geron's exclusive ownership of and restricted access to the hES cell technology by saying that "we know that Geron wants to reduce human suffering, but it also needs to respond to the pressures of the market and has an obligation to give its shareholders the best return on investment. Let's be candid. We should simply admit that access to medical resources, decent public health, and global justice cannot be easily attained if medical research is committed to private property and profit making." Others wanted the EAB to elucidate further on the moral status of embryonic and germ cells so that others could know, among other things, whether to treat the tissue as an end in itself or merely a means to an end.[97] Another article listed several reasons why a company-based advisory board was not able to exercise effective oversight.[98] Among these were the assertion that effective oversight must be located outside of the arena where the investigators work and must extend beyond the confines of the company. There is no assurance that the company would heed an inside board's recommendations or that any unpopular opinions of the board would become known. Further, if the board was composed of people with vested interests in the company, "rubber stamping" of the company actions is what could be expected. Finally, there would be no uniformity among inside ethics advisory boards—what would be acceptable to one board would not be to another, yet both companies would be able to claim that they had taken action based on sound ethics advice. To combat these problems, the author proposed that companies use common or "blue ribbon" panels of experts with no allegiance to one company, that deliberations be public, and that researchers oblige themselves to adhere to ethics guidelines developed by the panel.

Two articles focused on the timing of the EAB work. One author collected information on when the EAB was formed in relation to when the stem cell research was performed and concluded that "the ES cell lines had been cultured for as long as eight months, and that with additional time for preparatory steps, the donated embryos had to have been acquired no later than February 1998 [one month before the Geron EAB was formed]. Clearly most if not all of the scientific work had been completed before the EAB issued its ethical guidelines, even in their preliminary form."[99] Commenting further on her belief that the EAB work occurred simultaneously with the research, this author wondered whether any company ethics advisory board would disapprove of research that was nearly complete. Expounding on this point in a separate publication, three other prominent biomedical ethicists wrote:

> Geron Corporation, which funded both of the two published studies [on human stem cells] decided to set up its own ethics advisory board. The board's first statement, however, was not drafted until the research was complete and both papers had been accepted for publication. This seems more like "ethical cover" rather than ethics that can be taken seriously, especially as the board rewrote their statement after the publication of the study's results.[100]

The Geron EAB members disagreed with many of the criticisms, specifically about the timing, and discussed opening up their report process for further outside review. Eventually, however, the company decided against taking this step.

The company was also praised for how it managed the disclosures of the research it sponsored. Before the publication of the stem cell studies, Geron had sought the advice of the Biotechnology Industry Organization (BIO) to develop a strategy on how to deal with the public when the stem cell discovery announcements were made. According to BIO president Carl Feldbaum, Geron's announcements were not only very well received by the public but were a "textbook case of how it should be done." With this success, Feldbaum expected that BIO would assist other companies in handling ethically sensitive issues.[101]

FUTURE DIRECTIONS

The role of the EAB in Geron's future management decisions would likely remain important to the company. On May 4, 1999, Geron acquired Roslin Bio-Med—a commercial spin-off of the institution that cloned Dolly the sheep—in a $25.7 million transaction.[102] This action dramatically raised Geron's profile since it provided in-house capacity to clone tissues and animals using Roslin Bio-Med's somatic cell nuclear transfer technology. However, because this technology could potentially lead to the cloning of embryos and people, Geron could be faced with even more ethically controversial decisions in the future.

For its part, Geron's EAB was interested in exploring other issues beyond the stem cell research. These issues included how Geron would control access to its technology and how it would make important medical therapies available to poor people, whether the company should pursue gene enhancement, and whether it should resist the creation of perfect genes and the destruction of defective genes.[103] Given these developments, Okarma needed to consider the pros and cons of the EAB's activities, both inside the company and in the public ethical debate. Primarily, he had to consider whether there should be any changes in the timing of the EAB's statements or in its organization, governance, and composition to meet the ethical and practical challenges raised by new and future technologies.

Questions

1. Did Geron appropriately form and utilize the ethics advisory board, including how it managed its members, procedures, and publications?

2. What are the benefits and the risks to the company of using an ethics advisory board to advise on the stem cell research?

3. What should the company do if the ethics advisory board disagrees with Geron's intended activity?

4. Is an ethics advisory board important for a business venture like Geron's?

Discussion

This case can be used to discuss questions about the uses of ethics advice for a bioscience company. What purposes can ethics advice serve for a business enterprise? What people are best suited for the work and what relationship between the company and the ethicists is most appropriate? What benefits and risks to the company does such ethics advice pose? If the recommendations are of high quality, the company benefits. If the recommendations are poor or unrealistic or the company chooses to ignore them, then the company may be worse off, especially if it is seen as having undertaken a token effort with people predisposed to endorse company action. In such a case, the company can be seen as having acted unethically. Another difficulty involves the translation of philosophical and ethical insights into something useful to the company. Finally, what should the company do if the ethics advisory board disagrees with the company's intended activity?

TABLE 13.1

Geron Financial Data

(in thousands of dollars)

	Operations				
	1998	*1997*	*1996*	*1995*	*1994*
Revenues from collaborative agreements	6,706	7,175	5,235	5,490	—
License fees and royalties	91	78	58	—	—
Operating expenses—R & D	15,619	15,139	14,260	11,321	8,099
Operating expenses—general/ administration	3,769	3,120	3,161	2,888	2,397
Total operating expenses	19,388	18,259	17,421	14,209	10,496
Loss from operations	(12,591)	(11,006)	(12,128)	(8,719)	(10,496)
Interest and other income	2,666	1,757	1,826	919	638
Interest and other expenses	(907)	(392)	(385)	(399)	(320)
Net loss	(10,832)	(9,641)	(10,687)	(8,199)	(10,178)
Accretion of redemption value of redeemable convertible preferred stock	(578)				
Net loss applicable to common stockholders	(11,410)				

	Balance Sheet				
	1998	*1997*	*1996*	*1995*	*1994*
Cash and cash equivalents	24,469	21,597	24,269	15,553	13,915
Working capital	22,261	19,739	21,468	12,115	12,410
Total Assets	44,456	26,056	28,788	19,749	17,072
Nonrecurrent portion of liabilities	8,101	1,250	1,644	1,654	1,647
Accumulated deficit	(57,520)	(46,110)	(36,469)	(25,782)	(17,583)
Total stockholder equity	29,191	21,066	23,591	14,308	13,689

SOURCE: Geron Corporation financial reports, 1998

Notes

1. The Sentencing Reform Act of 1984 created the United States Sentencing Commission to develop guidelines to ensure uniformity and fairness for sentencing in federal felonies and most serious misdemeanors. The guidelines also include a definition of an effective corporate ethics program as one that is effective in preventing and detecting criminal conduct and lists what companies must do to ensure "due diligence" in preventing and detecting wrongdoing. For further information, see www.ussc.gov/guidelin.htm.

2. Boatright JR. Ethics in corporation. In *Ethics and the conduct of business*. 3rd ed. Upper Saddle River, NJ: Prentice-Hall; 2000. pp. 360–74.

3. Brower V. Biotech embraces bioethics; but are they being exemplary or expedient? And who are the bioethicists? BioSpace.com 1999 June 14. Available from www.biospace.com/b2/Articles/061499_bioethics.cfm and www.biospace.com/articles/ 061499_who_ethics.cfm.

4. Ibid.

5. Lambrecht B. World recoils at Monsanto's brave new crops. *St. Louis Post-Dispatch* 1998 Dec 27; Sect. A:1.

6. Kolata G. With cloning of a sheep, the ethical ground shifts. *New York Times* 1997 Feb 24; Sect. A:1.

7. See Note 3.

8. Brower V. Ethical culture: Millennium Pharmaceuticals, Inc. *HMS Beagle* 1999; 69. Available from http://news.bmn.com/hmsbeagle/69/notes/profile. Also, personal interviews, Steven Holtzman, 1998 Feb 2 and 2001 June 27.

9. Ibid.

10. Jacobs P. Labyrinth of ethics; panels of outside experts are asked to weigh social impact of research. *San Jose Mercury News* 2000 Oct 8; Sect. G:1.

11. Fleischer M. My kingdom for an ethics litmus test. *Genome Technology* 2001 Apr:24.

12. Kerr K. Research corporations hire ethicists to keep them honest. *San Jose Mercury News* 1999 June 5; Sect. RR:1E.

Gillis J. Scientists planning to make new form of life. *Washington Post* 2002 Nov 21; Sect. A:01.

13. See Note 10.

14. Ibid.

15. Weiss R. A cloning claim's controversies; Massachusetts firm says it created embryo out of human, cow cells. *Washington Post* 1998 Nov 13; Sect. A:03.

16. See Note 3.

17. Weiss R. Can scientists bypass stem cells' moral minefield? *Washington Post* 1998 Dec 14; Sect. A:03.

18. See Note 3.

19. Ibid.

20. Biotech companies seeking ethical advice. *Medical Industry Today* 1999 Dec 13.

21. See Note 10.

22. Hall S. The recycled generation. *New York Times Magazine* 2000 Jan 30; Sect. 6:30.

23. Stolberg SL. Bioethicists find themselves the ones being scrutinized. *New York Times* 2001 Aug 2; Sect. A:1.

24. Ibid.

25. See Note 3.

26. Agres T. Cloning capsized? Ethicists, company clash on cloning. *Scientist* 2001 Aug 20; 15:1. Available from www.the-scientist.com/yr2001/aug/agres_p1_010820.html; see also Note 23.

27. See Note 12, Kerr.

28. The initial case study was prepared by Clare Risa Ozawa and Gerald M. Farquharson under the guidance of and with later revisions by Margaret Eaton. The input and assistance of Tom Okarma and the members of the Geron Ethics Advisory Board is greatly appreciated. The events described in this case study occurred up until mid-1999.

29. Gearhart J. New potential for human embryonic stem cells. *Science* 1998; 282:1061–62.

30. Bodnar AG, Ouellette M, Frolkis M, et al. Extension of life-span by introduction of telomerase into normal human cells. *Science* 1998; 279:349–52.

Telomerase is an enzyme that prevents the shortening of telomeres—the stabilizing caps on the ends of chromosomes. Telomeres shorten whenever a cell divides; when the telomeres become very short, the cell stops dividing and dies. Telomerase is normally present only in certain rare cells that support tissue renewal, such as bone marrow stem cells that give rise to blood. Telomerase is always abnormally present at high levels in cancer cells. In most adult cells, telomerase is turned off, which is one reason that these cells can divide and replicate only a certain number of times before dying.

31. Thomson JA, Itskovitz-Eldor J, Shapiro SS, et al. Embryonic stem cell lines derived from human blastocysts. *Science* 1998; 282: 1145–47.

32. See www.geron.com.

33. Snyder EY, Vescovi AL. The possibilities/perplexities of stem cells. *Nature Biotechnology* 2000; 18:827.

34. Wade N. Senators hear of vast benefit in embryonic-cell work. *New York Times* 1998 Dec 3; Sect. A:29.

35. See Note 29.

36. Both the Wisconsin and Johns Hopkins groups received approval from their universities' institutional review boards for their methods of obtaining and using human embryos or fetuses for research purposes.

37. Marshall E. The business of stem cells. *Science* 2000; 287:1419–21.

38. Lewis R. Embryonic stem cells debut amid little media attention. *Scientist* 1997; 11:14. Available from www.the-scientist.library.upenn.edu.

Human embryonic germ cells were believed to behave much like hES cells and were often included in discussions as if they were hES cells. The science reporter for the *New York Times* described these cells as follows: "In the embryo, a small number of stem cells are set aside, before embryonic development begins, and protected from differentiation. These special cells, known as embryonic germ cells, migrate to the developing ovary or testis, where they generate the egg or sperm for the next generation. Thus there is a special lineage of cells that permanently resist terminal differentiation, cycling indefinitely from embryonic stem cell to embryonic germ cell, to oocyte or sperm, to fertilized egg and embryonic stem cell again. At each cycle the cells spin off a new body as the temporary vehicle to carry them forward on their unending journey." Wade NJ. Essay; immortality, of a sort, beckons to biologists. *New York Times* 1998 Nov 17; Sect. F:1.

39. See Note 38, Lewis.

40. Shamblott MJ, Axelman J, Wang S, et al. Derivation of pluripotent stem cells from cultured human primordial germ cells. *Proceedings of the National Academy of Sciences USA* 1998; 95:13726–731; see also Note 31.

41. Langreth R. Labs make a major advance in biotechnology. *Wall Street Journal* 1998 Nov. 6; Sect. A:3.

42. Marshall E. A versatile cell line raises scientific hopes, legal questions. *Science* 1998; 282:1014–15; Wade N. Primordial cells fuel debate on ethics. *New York Times* 1998 Nov 10; Sect. F:1; Rosin H. Outside laboratory, moral objections; abortion foes oppose embryo research. *Washington Post* 1998 Nov 6; Sect. A:14.

43. See Note 34.

44. The National Bioethics Advisory Commission, created in 1995 by executive order, was an advisory body composed of representatives from various disciplines. The commission's role was to provide guidance to the president on matters of biomedical ethical complexity, such as human cloning.

45. See Note 40, Shamblott, Axelman, Wang, et al.

46. The federal safeguards were meant to ensure that the researcher avoided participating in the abortion and did not influence the "timing, method, or procedures used to terminate the pregnancy." See 42 *United States Code* §289g-1(b)(2) and 45; *Federal Register*, Sect. 46.201–46.211.

47. Annas GJ, Caplan A, Elias S. The politics of human embryo research: Avoiding ethical gridlock. *New England Journal of Medicine* 1996; 334:1329–32.

48. See Note 31.

49. Geron's definition of blastocyst was "the preimplantation embryo of mammals

consisting of a sphere of cells with an outer cell layer that forms the placenta and a cluster of cells on the interior called the inner cell mass that forms the embryo." See the Glossary at http://geron.com.

50. The primary objections were raised by antiabortionists and religious groups, including the National Conference of Catholic Bishops, as well as by conservative members of Congress and some biomedical ethicists.

51. New laws for new tech; new biotechnologies should not be controlled by overly broad legislation [editorial]. *Los Angeles Times* 1998 Nov 9; Sect. B:4.

52. Friedrich ML. Debating pros and cons of stem cell research. *Journal of the American Medical Association* 2000; 284:681–82; see also Note 47.

53. Wade N. Scientists cultivate cells at root of human life. *New York Times* 1998 Nov 6; Sect. A:1.

54. See Note 42, Wade.

55. Kolata G. When a cell does an embryo's work, a debate is born. *New York Times* 1999 Feb 9; Sect. F:2.

56. Wertz DC. Human embryonic stem cells: A source of organ transplants. *Gene Letter* 1999 Feb. Available from www.geneletter.com.

57. See Note 53.

58. Fielding M. Life itself becomes another commodity [letters to the editor]. *Wall Street Journal* 1998 Nov 30; Sect. A:23.

59. Taking stock of spin science [editorial]. *Nature Biotechnology* 1998; 16:1291.

60. The panel recommended that research on methods of improving the chances of pregnancy; fertilization; egg activation, maturation, and freezing; genetic diagnosis before implantation; and the development of embryonic stem cells were acceptable for federal funding. Research on the cloning and use of human oocytes (eggs) without their transfer to the uterus for gestation was considered to warrant additional review. Unacceptable research included the cloning and use of oocytes followed by transfer to the uterus, and cross-species fertilization. The panel also made recommendations about the appropriate controls and oversight for such research. These recommendations included the following—that the research be conducted by a qualified researcher using a valid research design, which held the potential for major scientific or clinical benefits; that the research goals not be achievable with animals or gametes (eggs or sperm); that the number of embryos required for the research be kept to the minimum necessary to ensure valid results; that informed consent be obtained from gamete donors; that no gametes or embryos be purchased or sold for use in research; that the research protocol be reviewed by an institutional review board; that gamete donors be selected equitably; and that no research be conducted on embryos more than fourteen days after fertilization when the first evidence of a nervous system appears. *Report of the Human Embryo Research Panel*. Bethesda, MD: National Institutes of Health; 1994 Sept 27.

Other ethics commissions in Australia, the United Kingdom, and Denmark had approved research on human embryos up to fourteen days. A commission in Canada was studying the issue.

61. 45 *Code of Federal Regulations* 46.208(a)(2) and Public Health Service Act Sect. 498(b); Kreeger KY. Reproduction research held back by diffuse rules, charged politics. *Scientist* 1997 Mar 17. Available from www.the-scientist.library.upenn.edu.

62. Weiss R. A crucial human cell is isolated, multiplied; embryonic building block's therapeutic potential stirs debate. *Washington Post* 1998 Nov 6; Sect. A:1.

63. See Note 61, Kreeger.

64. Weiss R. Ban on "stem cell" testing reviewed; at Senate hearing, advocates offer evidence of research's medical promise. *Washington Post* 1998 Dec 3; Sect. A:2.

65. Cimons M. Groups renew call to lift embryo research ban. *Los Angeles Times* 1998 Dec 2; Sect. A:18.

66. Ibid.

67. Ibid.

68. Marshall E. Ruling may free NIH to fund stem cell studies. *Science* 1999 Jan 22; 283:465–67.

69. Wade N. Government says ban on human embryo research does not apply to cells. *New York Times* 1999 Jan 20; Sect. A:29.

70. Lanza RP, Arrow KJ, Axelrod J, et al. Science over politics. *Science* 1999; 283:1849–50.

71. *Ethical issues in human stem cell research.* Vol. 1. Report and recommendations of the National Bioethics Advisory Commission. Rockville, MD: National Bioethics Advisory Commission; 1999. Available from http://bioethics.gov/pubs.html.

72. U.S. government to fund controversial stem cell research. *CNN Interactive* 1999 Jan 19. Available from www.cnn.com.

73. Recer P. Prominent scientists support stem cell research. *Nando Media* 1999 Mar 18. Available from www.nandotimes.com.

74. Recer P. Work using fetal cells draws fire. *Boston Globe* 1999 Feb 18, Sect. A10.

75. Doerflinger RM. The ethics of funding embryonic stem cell research: A Catholic viewpoint. *Kennedy Institute of Ethics Journal* 1999; 9:137–50.

76. Weiss R. Panel drafts ethics plan for embryo cell studies; rules would guide federally funded research. *Washington Post* 1999 Apr 9; Sect. A:2.

77. See Note 42, Wade.

78. Geron's name came from the Greek word for "old man"—a tribute to the fact that the company's founding technology was related to controlling cellular aging.

79. Since cancers were characterized by excessive cell division, controlling telomerase's influence on cell division seemed a promising route to new and badly needed therapies. Geron estimated the worldwide cancer treatment market to be over $9 billion and growing at a rate of 8 percent annually. The company believed that other markets just as big existed for therapies related to controlling degenerative conditions and the aging process.

Pollack A. Small company gains high profile in the scientific world. *New York Times* 1998 Nov 6; Sect. A:24; see also Note 22.

80. Geron Corporation press release. Geron announces issuance of patent for human telomerase protein and ten other patents. 1998 Oct 5. Available from www.geron.com.

81. See Note 79, Pollack.

82. See Note 37.

83. Spalding BJ. Neural stem cell research on rise. BioSpace.com 2000 Mar 9. Available from www.biospace.com/articles/index.cfm.

84. Weiss R. Stem cell discovery grows into a debate. *Washington Post* 1999 Oct 9; Sect. A:1.

85. Vogel G. Harnessing the power of stem cells. *Science* 1999; 283:1432–34.

86. In 1997, Geron's stock price had fluctuated between $5.88 and $18.00. In 1998, Geron's stock price fluctuated between $4.20 and $17.00.

87. Veverka M. Some fear the recent run-up in Geron shares may be overdone. *Wall Street Journal* 1997 Aug 27; Sect. C:A2.

88. Ceron GF. Geron stock's gain reminiscent of January advances. *Dow Jones Newswires* 1998 Nov 6. Available from www.bis.dowjones.com.

89. Usdin S, Zipkin I. NIH wants in. *BioCentury* 1998 Nov 9; 6:1–14.

90. Layton BioScience, a small private company, worked with stem cells derived from fetal tissue and had already begun clinical trials successfully transplanting these cells into the brains of twelve stroke patients.

91. Pittenger MF, Mackay AM, Beck SC. Multilineage potential of adult human mesenchymal stem cells. *Science* 1999; 284:143–47; see also Note 85.

92. See Note 37.

93. See Note 75.

94. Geron Ethics Advisory Board. Research with human embryonic stem cells: Ethical considerations. *Hastings Center Report* 1999 Mar–Apr:31–36.

95. White GB. Foresight, insight, oversight. *Hastings Center Report* 1999 Mar–Apr:41–42; Tauer CA. Private ethics boards and public debate. *Hastings Center Report* 1999 Mar–Apr:43–45.

96. Knowles LP. Property, progeny, and patents. *Hastings Center Report* 1999 Mar–Apr; 29:38–40.

97. McGee G, Caplan AL. What's in the dish? *Hastings Center Report* 1999 Mar–Apr; 29:36–38.

98. See Note 95, White.

99. See Note 95, Tauer.

100. Annas GJ, Caplan A, Elias S. Stem cell politics, ethics and medical progress. *Nature Medicine* 1999; 5:1339–41.

101. See Note 3.

102. Jacobs P. Geron buys Scottish firm, spinoff of Dolly's maker. *Los Angeles Times* 1999 May 5; Sect. C:1.

103. See Note 12, Kerr.

Index

Alonso, Robert, 503
American Association for the Accreditation of Laboratory Animal Care-International (AAALAC-I), 120, 123
American Cancer Society, 443, 446
American Chemical Society, 441
American College of Medical Genetics, 349
American Cyanamid, 71–72
American Dietetic Association, 72
American Home Products (AHP), 261, 334
American Journal of Therapeutics, 118
American Life League, 495
American Medical Association (AMA), 72, 201, 204–5, 436, 440–41
American Society for Reproductive Medicine, 500
American Society of Clinical Oncology (ASCO), 348–49, 354, 451
American Society of Human Genetics, 349
Anchalee Soithong, 322
And the Band Played On (Shilts), 290
Angell, Marcia, 281, 283, 287
Animal research: animal model development in, 120–22; and animal welfare, 122–23; human applicability of, 120; modifications to, 123; public opinion on, 122–23; supply of animals for, 119–20
Animal rights movement, 122
Animal-to-human transplants, 211
Animal Welfare Act, 119
Animal welfare, rbST and, 72, 77–78, 79. *See also* Animal research
Annas, George, 489
Antiretroviral drugs, 142–43
Applied Immune Sciences, 502
Argentina, cardiac drug trials in, 284–85
Aristotle, 47
Army, 237
Aron, Joan, 3
Asilomar Conference Center, Pacific Grove, California, 4, 62
Association of University Technology Managers (AUTM), 168–69
Astra AB, 165

Autry, James A., 30
Aventis, 165, 285
Avoidance-of-harm reasoning, 27–28
AZT: AIDSVAX and, 317–18; Burroughs Wellcome and, 387–89, 403, 420n32; in combination therapy, 400, 401, 408; Crixivan compared to, 398; foreign drug trials for, 203–4, 280–82, 300, 321–22, 326n65; mice research for, 121; post-market problems with, 385

Baltimore, David, 298
Bangkok Metropolitan Administration, 306, 319
Barry, David, 387, 388
Baycol, 131
Bayer, 131
Bayh-Dole Act (1980), 167–69, 174
BCPT, *see* Breast Cancer Prevention Trial
Beecher, Henry K., 110–11, 196–200
Belmont Conference Center, Smithsonian Institution, 112
Belmont Report, 42, 110–14, 286
Ben & Jerry's Homemade, 76
Bendectin, 57
Benefit definition, 35–36
Bentham, Jeremy, 122
Berdahl, Robert, 178
Berring, Robert, 179–81
Best, Simon, 481
BIMO program, *see* Bioresearch Monitoring (BIMO) program
BIO, *see* Biotechnology Industry Organization
Biogen, 155
Bio-pharmaceutical companies, *see* Bioscience industry
Bioresearch Monitoring (BIMO) program, 136
Bioscience industry: case study of research collaboration with academia, 161–88; and compensation to research subjects, 236, 242–44; conflict of interest issue in, 115–17; corporate ethics programs in, 481–86; costs of research to, 164; definition of, 5; information evolution problems for, 335; mergers and acquisitions